High Bleeding Risk Patients in Interventional Cardiology

Bernardo Cortese • Stefano Rigattieri
Editors

High Bleeding Risk Patients in Interventional Cardiology

Springer

Editors
Bernardo Cortese
Harrington Heart & Vascular Institute
University Hospitals Cleveland
Ohio, OH, USA

Stefano Rigattieri
Cardiology Unit
Sant'Andrea University Hospital
Rome, Italy

ISBN 978-3-031-87301-0 ISBN 978-3-031-87302-7 (eBook)
https://doi.org/10.1007/978-3-031-87302-7

This Springer imprint is published by the registered company Springer Nature Switzerland AG
The registered company address is: Gewerbestrasse 11, 6330 Cham, Switzerland

Foreword

The field of interventional cardiology continues to evolve at a rapid pace, driven by technological advancements, innovative therapeutic strategies, and an ever-deepening understanding of patient complexity. Among the diverse challenges faced by practitioners, the management of high bleeding risk (HBR) patients has emerged as a critical area of focus. This unique subset of patients demands a careful balance between minimizing thrombotic risk and mitigating bleeding complications—a conundrum that lies at the heart of this comprehensive volume, *High Bleeding Risk Patients in Interventional Cardiology*.

Structured into five distinct parts, the book addresses the multifaceted dimensions of managing HBR patients with clarity and depth. The opening part explores the evolving phenotype of these patients, delving into their unique characteristics and prognostic implications. With contributions from leading experts, it traces the development of bleeding risk metrics, from global utilization of streptokinase and tissue plasminogen activator for occluded coronary arteries (GUSTO) and thrombolysis in myocardial infarction (TIMI) to the contemporary bleeding academic research consortium (BARC) criteria, while also grappling with the interplay of high thrombotic risk (HTR) and HBR—a pivotal consideration for clinicians.

The second part highlights revascularization strategies, including the challenges of treating elderly and frail patients, the role of drug-coated balloons (DCBs), and the selection of coronary stents. It offers a nuanced exploration of innovative approaches, such as hybrid coronary revascularization and protected percutaneous coronary intervention (PCI), underscoring the importance of tailoring interventions to the needs of this high-risk population.

Structural heart interventions form the focus of the third part, where the book addresses the intricacies of left atrial appendage closure, transradial balloon aortic valvuloplasty, and minimalist transcatheter aortic valve implantation (TAVI) setups for HBR patients. Each chapter combines evidence-based insights with practical guidance, equipping readers with the tools to navigate complex scenarios with confidence.

Antithrombotic therapy, a cornerstone of HBR patient management, is explored in detail in the fourth part. Topics range from intravenous and parenteral agents to de-escalation of double nti-platelet therapy (DAPT) and single antiplatelet therapy after DCB angioplasty. The authors provide a thorough examination of the latest evidence, bridging the gap between guideline recommendations and individualized patient care.

Finally, the book culminates in a discussion of bleeding management and prognostic implications, offering critical perspectives on post-TAVI bleeding, complex cases, and emerging therapies. These chapters serve as a roadmap for clinicians aiming to improve outcomes in HBR patients while addressing the broader challenges of modern interventional cardiology.

High Bleeding Risk Patients in Interventional Cardiology represents a landmark contribution to the field. It combines cutting-edge research with practical expertise, making it an invaluable resource for clinicians, researchers, and trainees alike. As the interventional cardiology landscape continues to evolve, this book provides a timely and authoritative guide to one of its most pressing challenges.

I congratulate Bernardo and Stefano and the many contributors for their remarkable effort in bringing this important work to fruition and am confident that it will inspire advancements in patient care for years to come.

Cardiology Division, Sant'Andrea University Hospital Department of Clinical and Molecular Medicine,
Sapienza University of Rome
Rome, Italy

Emanuele Barbato

Preface

When we started our careers as interventional cardiologists, in the early 2000s, the interest in powerful parenteral antiplatelet drugs, namely, glycoprotein IIb/IIIa receptor blockers, which were broadly used not only for acute coronary syndromes but also during elective PCI, was prominent. At that time, femoral approach was largely prevalent, despite the publication of the ACCESS trial in 1997 by Ferdinand Kiemeneij showing the safety of a transradial approach, and bleedings were not a matter of concern: rather, they were considered the demonstration that antithrombotic therapy was working. In those years it was also very infrequent to perform invasive procedures in elderly or sick patients.

In the last two decades the scenario has dramatically changed. The increase in the number of procedures performed in acute clinical settings and in patients with advanced age has been mirrored by a growing awareness of the prognostic implications of bleedings, which have been invariably linked to mortality. Consequently, this led the cardiological community to develop strategies, both pharmacological and non-pharmacological, to limit such complications. More recently, the diffusion of structural interventions and percutaneous left ventricle assist devices has determined an increased need for large-bore vascular accesses, which represent a relevant risk factor for access-related bleedings. A growing interest for a less invasive approach, aimed to avoid sternotomy and to reduce peri-operative complications, including bleedings, has also developed among cardiac surgeons leading to significant technical innovations such as Minimally Invasive Direct Coronary Artery Bypass (MIDCAB) and robotic surgery.

Having witnessed all these changes in our clinical and scientific activity, we conceived this book, which is focalized to high bleeding risk patients in interventional cardiology. With the valuable contribution of distinguished physicians from all over the globe, we tried to give a comprehensive, updated view on the issue of bleedings and bleeding prevention across a wide range of procedures (from coronary to structural) and of preventive strategies (pharmacological and non-pharmacological); our goal was to provide the reader with a useful and easy-to-use tool in clinical practice, and we truly hope we were able to get at least part of this goal.

In Latin, the language of our ancestors, the sentence *primum non nocere* means that, as doctors, first we need to avoid harm to the patient. Bleedings undoubtedly represent a harm for cardiac patients, especially for the elderly and frail ones, therefore we are committed to develop and apply all possible preventive strategies during our professional activity.

Cleveland, OH, USA Bernardo Cortese
Rome, Italy Stefano Rigattieri

Contents

Part I

General Concepts

1 The Evolving Phenotype of the Patient Undergoing Interventional Cardiology Procedures

Sindhuri Gollamudi and Bernardo Cortese

1.1 Historical Background of the Interventional Patient (40 Years Ago, 20 Years Ago, and Now) in Comparisons of High Bleeding Risk and Thrombotic Risk

Coronary artery disease (CAD) stands as the leading cause of death in the United States, responsible for approximately 610,000 deaths annually. Globally, it ranks as the third leading cause of mortality, associated with 17.8 million deaths each year [5]. However, since 1965, there has been a remarkable 60% decline in mortality from coronary heart disease, a testament to advancements in medical and surgical interventions, as well as positive lifestyle changes within the population [3].

The field of interventional cardiology has undergone significant evolution, starting from the early days of percutaneous transluminal coronary angioplasty (PTCA) in 1964, initially studied in elective patients deemed low risk for surgery, to the present-day treatment of high-risk patients with extensive comorbidities using drug-eluting stents (DES). This journey of innovation can be encapsulated in four major revolutions: the first being the nonoperative dilation of coronary artery stenosis through PTCA, the second marked by the introduction of coronary stent placement, and the third revolutionized by the advent of DES, with studies encompassing high-bleeding risk populations. More recently, the "leave nothing behind" philosophy (the Forth Revolution) encompassed the use of bio-resorbable scaffolds and, mostly, drug-coated balloons, without the need for permanent prosthesis implant.

Each of these milestones has significantly contributed to the advancement and efficacy of CAD treatment. We will go through these steps with a specific attention to the evolution of patients' phenotype.

S. Gollamudi
Brooklyn Hospital Center, Brooklyn, NY, USA

B. Cortese (✉)
University Hospitals Harrington Heart & Vascular Institute, Cleveland, OH, USA

Fondazione Ricerca e Innovazione Cardiovascolare, Milan, Italy

DCB Academy, Milan, Italy

1.2 The First Revolution: Plain Old Balloon Angioplasty

Plain old balloon angioplasty (POBA) was the first interventional treatment before the development of stents. Its origin was from an accidental "recanalization" of an occluded iliac artery while performing an abdominal aortogram. In 1964, the first successful percutaneous

B. Cortese, S. Rigattieri (eds.), *High Bleeding Risk Patients in Interventional Cardiology*,
https://doi.org/10.1007/978-3-031-87302-7_1

transluminal peripheral angioplasty was performed. A decade later, in 1977, the first balloon percutaneous transluminal coronary angioplasty or plain old balloon angioplasty (POBA) was performed. The balloon caused the intimal layer to uncover and the medial layer to tear, exposing the subendothelial matrix to blood. This process promoted platelet aggregation and thrombosis in the short term, and led to chronic negative changes in vascular structure, including neointimal hyperplasia and remodeling. Due to insufficient initial gain as well as restenosis, there was loss of clinical benefit in 30–40% of patients in the first 6–9 months. Due to these limitations, further technological advancements were discovered which led to development of coronary stents [4].

In 1979, Andreas Gruntzig pioneered the field of interventional cardiology with his study on the nonoperative dilation of coronary artery stenosis using percutaneous transluminal coronary angioplasty. This groundbreaking technique marked the first revolution in the field. The study focused on patients with single-vessel disease, a short history of chest pain indicating a likely responsive soft atheroma, and low operative risk. Of the 50 patients included, 32 experienced successful dilation. However, this method faced limitations due to anatomical factors such as vessel tortuosity, sharply angled arteries, cul-de-sac lesions, fibrotic or calcified lesions, and stenotic main stems of the left coronary arteries [1]. Patients received aspirin for the first 3 days starting from the day of the procedure and heparin and low-molecular-weight dextran during dilation, followed by warfarin for 6–9 months post-procedure. It is crucial to note that this study's population comprised relatively young, low-risk individuals without comorbidities (age <65) [1]. For high-bleeding-risk patients, the standard procedure remained open-heart surgery. Due to the high rate of restenosis in these patients, a study was conducted by Dr. Fischman comparing coronary stent placement with balloon angioplasty, heralding the second revolution in interventional cardiology.

1.3 The Second Revolution: Coronary Stents

The first expanding coronary stent was discovered in 1986 by Peul and Sigwart followed by the first balloon expandable stent, which became the first FDA-approved stent in the United States. These stents were made from stainless steel and were quite thick with poor flexibility. They were superior to the plain old balloon angioplasty as they eliminated abrupt occlusion and reduced the rate of restenosis. The limitation with these stents were their high incidence of acute and subacute stent thrombosis which required high doses of anticoagulant drugs, leading to high rates of bleeding. Moreover, these stents were still at a significant risk of in-stent restenosis (ISR), reported in 15–30% of treated lesions at mid- and long-term follow-up [7]. Given the in-stent restenosis and neointimal hyperplasia being the major determinant of ISR, application of antiproliferative agents seems to be the next step. Thus in 1999 came the next revolution in interventional cardiology, the first drug-eluting stent.

In 1994, Dr. Fischman and colleagues demonstrated through a study that coronary stent placement was superior to balloon angioplasty, with lower restenosis rates and reduced myocardial infarction incidents post-procedure. This study included patients with single-vessel disease, excluding those with recent myocardial infarction (within 7 days), contraindications to aspirin, dipyridamole, or warfarin, left ventricular ejection fraction below 40%, coronary thrombus, multiple focal lesions or diffuse disease, severe left main coronary artery disease, ostial lesions, and severe vessel tortuosity. Despite its success, stent placement presented increased thrombotic risks and complications due to the intense anticoagulation and antiplatelet regimens required [7]. Notably, high-bleeding-risk patients were not included in this study due to the associated bleeding risks of the anticoagulation and antiplatelet regimens.

1.4 The Third Revolution: DES

The third revolution brought the advent of first-generation drug-eluting stents, which initially faced limitations due to increased risks of death and myocardial infarction (MI) related to late and very late stent thrombosis. This was possibly due to delayed endothelialization secondary to antiproliferative drug elution and hypersensitivity reactions to the polymer coating. In response, second-generation drug-eluting stents were developed and have since become the widely accepted percutaneous treatment of choice for coronary artery disease (CAD). Nearly 50 years after the inception of interventional cardiology, the field witnessed the LEADERS FREE trial, which studied high-bleeding-risk groups using drug-eluting stents versus bare-metal stents. The LEADERS FREE trial included patients at increased bleeding risk or those eligible for bare-metal stents due to the need to terminate dual antiplatelet therapy after 1 month. Inclusion criteria encompassed age ≥75 years, hemoglobin <11 g/dL, platelet count <100,000, recent hospital admission for bleeding, recent stroke or intracerebral hemorrhage, severe chronic liver disease, creatinine clearance <40 ml/min, recent cancer, planned major surgery, long-term glucocorticoid or NSAID use, and expected nonadherence to dual antiplatelet therapy for over 30 days. The study concluded that drug-eluting stents were superior to bare-metal stents regarding the primary safety endpoint of cardiac death, myocardial infarction, or stent thrombosis [13].

Jose Eduardo Sousa implanted the first drug-eluting stent (DES) in Brazil. This first-generation stents, CYPHER and TAXUS, used sirolimus and paclitaxel as the antiproliferative drugs. They were made of stainless steel and a strut thickness greater than 130 μm. These stents were shown to have a significant reduction in ISR, late lumen loss, and rate of target lesion/vessel revascularization compared with BMS. The drawbacks of the DES stents were increased risk of death and myocardial infarction (MI) related to late and very late stent thrombosis, delayed endothelialization secondary to antiproliferative drug elution, and a hypersensitivity reaction to the polymer coating. These drawbacks provoked the evolution from first-generation DES to second-generation DES, offering improved clinical outcomes and greater acceptance in the treatment of coronary artery disease [4].

Second-generation drug-eluting stents began to emerge in the mid-2000s, with significant advancements continuing into the following decade. These new stents featured platforms made from metal alloys, which allowed for thinner struts and increased flexibility. Additionally, the polymers used in these stents were developed from more biocompatible molecules, including zotarolimus, everolimus, and novolimus (the "limus family" drugs). These advancements led to faster drug elution and earlier endothelial coverage. As a result, second-generation stents significantly reduced rates of myocardial infarction (MI), target lesion revascularization, and stent thrombosis (ST) compared to their first-generation counterparts. Given their clinical benefits, second-generation drug-eluting stents have become widely used and are now considered the percutaneous treatment of choice for coronary artery disease (CAD) [4]. While second-generation drug-eluting stents marked a significant advancement with their improved materials and reduced complication rates, ongoing research revealed new challenges related to their polymer coatings. This led to the exploration and development of polymer-free drug-eluting stents, aimed at addressing these issues and further enhancing patient outcomes.

The polymer coating was identified as the cause of long-term stent failure due to its potential to induce a chronic inflammatory response, leading to delayed endothelial coverage and stent thrombosis (ST). This realization sparked the development of polymer-free drug-eluting stents (DES). However, since the polymer serves as a drug carrier and regulates the controlled release of the drug over time, creating polymer-free DES required a different approach to maintain adequate levels of antiproliferative drugs. This led to the development of stents with a porous metallic surface, with pore sizes ranging from 5 to 15 nanometers. These pores were loaded with the antiproliferative drug during the manufacturing process. The major drawback of this design was the lack of control over drug release. Randomized controlled trials comparing porous stents to second-generation DES showed no improvement in clinical outcomes. Besides the porous metallic stent surface, other variations of polymer-free DES emerged, including stents incorporating nanoparticles in a matrix compound (such as the Cre8 and BioFreedom stents) or microdrops by crystallization (such as the VESTAsync stent). Very few randomized controlled trials have evaluated the clinical outcomes of polymer-free DES, indicating the need for larger trials to assess their long-term efficacy and safety [12].

Another promising advancement in the realm of stents is the development of biodegradable polymer stents. These DES, coated with biodegradable polymers such as poly-DL-lactide-co-glycolide, initially function as DES and later as bare-metal stents (BMS). In the early phase, the antiproliferative drug is released, while the bioresorbable polymer degrades, leaving the metallic platform in the coronary artery [12]. The primary advantage of these stents is their lower rates of very late ST compared to first-generation DES, and their safety and efficacy are comparable to second-generation DES. However, more trials are needed to establish long-term results.

1.5 The Fourth Revolution: BVS and DCB and Inclusiveness of High-Bleeding-Risk Patients

Building on the success of biodegradable polymer stents, fully bioresorbable scaffolds were developed over the past 15 years as a solution to late adverse events associated with the persistence of metallic platforms in the coronary vessels. These devices provide local drug delivery and mechanical support similar to permanent metallic DES during the first months, and they fully absorb within 24–36 months. This absorption allows for the restoration of normal luminal diameter and vasomotor function, eliminates the focus for late adverse events, reduces the need for long-term dual antiplatelet therapy (DAPT), and permits surgical revascularization if necessary [4].

Bioresorbable scaffolds can be made from metallic alloys or an L-isomer of PLLA polymeric platforms, and they are typically covered with a polymer and an antiproliferative drug. Since the first drug-eluting bioresorbable scaffold (BRS) was implanted in 1995, approximately nine BRS have been studied in clinical trials. The most extensively studied device, the BVS ABSORB, was withdrawn from the market due to issues with radial force and higher rates of device thrombosis and myocardial infarction (MI) at 1 year, higher than currently available DES platforms [4]. To address these limitations, metallic bioabsorbable stents were designed. These stents offer more radial force and thinner struts, helping to maintain radial length and overcome the limitations of biodegradable polymer stents.

Much like bioresorbable scaffolds, drug-coated balloon (DCB) technology was designed to deliver antiproliferative drugs to the vessel wall without leaving a permanent prosthesis or durable polymers. DCB serve as an alternative to DES, directly delivering antiproliferative drugs to the vessel wall through a matrix which helps the drug entering the vessel wall and persisting there for weeks, in order to counteract the restenotic process. This approach negates the need for a permanent metallic prosthesis or durable polymer [15]. Presently, DCB technology is primarily used for patients with in-stent restenosis or de novo small vessel lesions. While there is initial evidence regarding DCB use in de novo lesions with larger reference vessel diameters ($\geq$3.0 mm), studies have demonstrated its angiographic superiority vs DES and comparable clinical outcome at 1 and 2 years [16]. Interestingly, there are initial advantages vs DES on the long term [17, 18]. As regards HBR patients, DCB have shown their superiority over BMS, suggesting it as a potential alternative treatment for this group [15, 20].

Several trials like LEADERS FREE and DEBUT trials have become trailblazers in studying alternative strategies for high-bleeding-risk patients undergoing interventions. Both DCS (in LEADERS FREE trial) and DCB (in DEBUT trial) showed superior efficacy compared to BMS in reducing the need for revascularization and in decreasing the incidence of major adverse cardiac events [12, 15]. Overall, the results from these trials advocate for a paradigm shift in treating HBR patients, emphasizing the efficacy and safety of drug-coated technologies with short-term DAPT. This approach helps balance the need to minimize bleeding risk while ensuring effective prevention of restenosis and other cardiac events.

1.6 Structural Procedures and Their Advances

1.6.1 Aortic Valve Replacement Advances

Aortic stenosis, a common valvular heart disease, affects between 2% and 9% of the elderly population. Surgical aortic valve replacement (SAVR) remains the gold standard treatment. However, this approach poses significant risks for patients with poor ventricular ejection fraction, advanced age, heart failure, elevated serum creatinine levels, severe mitral regurgitation, pulmonary hypertension, and systemic hypertension. For these high-risk patients, transcatheter aortic valve implantation (TAVI) and sutureless aortic valve replacement present viable alternatives. The use of balloon-expandable or self-expandable transcatheter valves has proven to be noninferior to conventional SAVR in two major prospective randomized trials. These findings have led to the inclusion of the transcatheter approach in the most recent guidelines and consensus statements on valvular heart disease as an additional therapeutic option for high-risk or inoperable patients (please see the relative chapter in this book). Additionally, the efficacy of the transcatheter approach is being evaluated in patients with severe aortic stenosis and an intermediate-to-high-risk profile for conventional surgery through several randomized CESANA IDEM trials [6].

1.6.2 Mitral Valve Transcatheter Therapies

Following the advances in aortic valve replacement, transcatheter edge-to-edge repair has become the established treatment for mitral regurgitation. However, this method excludes certain anatomies and does not consistently achieve sustained reductions in regurgitation. To address these limitations, transcatheter mitral valve replacement (TMVR) has been developed, offering a greater and more sustained reduction in regurgitation postimplantation. Nonetheless, the development of TMVR systems faces challenges due to the complex anatomy of the mitral valve and the various pathologies causing regurgitation and/or stenosis. Mitral regurgitation can be classified as functional, degenerative, or mixed, each requiring different treatment approaches. The intricate anatomy and disease pathologies complicate valve delivery, positioning, anchoring, and sealing. Additionally, due to the proximity of the aortic valve and the left ventricular outflow tract, left ventricular outflow obstruction (LVOTO) is a potential complication of TMVR, associated with poor prognosis. The transapical approach, commonly used for TMVR, has been linked to substantial morbidity and mortality. Consequently, current research focuses on transseptal TMVR, which presents procedural and engineering challenges. Despite these obstacles, transcatheter repair remains the mainstay treatment for mitral regurgitation. TMVR is reserved for suboptimal anatomies, but improved outcomes are being seen with current devices due to a better understanding of anatomic limitations, procedural advancements like anterior mitral valve leaflet laceration to prevent LVOTO, septal ablation, development of maneuverable low-profile delivery systems, and recapturable and repositionable valves [9].

1.6.3 Left Atrial Appendage Occlusion (LAAO)

In addition to advancements in valve therapies, left atrial appendage occlusion (LAAO) has emerged as an alternative to oral anticoagulation therapy for stroke prevention in nonvalvular atrial fibrillation. Although data comparing LAAO and anticoagulation therapy are sparse, three randomized controlled trials suggest that LAAO is not inferior to anticoagulation (please see the relative chapter in this book). Despite this, concerns persist regarding the limited efficacy data, potential adverse long-term sequelae such as device-related thrombosis (DRT) and peridevice leak (PDL), and the need for procedural simplification and optimization. Ongoing clinical investigations aim to address these challenges and further clarify the role of LAAO in stroke prevention [11].

1.7 Overview of Antithrombotic Regimens in Each Intervention Type

Antithrombotic regimens for coronary interventions have evolved significantly over the years, reflecting advancements in stent technology and an improved understanding of thrombotic risks associated with different clinical scenarios. For POBA, antithrombotic therapy primarily involved warfarin usage to prevent acute vessel closure and restenosis. BMS then necessitated a more aggressive approach with DAPT for at least 1 month to mitigate the risk of stent thrombosis, with a subsequent transition to single antiplatelet therapy. The advent of first-generation DES introduced the challenge of late stent thrombosis, necessitating prolonged DAPT, typically for 12 months, to ensure adequate endothelialization and minimize thrombotic complications [14]. Newer DES have further refined the antithrombotic regimen, balancing efficacy in preventing restenosis with a reduced need for extended DAPT, tailored to the individual patient's risk profile and clinical presentation, such as stable coronary artery disease (CAD) or acute coronary syndrome (ACS). In the context of stable angina, the antithrombotic strategy is calibrated to maintain long-term vessel patency and minimize ischemic events, balancing the risks of bleeding with the benefits of sustained antiplatelet activity [14]. Philosophically, these evolving regimens underscore a broader shift toward personalized medicine, where therapeutic strategies are increasingly tailored to the nuanced interplay of stent characteristics, patient-specific factors, and the dynamic nature of thrombotic risk. See below figures for panoramic view of the antithrombotic regimens.

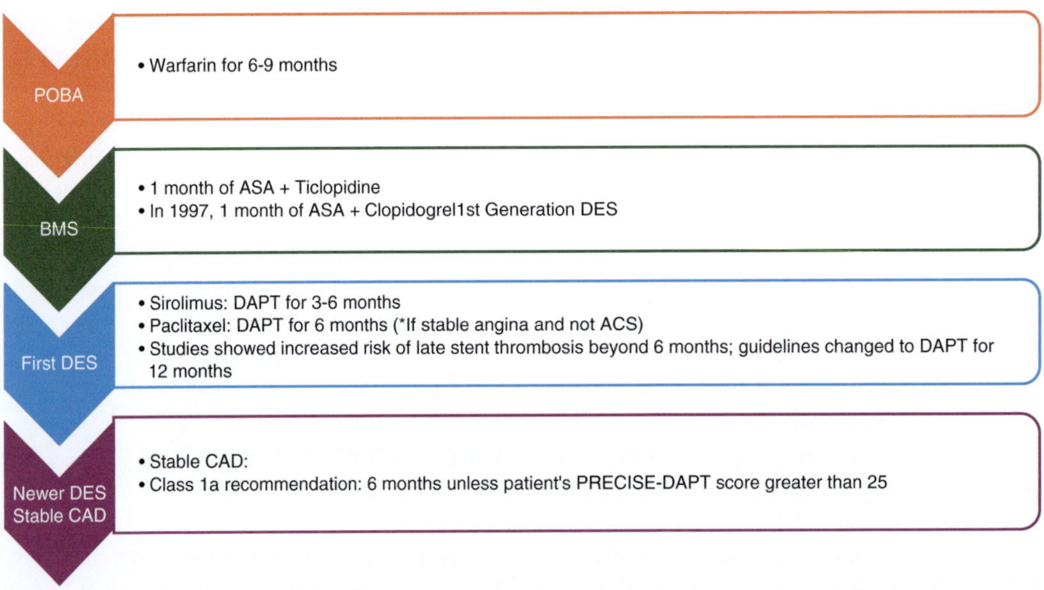

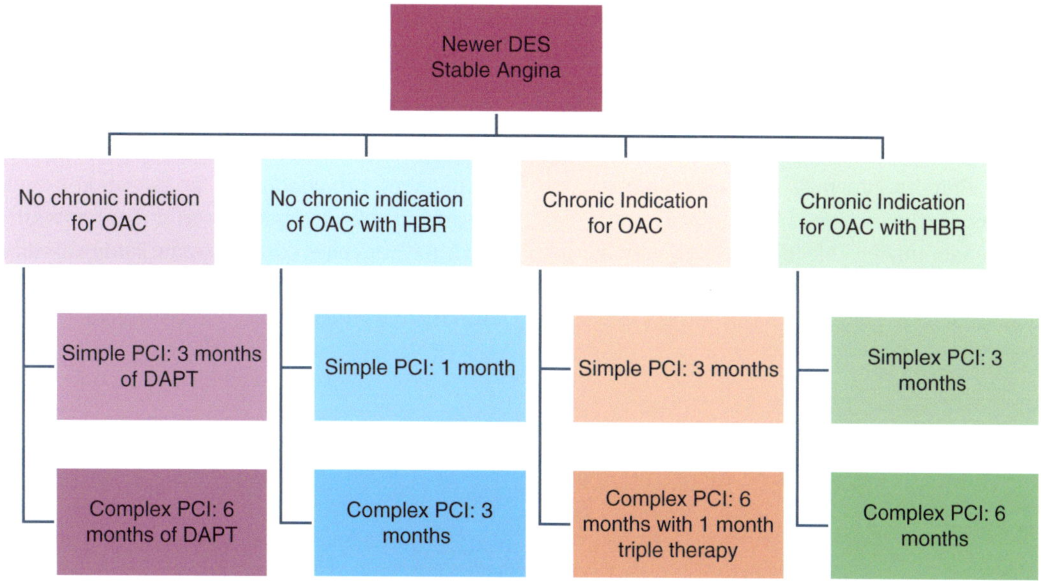

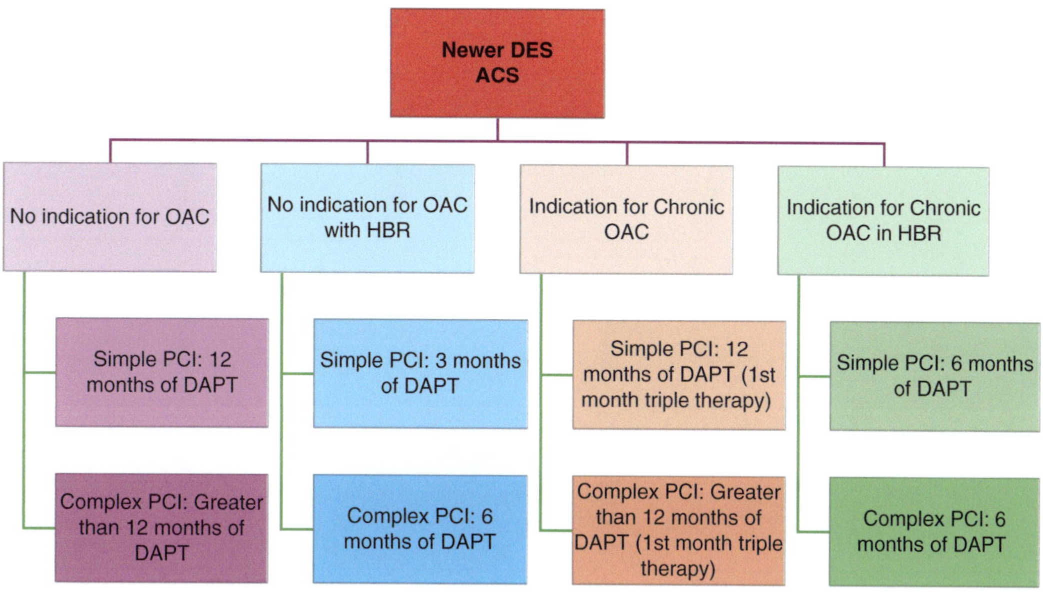

The landscape of antithrombotic regimens in the context of advanced cardiac interventions such as TAVR, TMVR, mitral transcatheter edge-to-edge repair (m-TEER), transcatheter tricuspid valve replacement (TTVR), and LAAO reflects a nuanced balance between thrombosis prevention and bleeding risk management. In TAVR, DAPT is typically employed initially to mitigate the risk of thromboembolic events, followed by a transition to single antiplatelet therapy, especially in patients with higher bleeding risks [10]. TMVR and m-TEER procedures, which address mitral valve pathologies, often necessitate *individualized* antithrombotic strategies, including anticoagulation or DAPT, depending on the patient's atrial fibrillation status and bleeding propensity. For TTVR, an emerging field with evolving protocols, antithrombotic regimens are largely extrapolated from TAVR experiences, emphasizing the need for personalized approaches [2]. LAAO, designed to prevent stroke in atrial fibrillation patients, often leads to a tailored regimen of anticoagulation or antiplatelet therapy, aimed at reducing stroke risk while minimizing bleeding complications [8]. Philosophically, the evolution of these regimens underscores a paradigm shift toward precision medicine, where therapeutic decisions are increasingly guided by a comprehensive assessment of procedural characteristics, patient-specific thrombotic and hemorrhagic profiles, and the dynamic interplay of individual risks and benefits. This holistic approach epitomizes the transition from a one-size-fits-all methodology to a more sophisticated, patient-centered strategy in cardiovascular care. See figures below for overview for antithrombotic regimen for each intervention.

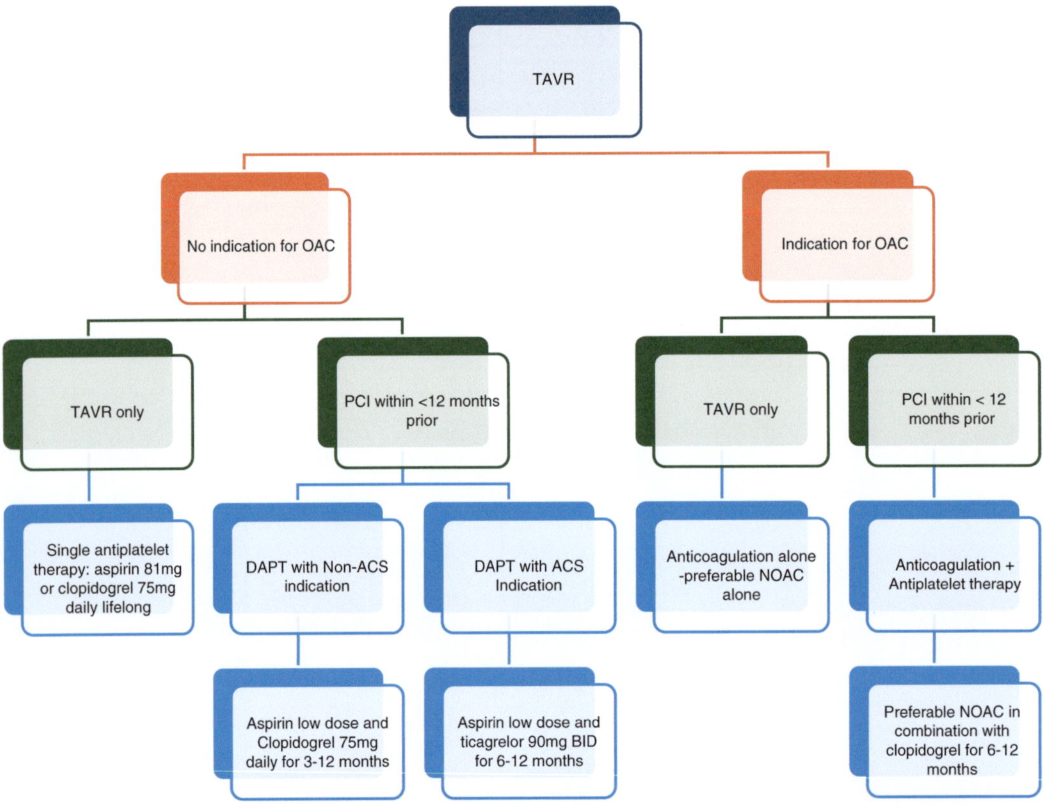
TAVR
No indication for OAC
Indication for OAC
TAVR only
PCI within <12 months prior
TAVR only
PCI within < 12 months prior
Single antiplatelet therapy: aspirin 81mg or clopidogrel 75mg daily lifelong
DAPT with Non-ACS indication
DAPT with ACS Indication
Anticoagulation alone -preferable NOAC alone
Anticoagulation + Antiplatelet therapy
Aspirin low dose and Clopidogrel 75mg daily for 3-12 months
Aspirin low dose and ticagrelor 90mg BID for 6-12 months
Preferable NOAC in combination with clopidogrel for 6-12 months

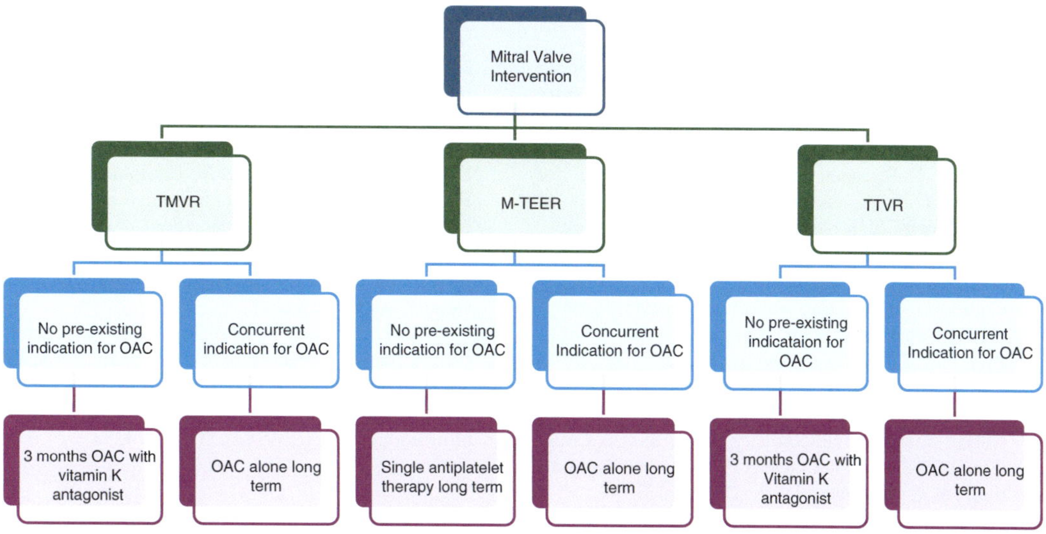

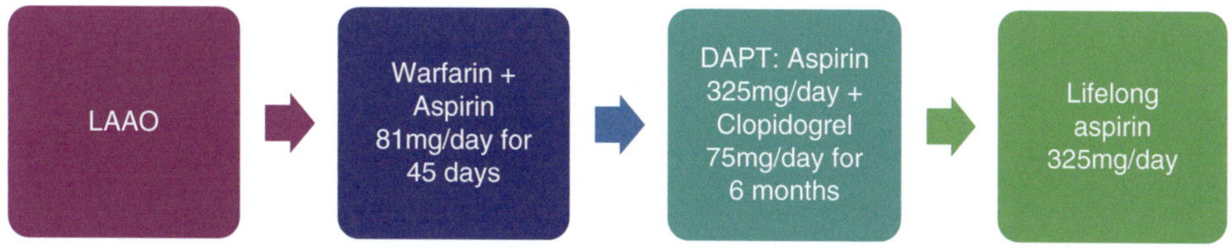
LAAO
Warfarin + Aspirin 81mg/day for 45 days
DAPT: Aspirin 325mg/day + Clopidogrel 75mg/day for 6 months
Lifelong aspirin 325mg/day

Bibliography

1. Andreas R, Gruntzig MD, Senning Å. Nonoperative dilation of coronary artery stenosis percutaneous transluminal coronary angioplasty. N Engl J Med. 1979;301:61–8.
2. Maznyczka A, Pilgrim T. Antithrombotic treatment after transcatheter valve interventions: current status and future directions. Clin Ther. 2024;46:122–33.
3. Beller GA. Coronary heart disease in the first 30 years of the 21st century: challenges and opportunities. Circulation. 2001;103:2428–35.
4. BenedettaTomberli A. A brief history of coronary artery stents. Rev Esp Cardiol. 2018;71:312–9.
5. Brown JC, Gerhardt TE, Kwon E (2024, January). Risk factors for coronary artery disease. Retrieved from StatPearls: https://www.ncbi.nlm.nih.gov/books/NBK554410/.
6. Muneretto C, Alfieri O, Cesana BM, Bisleri G, De Bonis M, Di Bartolomeo R, Savini C, Folesani G, Di Bacco L, Rambaldini M, Maureira JP. A comparison of conventional surgery, transcatheter aortic valve replacement, and sutureless valves in "real-world" patients with aortic stenosis and intermediate- to high-risk profile. J Thorac Cardiovasc Surg. 2015;150:1570–9.
7. Fischman DL, Leon MB, Baim DS, Schatz RA, Savage MP, Penn I, Detre K, Veltri L, Ricci D, Nobuyoshi M, Cleman M. A randomized comparison of coronary-stent placement and balloon angioplasty in the treatment of coronary artery disease. N Engl J Med. 1994;331:496–501.
8. Jules Mesnier PC-G-U-C. Antithrombotic management after left atrial appendage closure: current evidence and future perspectives. Circ Cardiovasc Interv. 2023;16:e012812.
9. Mark Hensey MB. Transcatheter mitral valve replacement. JACC Cardiovasc Interv. 2021;14: 489–500.
10. Hindi MN, et al. Antithrombotic therapy after transcatheter aortic valve replacement: an overview. Struct Heart. 2022;6:100085.
11. Mohamad Alkhouli CR-K. Left atrial appendage occlusion: current advances and remaining challenges. JACC Adv. 2022;1:1–18.
12. Philip Urban MI. Polymer-free drug-coated coronary stents in patients at high bleeding risk. N Engl J Med. 2015;373:2038–47.
13. Ruiz-Nodar JM. High bleeding risk patients undergoing percutaneous coronary intervention: still a

large margin left for improvement. Rev Esp Cardiol. 2020;73:521–3.
14. Camarero TG, de la Torre Hernández JM. Antithrombotic treatment after coronary intervention: agreement and controversy. Eur Cardiol Rev. 2020;15:e07.
15. Tuomas T, Rissanen MS. Drug-coated balloon for treatment of de-novo coronary artery lesions in patients with high bleeding risk (DEBUT): a single-blind, randomised, non-inferiority trial. Lancet. 2019;394:230–9.
16. Cortese B, et al. Drug-coated balloon versus drug-eluting stent for small coronary vessel disease. PICCOLETO II randomized clinical trial. JACC Cardiovasc Interv. 2020:2020.
17. Cortese B, et al. Drug-coated balloon versus drug-eluting stent for small coronary vessel disease. Long-term follow up of PICCOLETO II randomized clinical trial. JACC Cardiovasc Interv. 2023:2023.
18. Cortese B, et al. ANDROMEDA, a patient level meta-analysis of the long-term outcome of DCB vs DES in small coronary arteries. Oral presentation at the lete breaking clinical trials session, CRT 2024, Washington
19. Urban P, Mehran R, Colleran R, Angiolillo DJ, Byrne RA, Capodanno D, Cuisset T, Cutlip D, Eerdmans P, Eikelboom J, Farb A. Defining high bleeding risk in patients undergoing percutaneous coronary intervention: a consensus document from the Academic Research Consortium for High Bleeding Risk. Eur Heart J. 2019;40:2632–53.
20. Cortese B, Di Palma G, Guimaraes MG, et al. Drug-coated balloon versus drug-eluting stent for small coronary vessel disease: PICCOLETO II randomized clinical trial. JACC Cardiovasc Interv. 13(28):2840–9. https://doi.org/10.1016/j.jcin.2020.08.035.

Prognostic Impact of Bleeding in Interventional Cardiology

2

Felice Gragnano, Vincenzo De Sio, Arturo Cesaro, Silvio Coletta, Elisabetta Moscarella, and Paolo Calabrò

2.1 Impact of Bleeding in Patients Undergoing PCI

In patients undergoing percutaneous coronary intervention (PCI) with drug-eluting stent (DES) implantation, dual antiplatelet therapy (DAPT) is the current standard strategy to reduce the risk of adverse ischemic events including stent thrombosis and spontaneous atherothrombotic complications [1]. Current guidelines recommend 12 and 6 months of DAPT in patients undergoing PCI for acute coronary syndrome (ACS) and chronic coronary syndrome (CCS), respectively, followed by single-antiplatelet therapy with aspirin or clopidogrel for long-term secondary prevention [2, 3]. However, the use of longer and more intense DAPT regimens has been shown to increase the risk of bleeding, which may offset the benefit of anti-ischemic protection [1, 4, 5]. Bleeding has long been considered less clinically relevant than ischemic events, and its prognostic impact has often been underestimated in the past [6]. Yet, in recent years, bleeding has received growing attention as it is the most common non-cardiac adverse event after PCI and is associated with a worse prognosis, prolonged hospital stay, and higher healthcare costs [1]. In the first year after PCI, major bleeding can occur in approximately 2–4% of patients in the absence of high bleeding risk and in more than 4% of patients with high bleeding risk [7, 8]. Moreover, bleeding events occur more frequently in patients presenting with ACS than in those undergoing elective PCI [9].

Patients who experience bleeding have a worse prognosis and a higher risk of short- and long-term mortality [7, 8]. Several mechanisms have been proposed to explain this adverse association, such as hypotension, hemodynamic compromise, myocardial ischemia, and arrhythmias. The use of blood transfusions has also been associated with detrimental effects, including vasoconstriction, systemic inflammation, and increased platelet activation and aggregation, which may further increase mortality risk and should be considered only when necessary [10]. In addition, discontinuing DAPT (especially in the first 1–3 months after PCI) and other cardiac medications (e.g., beta-blockers and angiotensin-converting enzyme inhibitors) may help control bleeding and hypotension but may adversely affect long-term prognosis.

The prognostic impact of bleeding after PCI depends on the timing of its occurrence (early vs. late bleeding) and its severity. Several classifica-

F. Gragnano · V. De Sio · A. Cesaro · S. Coletta · E. Moscarella · P. Calabrò (✉)
Department of Translational Medical Sciences, University of Campania "Luigi Vanvitelli", Caserta, Italy

Division of Clinical Cardiology, A.O.R.N. "Sant'Anna e San Sebastiano", Caserta, Italy
e-mail: paolo.calabro@unicampania.it

B. Cortese, S. Rigattieri (eds.), *High Bleeding Risk Patients in Interventional Cardiology*, https://doi.org/10.1007/978-3-031-87302-7_2

tions have been proposed to define the severity of bleeding and to distinguish prognostically relevant events from those with minimal clinical impact, including the Bleeding Academic Research Consortium (BARC), Thrombolysis in Myocardial Infarction (TIMI), International Society on Thrombosis and Haemostasis (ISTH), Global Utilization of Streptokinase and Tissue Plasminogen Activator for Occluded Arteries (GUSTO), and Acute Catheterization and Urgent Intervention Triage Strategy (ACUITY) classifications [7]. To date, the BARC scale has been widely used to standardize the definition of bleeding and stratify bleeding risk after PCI in contemporary trials and clinical practice [7].

2.1.1 Early Bleeding Events

Early bleeding, generally defined as a hemorrhagic event occurring within 30 days of PCI, is relatively common in practice, particularly in high-risk subgroups [7, 11]. Older age, female sex, lower body weight, and renal insufficiency have been shown to consistently predict early bleeding complications after PCI. Patients with advanced age are at higher risk for in-hospital bleeding, with an estimated increase of approximately 30% per decade, likely due to arterial aging and altered hemostatic vasoconstrictor response [7, 11]. Women undergoing PCI also have a higher likelihood of developing in-hospital major bleeding than men, mainly because of differences in vascular anatomy and pharmacologic response to antithrombotic drugs [12, 13]. In a recent study, female sex was an independent predictor of access site bleeding after PCI but not of spontaneous bleeding [13]. Renal function is also widely recognized as an essential determinant of early post-PCI complications. In large studies, the estimated risk of in-hospital major bleeding in ACS patients was increased by ≈50% in patients with renal failure, with the magnitude depending on the decrease of renal function [7].

Several studies have shown an independent association between early bleeding and subsequent prognosis. A recent sub-analysis of the Minimizing Adverse Haemorrhagic Events by Transradial Access Site and Systemic Implementation of Angiox (MATRIX) trial focused on 7781 patients with ACS, of whom 748 (11.5%) had in-hospital bleeding [14]. In this study, minor bleeding (hemoglobin drop: ≥3 and <5 g/dl) and major bleeding (hemoglobin drop: ≥5 g/dl) were independently associated with a threefold and tenfold increased risk of 1-year mortality, respectively. Of note, an in-hospital hemoglobin drop of ≥3 g/dl, even in the absence of overt bleeding, was common and independently associated with a twofold greater risk of 1-year mortality. Several mechanisms may be responsible for the in-hospital hemoglobin drop in the absence of overt bleeding, such as the inflammatory status, stress polycythemia, hemodilution secondary to volume repletion, and impaired bone marrow activity, but their individual contribution to this phenomenon and subsequent prognosis remains unclear [14].

Early post-procedural bleeding appears to have a similar or even stronger association with mortality than recurrent myocardial infarction (MI), underscoring the importance of implementing prevention strategies. A recent meta-analysis [15] evaluated the prognostic value of early adverse events in 51,934 patients undergoing PCI from 7 studies. The median risk of early bleeding was 3.5%; the median risk of early MI was 5.2%; the median risk of death in patients with early bleeding or early MI was 15.3% and 8.6%, respectively. In this pooled analysis, the risk of all-cause mortality was increased to a greater extent after early bleeding (hazard ratio [HR]: 3.77; 95% CI: 3.23–4.41) than after early MI (HR: 2.45; 95% CI: 1.98–3.02), resulting in a significant 46% higher relative risk of death after early bleeding than after early MI, with relevant implications for practice [15].

2.1.2 Access Site Bleeding

In patients undergoing PCI, approximately half of all early bleeding events occur at the arterial access site, ranging from mild subcutaneous hematoma to potentially life-threatening bleeding (e.g., retroperitoneal hemorrhage) [6].

Arterial access site selection and management significantly impact access site complications, and radial access has been shown to have a superior safety profile compared to femoral access. In the MATRIX trial, which included 8404 patients with ACS undergoing invasive management, radial access significantly reduced the relative risk of net adverse clinical events by 20% compared to femoral access. This benefit was driven by a significant 33% reduction in BARC type 3 or 5 bleeding and a 28% reduction in all-cause mortality [16]. In a sub-analysis of the trial, the use of vascular closure devices for femoral access did not reduce the risk of bleeding, confirming the benefit of radial access regardless of the technique used to close the femoral access [17].

In a recent patient-level meta-analysis of 21,600 patients undergoing coronary angiography and PCI from 7 randomized trials, all-cause mortality (1.6% vs. 2.1%; HR: 0.77; 95% CI: 0.63–0.95; $p = 0.012$) and major bleeding (1.5% vs. 2.7%; odds ratio: 0.55; 95% CI: 0.45–0.67; $p < 0.001$) were both lower with radial access compared to femoral access. Interestingly, mediation analysis showed that the mortality benefit of radial access was only partially driven by bleeding prevention and that additional mechanisms are needed to fully explain the causal association [18]. In this context, it is essential to note that the prognostic impact of post-PCI bleeding events may differ depending on whether they are access site-related or not. Patients with major spontaneous bleeding have a twofold higher risk of mortality than patients with major access site bleeding [19].

2.1.3 Late Bleeding Events

Late bleeding events (>30 days after PCI) are also common in patients undergoing PCI and have a significant impact on patient prognosis [15, 20]. Several clinical and treatment factors have been associated with an increased risk of late bleeding. Among these, the type of antiplatelet regimen beyond 1 month after PCI has a significant impact on this risk and possibly on mortality. A short duration of DAPT (1–3 months) after PCI has been shown to significantly reduce the risk of major bleeding compared to standard DAPT, with an effect that is more relevant in patients with high bleeding risk [4, 21]. In a recent meta-analysis, ticagrelor monotherapy after a short course of DAPT was associated with a significant 28% lower mortality risk than standard DAPT, which may be related to the substantial reduction in major bleeding observed with this strategy [22].

The association between late bleeding events and mortality has been evaluated in several studies, including large observational registries and sub-analyses of randomized controlled trials. An analysis of the Assessment of Dual AntiPlatelet Therapy With Drug Eluting Stents (ADAPT-DES) study examined the incidence and prognostic impact of clinically relevant post-discharge bleeding in 8577 all-comer patients undergoing PCI [20]. Post-discharge bleeding was defined as bleeding requiring medical attention according to various classifications (e.g., TIMI major or minor bleeding, GUSTO severe or moderate bleeding, and ACUITY major bleeding). During 2 years of follow-up, 535 (6.2%) patients experienced post-discharge bleeding, with approximately 90% of events occurring beyond 30 days after discharge (median time: 300 days (130–509 days)); the site of bleeding was the gastrointestinal tract in 62% of cases. Patients who experienced post-discharge bleeding had higher rates of all-cause mortality (13.0% vs. 3.2%; $p < 0.0001$) and higher rates of cardiac mortality (5.1% vs. 1.9%; $p < 0.0001$); bleeding occurring between 30 days and 1 year or between 1 and 2 years were similarly associated with an increased risk of death. Patients who bled and received blood transfusions had the highest rates of all-cause and cardiac mortality. At multivariate analysis, post-discharge bleeding was strongly associated with 2-year mortality (HR: 5.03; 95% CI: 3.29–7.66; $p < 0.0001$). Noteworthy, the effect of post-discharge bleeding on subsequent mortality was approximately twofold greater than that of post-discharge MI, suggesting the clinical relevance of such events [20].

The prognostic impact of late bleeding and MI was also evaluated using data from 12,944 patients with non-ST-segment elevation ACS from the

Thrombin Receptor Antagonist for Clinical Event Reduction in Acute Coronary Syndrome (TRACER) trial [23]. In this study, 500 patients (3.9%) died. A total of 718 patients (5.6%) had a recurrent MI >30 days after the index coronary event, and these patients had a fivefold increased risk of death compared to patients without recurrent MI (adjusted HR: 5.36; 95% CI: 4.26–6.74; $p < 0.001$). Late bleeding events were distributed by severity as follows: BARC 1 in 878 patients (6.9%); BARC 2 in 712 patients (5.6%); and BARC 3 in 346 patients (2.7%). During follow-up, BARC 1 bleeding did not affect subsequent survival (adjusted HR: 0.89; CI 95%: 0.61–1.31; $p = 0.551$). Both BARC 2 bleeding (adjusted HR: 1.70; 95% CI: 1.23–2.36; $p = 0.001$) and BARC 3 bleeding (HR: 5.73; 95% CI: 4.32–7.59; $p < 0.001$) were associated with a significant increase in the risk of death. When the relative impact of MI versus bleeding was assessed, recurrent MI was associated with a threefold and twofold higher risk of death compared with BARC 2 and BARC 3a bleeding, respectively, and a risk similar to that of BARC 3b bleeding. The risk of death following MI was significantly lower than after BARC 3c bleeding (which includes intracranial and intraocular bleeding) (relative risk: 0.22; CI 95%: 0.13–0.36; $p < 0.001$). These results indicate that late bleeding significantly affects mortality risk after ACS, with an effect similar to that of late MI for more severe events, supporting the concept that "irreparable" injury is dangerous regardless of whether it results from ischemia or bleeding [24].

Recently, an updated meta-analysis comprehensively evaluated the prognostic impact of late bleeding versus MI using available evidence from 8 studies involving 94,196 patients with CAD [15]. In this analysis, the median risk of late bleeding was 3.1% (IQR: 2.2%–5.8%), and the median risk of late MI was 2.9% (IQR: 2.5%–4.7%). The median risk of death in patients with late bleeding or late MI was 17.6% (IQR: 13.4%–22.1%) and 17.2% (IQR: 10.9%–21.3%), respectively. Mortality risk was significantly higher in patients with late bleeding (HR: 5.51; 95% CI: 3.13–9.68; I^2=95%) and late MI (HR: 4.67; 95% CI: 2.85–7.63; I^2=94%) compared to patients without bleeding or MI. Furthermore, the impact of late bleeding and late MI on mortality was similar, suggesting a prognostic equivalence of the two adverse events in the long term after PCI [15].

2.2 Impact of Bleeding in Patients Undergoing TAVI

For patients with severe aortic stenosis, transcatheter aortic valve implantation (TAVI) is a less invasive treatment option than surgical aortic valve replacement (SAVR), halving the risk of major bleeding, one of the major benefits of the percutaneous route [25]. Recently, the incidence of bleeding has been reduced by advances in procedural techniques, smaller sheaths, improved operator experience, and expanded recommendations for TAVI in younger and lower surgical risk patients. Nevertheless, TAVI still carries a high rate of procedural and spontaneous bleeding, with a 5-year incidence of approximately 30% in some studies [25]. Even in contemporary cohorts of low-risk patients, the risk of life-threatening, disabling, or major bleeding remains significant, exceeding 7% at 1 year, with some patients experiencing recurrent events [26]. The risk of bleeding after TAVI is particularly high in patients with advanced age, anemia, frailty, low body mass index, chronic kidney disease, acquired von Willebrand factor deficiency, and thrombocytopenia [25].

According to the time of onset, bleeding events are commonly classified as early (within 30 days of TAVI) or late (after 30 days of TAVI) [25]. Hemorrhagic events can occur at the vascular access site (mainly in the periprocedural period) or at other sites (generally occurring later in the follow-up period). Like the PCI setting, bleeding is associated with poor short- and long-term prognosis, regardless of the timing of occurrence [27–29]. The Valve Academic Research Consortium (VARC)-3 criteria are currently used to define bleeding occurring after valve implantation and distinguish four types of bleeding with increasing severity and progressively greater prognostic impact [30].

The bleeding site also has a relevant impact on the prognosis of patients undergoing TAVI. In the Swiss TAVI Registry [31], there was an increased 5-year risk of mortality in patients who experienced access site bleeding (adjusted HR: 1.34; 95% CI: 1.01–1.76; $p = 0.04$) or nonaccess site bleeding (adjusted HR: 2.08; CI 95%: 1.60–2.71; $p < 0.001$) as compared to those who were free of bleeding events. Similar to PCI patients, nonaccess site bleeding was shown to have a greater impact on mortality (approximately 1.5 times higher risk compared to access site bleeding). Of note, more than one-third of patients undergoing TAVI are anemic and often require red blood cell transfusions. Yet, post-TAVI transfusions have been associated with an increased mortality risk, regardless of whether they are given in the presence or absence of major hemorrhagic complications [31, 32].

2.2.1 Early Bleeding Events

Early bleeding is the most common complication following TAVI. Approximately 80% of all bleeding events after TAVI occur within the first 30 days and are associated with a poor prognosis [27, 33]. In a meta-analysis including 3519 high-risk patients undergoing TAVI from 16 studies, the 30-day major and life-threatening bleeding rates were 22.3% and 15.5%, respectively [34]. Early bleeding complications after TAVI are mainly related to vascular complications [35]. The risk of periprocedural bleeding is particularly high in patients receiving transaortic and transapical approaches, which have been gradually abandoned due to higher complication rates; among alternative approaches to the transfemoral access, the use of trans-carotid and trans-subclavian approaches is preferred because they are generally safer [36, 37]. Female sex is also associated with early access site bleeding, likely due to small femoral arteries with and consequently lower sheath-femoral artery ratio [38]. Patients with chronic kidney disease have an increased risk of major in-hospital bleeding (OR: 1.35; CI 95%: 1.27–1.44) [39].

2.2.2 Late Bleeding Events

Late bleeding is a common complication in patients undergoing TAVI, ranging from 10% to 25%, with relevant prognostic impact [25]. Predictors of late bleeding include advanced age, cardiovascular and non-cardiovascular comorbidities, long-term anticoagulation, and moderate to severe paravalvular leak after TAVI [35].

In a pooled analysis of 2401 patients undergoing TAVI in the Placement of Aortic Transcatheter Valves (PARTNER) program, bleeding occurring beyond 30 days after TAVI was associated with a fourfold increased risk of mortality between 30 days and 12 months (adjusted HR: 3.91; CI 95%: 2.67–5.71; $p < 0.001$) [27]. In this cohort, the most common types of bleeding were gastrointestinal (40.8%, mainly from upper gastrointestinal tract) and neurological (15.5%). These data were consistent with another study that reported that major late bleeding was associated with a worse prognosis, including a higher risk of all-cause mortality (HR: 5.66; CI 95%: 3.10–10.31; $p < 0.001$), cardiac mortality (HR: 11.62; CI 95%: 4.59–29.37; $p < 0.001$), transfusion, and rehospitalization [40].

Patients with severe aortic stenosis often have concomitant coronary artery disease (approximately 30% of patients), and some of them (approximately 20%) undergo PCI before TAVI requiring DAPT, which may further increase the risk of late bleeding [41]. In a recent multicenter TAVI registry including 1457 PCI-TAVI patients (PCI performed within 3 months before TAVI), late bleeding was found to be associated with a higher rate of all-cause death (HR: 1.39; 95% CI: 1.05–1.83), with early major bleeding (HR: 2.00; 95% CI: 1.10–3.62) and the combination of antiplatelet and anticoagulation therapy (HR: 1.72; 95% CI: 1.19–2.49) both emerging as independent predictors of late bleeding [42, 43].

2.3 Conclusions

In current practice, bleeding remains a common complication in patients undergoing PCI or TAVI. The occurrence of early bleeding (mainly procedure-related) or late bleeding (mainly spontaneous) has been associated with more complex management and adverse prognosis in these patients, with a prognostic impact similar to that of ischemic complications. Routine implementation of bleeding avoidance strategies is therefore essential to minimize the risk of major bleeding and improve patient management and outcomes after PCI or TAVI (Figs. 2.1 and 2.2).

Relationships with Industry and Other Entities The authors have no relevant relationships to the contents of this paper to disclose.

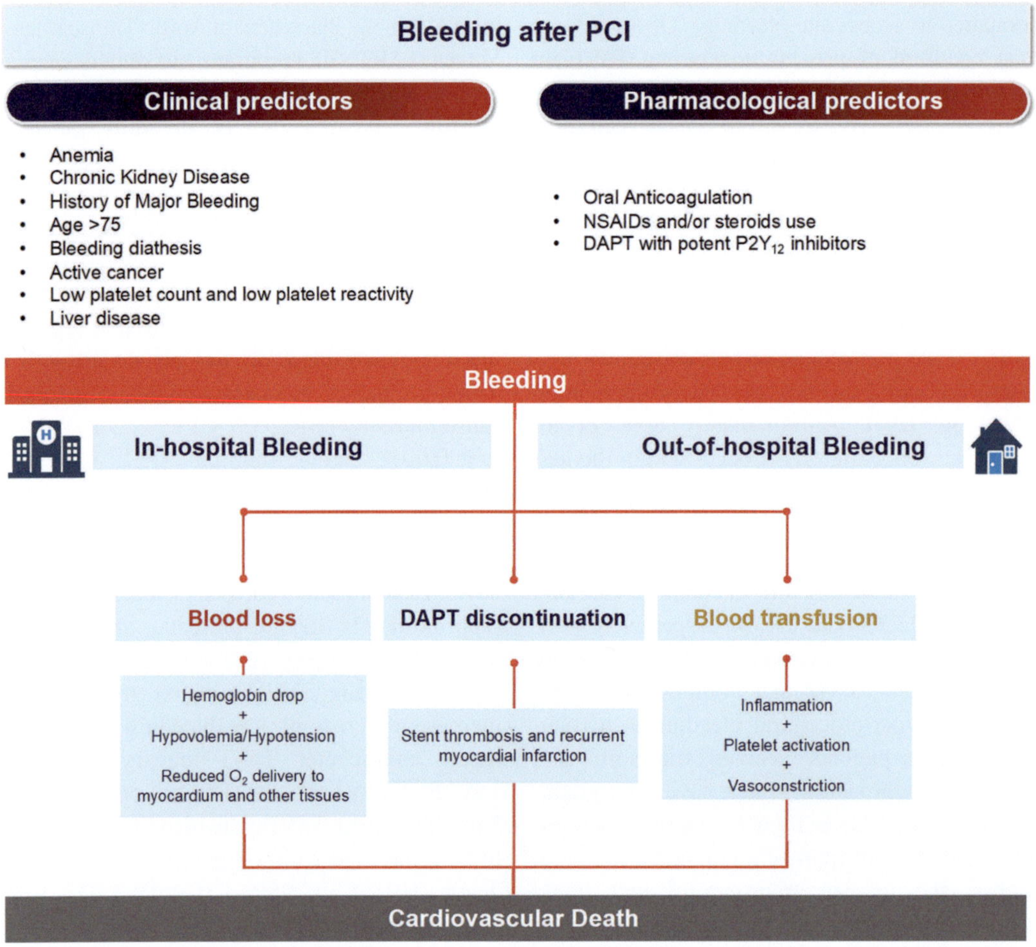

Fig. 2.1 Predictors and prognostic impact of bleeding events after percutaneous coronary intervention (PCI). *PCI* percutaneous coronary intervention, *NSAID* nonsteroidal anti-inflammatory drug, *DAPT* dual antiplatelet therapy

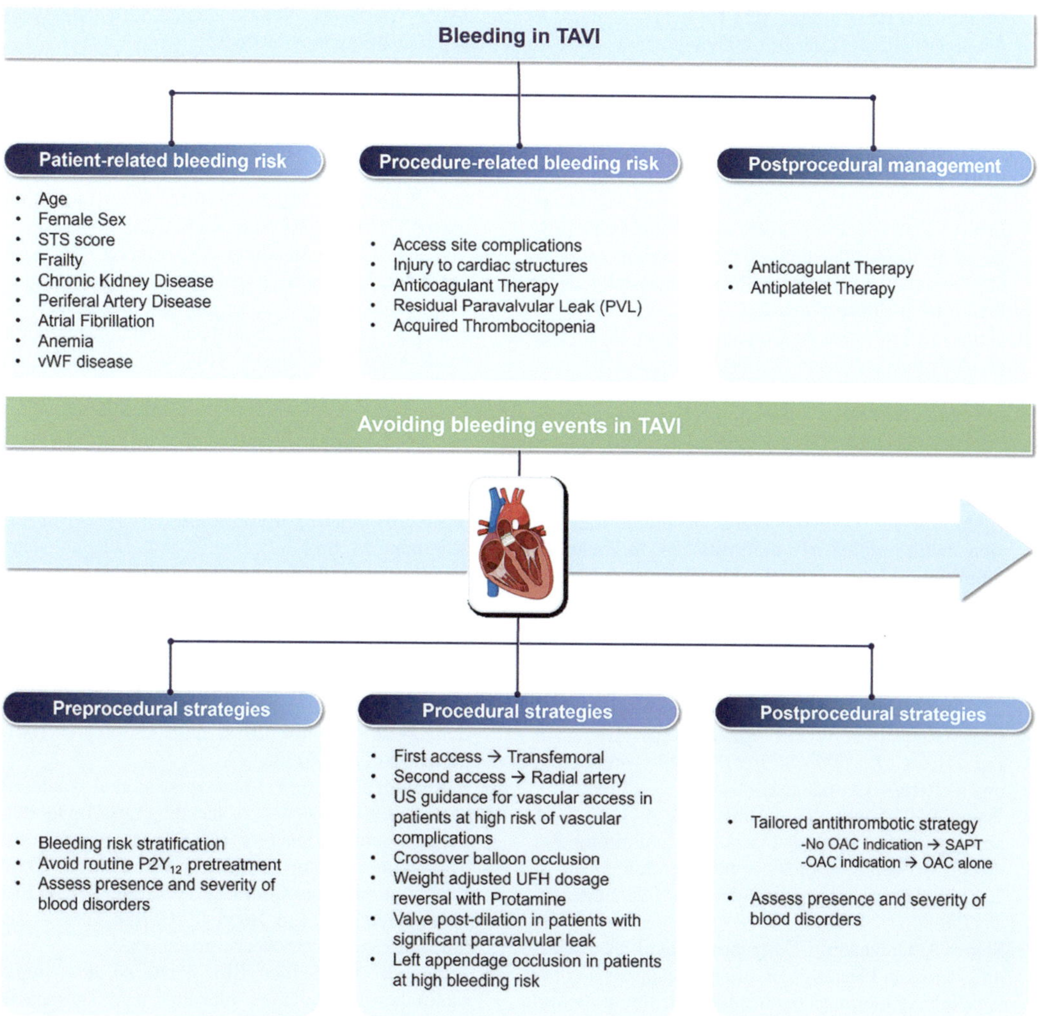

Fig. 2.2 Factors related to bleeding events in patients undergoing transcatheter aortic valve implantation (TAVI) and potential preventive strategies. *TAVI* transcatheter aortic valve implantation, *vWF* von Willebrand factor, *UFH* unfractionated heparin

References

1. Angiolillo DJ, Galli M, Collet J-P, Kastrati A, O'Donoghue ML. Antiplatelet therapy after percutaneous coronary intervention. EuroIntervention. 2022;17(17):e1371–96. https://doi.org/10.4244/EIJ-D-21-00904.
2. Byrne RA, Rossello X, Coughlan JJ, et al. 2023 ESC guidelines for the management of acute coronary syndromes. Eur Heart J. 2023;44(38):3720–826. https://doi.org/10.1093/eurheartj/ehad191.
3. Vrints C, Andreotti F, Koskinas KC, et al. 2024 ESC guidelines for the management of chronic coronary syndromes. Eur Heart J. 2024;45(36):3415–537. https://doi.org/10.1093/eurheartj/ehae177.
4. Valgimigli M, Gragnano F, Branca M, et al. P2Y12 inhibitor monotherapy or dual antiplatelet therapy after coronary revascularisation: individual patient level meta-analysis of randomised controlled trials. BMJ. 2021;373:n1332. https://doi.org/10.1136/bmj.n1332.
5. Gragnano F, Mehran R, Branca M, et al. P2Y12 inhibitor monotherapy or dual antiplatelet therapy after complex percutaneous coronary interventions. J Am Coll Cardiol. 2023;81(6):537–52. https://doi.org/10.1016/j.jacc.2022.11.041.
6. Capodanno D, Bhatt DL, Gibson CM, et al. Bleeding avoidance strategies in percutaneous coronary inter-

vention. Nat Rev Cardiol. 2022;19(2):117–32. https://doi.org/10.1038/s41569-021-00598-1.
7. Urban P, Mehran R, Colleran R, et al. Defining high bleeding risk in patients undergoing percutaneous coronary intervention. Circulation. 2019;140(3):240–61. https://doi.org/10.1161/CIRCULATIONAHA.119.040167.
8. Corpataux N, Spirito A, Gragnano F, et al. Validation of high bleeding risk criteria and definition as proposed by the academic research consortium for high bleeding risk. Eur Heart J. 2020;41(38) https://doi.org/10.1093/eurheartj/ehaa671.
9. Gragnano F, Spirito A, Corpataux N, et al. Impact of clinical presentation on bleeding risk after percutaneous coronary intervention and implications for the ARC-HBR definition. EuroIntervention. 2021;17(11):e898–909. https://doi.org/10.4244/EIJ-D-21-00181.
10. Chatterjee S, Wetterslev J, Sharma A, Lichstein E, Mukherjee D. Association of blood transfusion with increased mortality in myocardial infarction: a meta-analysis and diversity-adjusted study sequential analysis. JAMA Intern Med. 2013;173(2):132–9. https://doi.org/10.1001/2013.jamainternmed.1001.
11. Moscucci M, Fox KAA, Cannon CP, et al. Predictors of major bleeding in acute coronary syndromes: the Global Registry of Acute Coronary Events (GRACE). Eur Heart J. 2003;24(20):1815–23. https://doi.org/10.1016/s0195-668x(03)00485-8.
12. Wang WT, James SK, Wang TY. A review of sex-specific benefits and risks of antithrombotic therapy in acute coronary syndrome. Eur Heart J. 2017;38(3):165–71. https://doi.org/10.1093/eurheartj/ehv758.
13. Spirito A, Gragnano F, Corpataux N, et al. Sex-based differences in bleeding risk after percutaneous coronary intervention and implications for the academic research consortium high bleeding risk criteria. J Am Heart Assoc. 2021;10(12):e021965. https://doi.org/10.1161/JAHA.121.021965.
14. Leonardi S, Gragnano F, Carrara G, et al. Prognostic implications of declining hemoglobin content in patients hospitalized with acute coronary syndromes. J Am Coll Cardiol. 2021;77(4):375–88. https://doi.org/10.1016/j.jacc.2020.11.046.
15. Piccolo R, Oliva A, Avvedimento M, et al. Mortality after bleeding versus myocardial infarction in coronary artery disease: a systematic review and meta-analysis. EuroIntervention. 2021;17(7):550–60. https://doi.org/10.4244/EIJ-D-20-01197.
16. Valgimigli M, Gagnor A, Calabró P, et al. Radial versus femoral access in patients with acute coronary syndromes undergoing invasive management: a randomised multicentre trial. Lancet. 2015;385(9986):2465–76. https://doi.org/10.1016/S0140-6736(15)60292-6.
17. Gragnano F, Manavifar N, Gargiulo G, et al. Femoral access with or without vascular closure device or radial access in acute coronary syndrome. JACC Cardiovasc Interv. 2019;12(20) https://doi.org/10.1016/j.jcin.2019.06.027.
18. Gargiulo G, Giacoppo D, Jolly SS, et al. Effects on mortality and major bleeding of radial versus femoral artery access for coronary angiography or percutaneous coronary intervention: meta-analysis of individual patient data from 7 multicenter randomized clinical trials. Circulation. 2022;146(18):1329–43. https://doi.org/10.1161/CIRCULATIONAHA.122.061527.
19. Verheugt FWA, Steinhubl SR, Hamon M, et al. Incidence, prognostic impact, and influence of antithrombotic therapy on access and nonaccess site bleeding in percutaneous coronary intervention. JACC Cardiovasc Interv. 2011;4(2):191–7. https://doi.org/10.1016/j.jcin.2010.10.011.
20. Généreux P, Giustino G, Witzenbichler B, et al. Incidence, predictors, and impact of post-discharge bleeding after percutaneous coronary intervention. J Am Coll Cardiol. 2015;66(9):1036–45. https://doi.org/10.1016/j.jacc.2015.06.1323.
21. Valgimigli M, Frigoli E, Heg D, et al. Dual antiplatelet therapy after PCI in patients at high bleeding risk. N Engl J Med. 2021;385(18):1643–55. https://doi.org/10.1056/NEJMoa2108749.
22. Valgimigli M, Gragnano F, Branca M, et al. Ticagrelor or clopidogrel monotherapy vs dual antiplatelet therapy after percutaneous coronary intervention. JAMA Cardiol. 2024; https://doi.org/10.1001/jamacardio.2024.0133.
23. Valgimigli M, Costa F, Lokhnygina Y, et al. Trade-off of myocardial infarction vs. bleeding types on mortality after acute coronary syndrome: lessons from the Thrombin Receptor Antagonist for Clinical Event Reduction in Acute Coronary Syndrome (TRACER) randomized trial. Eur Heart J. 2017;38(11):804–10. https://doi.org/10.1093/eurheartj/ehw525.
24. Bergmark BA, Scirica BM. First, do no (irreparable) harm: infarction, bleeding, and subsequent risk of death. The dangers of false equivalency. Eur Heart J. 2017;38(11):811–3. https://doi.org/10.1093/eurheartj/ehw639.
25. Avvedimento M, Nuche J, Farjat-Pasos JI, Rodés-Cabau J. Bleeding events after transcatheter aortic valve replacement: JACC state-of-the-art review. J Am Coll Cardiol. 2023;81(7):684–702. https://doi.org/10.1016/j.jacc.2022.11.050.
26. Mack MJ, Leon MB, Thourani VH, et al. Transcatheter aortic-valve replacement with a balloon-expandable valve in low-risk patients. N Engl J Med. 2019;380(18):1695–705. https://doi.org/10.1056/NEJMoa1814052.
27. Généreux P, Cohen DJ, Mack M, et al. Incidence, predictors, and prognostic impact of late bleeding complications after transcatheter aortic valve replacement. J Am Coll Cardiol. 2014;64(24):2605–15. https://doi.org/10.1016/j.jacc.2014.08.052.
28. Siemieniuk RA, Agoritsas T, Manja V, et al. Transcatheter versus surgical aortic valve replacement in patients with severe aortic stenosis at low and intermediate risk: systematic review and meta-analysis.

BMJ. 2016;354:i5130. https://doi.org/10.1136/bmj.i5130.
29. Siontis GCM, Overtchouk P, Cahill TJ, et al. Transcatheter aortic valve implantation vs. surgical aortic valve replacement for treatment of symptomatic severe aortic stenosis: an updated meta-analysis. Eur Heart J. 2019;40(38):3143–53. https://doi.org/10.1093/eurheartj/ehz275.
30. Généreux P, Piazza N, et al. Valve academic research consortium 3: updated endpoint definitions for aortic valve clinical research. J Am Coll Cardiol. 2021;77(21):2717–46. https://doi.org/10.1016/j.jacc.2021.02.038.
31. Piccolo R, Pilgrim T, Franzone A, et al. Frequency, timing, and impact of access-site and non-access-site bleeding on mortality among patients undergoing transcatheter aortic valve replacement. JACC Cardiovasc Interv. 2017;10(14):1436–46. https://doi.org/10.1016/j.jcin.2017.04.034.
32. Zimarino M, Barbanti M, Dangas GD, et al. Early adverse impact of transfusion after transcatheter aortic valve replacement: a propensity-matched comparison from the TRITAVI Registry. Circ Cardiovasc Interv. 2020;13(12):e009026. https://doi.org/10.1161/CIRCINTERVENTIONS.120.009026.
33. Pilgrim T, Stortecky S, Luterbacher F, Windecker S, Wenaweser P. Transcatheter aortic valve implantation and bleeding: incidence, predictors and prognosis. J Thromb Thrombolysis. 2013;35(4):456–62. https://doi.org/10.1007/s11239-012-0842-3.
34. Généreux P, Head SJ, Van Mieghem NM, et al. Clinical outcomes after transcatheter aortic valve replacement using valve academic research consortium definitions: a weighted meta-analysis of 3,519 patients from 16 studies. J Am Coll Cardiol. 2012;59(25):2317–26. https://doi.org/10.1016/j.jacc.2012.02.022.
35. Généreux P, Webb JG, Svensson LG, et al. Vascular complications after transcatheter aortic valve replacement: insights from the PARTNER (Placement of AoRTic TraNscathetER Valve) trial. J Am Coll Cardiol. 2012;60(12):1043–52. https://doi.org/10.1016/j.jacc.2012.07.003.
36. Chamandi C, Abi-Akar R, Rodés-Cabau J, et al. Transcarotid compared with other alternative access routes for transcatheter aortic valve replacement. Circ Cardiovasc Interv. 2018;11(11):e006388. https://doi.org/10.1161/CIRCINTERVENTIONS.118.006388.
37. Faroux L, Junquera L, Mohammadi S, et al. Femoral versus nonfemoral subclavian/carotid arterial access route for transcatheter aortic valve replacement: a systematic review and meta-analysis. J Am Heart Assoc. 2020;9(19):e017460. https://doi.org/10.1161/JAHA.120.017460.
38. O'Connor SA, Morice M-C, Gilard M, et al. Revisiting sex equality with transcatheter aortic valve replacement outcomes: a collaborative, patient-level meta-analysis of 11,310 patients. J Am Coll Cardiol. 2015;66(3):221–8. https://doi.org/10.1016/j.jacc.2015.05.024.
39. Gupta T, Goel K, Kolte D, et al. Association of chronic kidney disease with in-hospital outcomes of transcatheter aortic valve replacement. JACC Cardiovasc Interv. 2017;10(20):2050–60. https://doi.org/10.1016/j.jcin.2017.07.044.
40. Kibler M, Marchandot B, Messas N, et al. Primary hemostatic disorders and late major bleeding after transcatheter aortic valve replacement. J Am Coll Cardiol. 2018;72(18):2139–48. https://doi.org/10.1016/j.jacc.2018.08.2143.
41. Tarantini G, Tang G, Nai FL, et al. Management of coronary artery disease in patients undergoing transcatheter aortic valve implantation. A clinical consensus statement from the European Association of Percutaneous Cardiovascular Interventions in collaboration with the ESC Working Group on Cardiovascular Surgery. EuroIntervention. 2023;19(1):37–52. https://doi.org/10.4244/EIJ-D-22-00958.
42. Avvedimento M, Campelo-Parada F, Munoz-Garcia E, et al. Late bleeding events in patients undergoing percutaneous coronary intervention in the workup pre-TAVR. JACC Cardiovasc Interv. 2023;16(17):2153–64. https://doi.org/10.1016/j.jcin.2023.06.037.
43. Calabrò P, Gragnano F. Bleeding in patients undergoing PCI and TAVR: combining coronary and valve procedures raises new challenges. JACC Cardiovasc Interv. 2023;16(17):2165–8. https://doi.org/10.1016/j.jcin.2023.07.036.

From GUSTO to TIMI to BARC

3

Tsung-Ying Tsai, Mick Renkens, Bo Wang, Scot Garg, Davide Capodanno, Dominick J. Angiolillo, Yoshinobu Onuma, and Patrick W. Serruys

3.1 The Need/Rationale for Bleeding Classification

In 1977, Andreas Grüntzig performed the first coronary balloon angioplasty (POBA), introducing the world to percutaneous coronary intervention (PCI) and paving the way for the advancements in techniques and devices that are integral to modern interventional cardiology [1, 2]. In parallel, this iatrogenic ischemia caused by the intended manipulation of epicardial coronary arteries, drove the development of antithrombotic therapies to mitigate this ischemic risk. The use of intravenous thrombolysis (IVT) with agents such as streptokinase, alteplase, and tPA, and later, the use of antiplatelet therapies during the stent era, demonstrated that while these treatments were effective in reducing ischemic risk, they also increased the risk of bleeding which negatively impacts a patient's prognosis [3]. Over the years, there has been a continual endeavor to balance the risks of ischemia and bleeding, and

T.-Y. Tsai
Corrib Research Centre for Advanced Imaging and Core Laboratory, University of Galway, Galway, Ireland

Taichung Veterans General Hospital, Taichung, Taiwan

M. Renkens
Corrib Research Centre for Advanced Imaging and Core Laboratory, University of Galway, Galway, Ireland

Amsterdam University Medical Centers, Heart Center, University of Amsterdam, Amsterdam, The Netherlands

B. Wang · Y. Onuma
Corrib Research Centre for Advanced Imaging and Core Laboratory, University of Galway, Galway, Ireland

S. Garg
Department of Cardiology, Royal Blackburn Hospital, Blackburn, UK

D. Capodanno
A.O.U. Policlinico "G. Rodolico - San Marco", University of Catania, Catania, Italy

D. J. Angiolillo
Division of Cardiology, University of Florida College of Medicine, Jacksonville, FL, USA

P. W. Serruys (✉)
Corrib Research Centre for Advanced Imaging and Core Laboratory, University of Galway, Galway, Ireland

Interventional Medicine and Innovation at the University of Galway, Research Centre for Advanced Imaging and Core Lab (CORRIB) Research Centre, Galway, Ireland

Science Foundation of Ireland (SFI), Dublin, Ireland
e-mail: patrick.serruys@universityofgalway.ie

B. Cortese, S. Rigattieri (eds.), *High Bleeding Risk Patients in Interventional Cardiology*,
https://doi.org/10.1007/978-3-031-87302-7_3

over the past decade, advancements in devices and antithrombotic strategies have led to substantial reductions in the absolute risks for both. This has ushered in the current era, characterized by the pursuit of equipoise in ischemic and bleeding risk, where this risk is dynamic with a gradual shift in concern toward bleeding risk [3–6].

3.2 History of Bleeding Classification

IVT was the first therapy proven to reduce mortality in patients with acute ST-elevation myocardial infarction (STEMI) [7–9]; and notably while bleeding events were frequently observed in these primary studies, they were not systematically recorded. In 1993 the GUSTO trial showed a 30-day survival benefit (14% risk reduction, $p = 0.001$) by using an aggressive short-acting thrombolytic (accelerated t-PA) compared to conventional streptokinase [10]. Prior to this study, the US Federal Drug Administration (FDA) had already requested a 100-patient pilot study to assess the safety profile of this more aggressive thrombolytic, recognizing the important adverse impact from severe bleeding [11].

This pilot study led to the development of the GUSTO Bleeding criteria, a clinical classification without laboratory components or the requirement for medical treatment in response to the bleed [10]. The GUSTO trial was among the first to simultaneously report ischemic and bleeding risks, highlighting that the mortality benefit of aggressive IVT came at the cost of higher bleeding risk. The GUSTO Bleeding criteria, while practical, lack objective criteria, making independent adjudication by clinical event committees (CEC) difficult.

The TIMI group later classified bleeding severity by the laboratory-focused TIMI classification, with the necessity for clinical intervention added later. This classification was first used in patients with STEMI treated with recombinant t-PA, aspirin, and heparin who were randomly assigned to POBA or conservative medical treatment [12–15].

The indication and success rate of PCI was revolutionized with the introduction of coronary stents; however, these initial bare metal stents (BMS) and later, the early generation drug-eluting stents (DES), were blighted by the 2–3% risk of stent thrombosis (ST), which had an associated mortality rate of up to 50% [16]. Since 1984, aspirin has been pivotal in antithrombotic therapy regimes [17]. In 1996, Schömig et al. demonstrated that dual antiplatelet therapy (DAPT) with ticlopidine and aspirin was superior to conventional anticoagulation with aspirin in reducing the risk of ST (RR 0.14, 95%CI, 0.02–0.31) [18], which laid the foundations for the routine use of DAPT at the expense of IVT and anticoagulation [19]. Unfortunately, delayed reendothelialization with DES resulted in a risk of late ST following the cessation of DAPT, which triggered a pragmatic extension of DAPT from 6 to 12 months, which consequently extended the duration of higher bleeding risk [20]. Subsequent improvements in device technology and potent antithrombotic therapies have led to re-evaluations of the ischemic-bleeding risk trade-off (Fig. 3.1) [3, 4], which are supported by seminal papers reporting the substantial increase in mortality and ischemic events following even mild bleeding.

The GUSTO and TIMI classifications were defined in the fibrinolytic era and were not designed to capture contemporary bleeding events [21], resulting in trialists introducing multiple bleeding definitions. This heterogeneity lead to the development of a refined, standardized and comprehensive bleeding classification—the

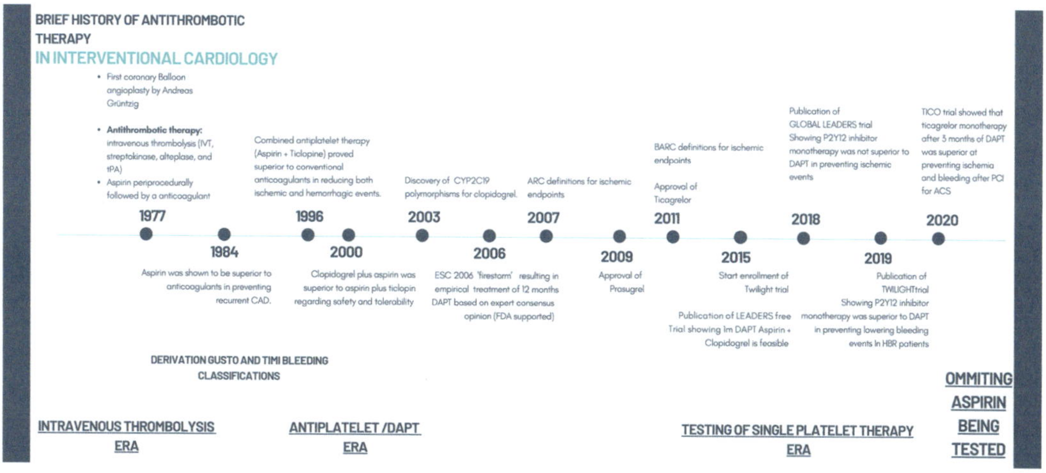

Fig. 3.1 Development of antithrombotic therapies and bleeding risk in percutaneous coronary interventions including re-evaluations of the ischemic-bleeding risk trade-off

Bleeding Academic Research Consortium (BARC) classification [21]—which facilitates a comparative evaluation of the safety profiles of different antithrombotic drugs and streamlines CEC adjudication. In this chapter, we will delve into the different bleeding classifications, compare their validations in prospective cohorts, and explore future directions.

3.3 Definitions of Bleeding Classification in Clinical Trials

The classification of bleeding has evolved in parallel with antithrombotic treatment strategies, resulting in numerous definitions, which make interpretation and comparison between studies difficult, if not impossible. For example, the Superior Yield of the New Strategy of Enoxaparin, Revascularization and Glycoprotein IIb/IIIa Inhibitors (SYNERGY) trial compared enoxaparin with unfractionated heparin in 10,027 patients with non–ST-segment elevation acute coronary syndrome (ACS) [22]. The enoxaparin strategy was associated with a significantly higher rate of TIMI major bleeding, while GUSTO bleeding was not statistically different; hence, the conclusion of bleeding risk depended entirely on the bleeding definition. To resolve this and other issues, bleeding classifications have been updated, and largely superseded by the BARC classification.

Table 3.1 shows the bleeding definitions among previous trials and the BARC classification [23, 24].

The *Global Use of Strategies to Open Occluded Arteries* (*GUSTO*) was developed in the IVT era and was the first bleeding classification to be used, categorizing bleedings as severe/life-threatening, moderate or minor (Table 3.1). The GUSTO classification is only clinical, is easy to use, and its severity aligns well with the

Table 3.1 Heterogeneity in bleeding definitions used in clinical trials

Classification	Bleeding definition
BARC	***Type 1***: Bleeding that is not actionable and does not cause the patient to seek an unscheduled performance of studies, hospitalization, or treatment by a healthcare professional; it may include episodes leading to self-discontinuation of medical therapy by the patient without consulting a health care professional ***Type 2***: Any overt, actionable sign of hemorrhage (e.g., more bleeding than would be expected for a clinical circumstance, including bleeding found by imaging alone) that does not fit the criteria for type 3, type 4, or type 5 but does meet at least one of the following criteria: requiring nonsurgical, medical intervention by a healthcare professional; leading to hospitalization or increased level of care; or prompting evaluation ***Type 3a***: Overt bleeding plus a hemoglobin drop of 3–5 g/dL* (provided the hemoglobin drop is related to bleed); any transfusion with overt bleeding ***Type 3b***: Overt bleeding plus a hemoglobin drop of 5 g/dL (provided the hemoglobin drop is related to bleed); cardiac tamponade; bleeding requiring surgical intervention for control (excluding dental, nasal, skin, and hemorrhoid); bleeding requiring intravenous vasoactive agents ***Type 3c***: Intracranial hemorrhage (does not include microbleeds or hemorrhagic transformation, does include intraspinal); subcategories confirmed by autopsy or imaging, or lumbar puncture; intraocular bleed compromising vision ***Type 4***: Coronary artery bypass grafting-related bleeding; perioperative intracranial bleeding within 48 h; reoperation after closure of sternotomy for the purpose of controlling bleeding; transfusion of 5 U of whole blood or packed red blood cells within a 48-h period; chest tube output 2 L within a 24-h period ***Type 5a***: Probable fatal bleeding; no autopsy or imaging confirmation but clinically suspicious ***Type 5b***: Definite fatal bleeding; overt bleeding or autopsy, or imaging confirmation
ISTH-SSC (International Society on Thrombosis and Haemostasis, Scientific and Standardization Committee)	*Major* Fatal bleeding Bleeding in a critical area or organ, such as intracranial, intraspinal, intraocular, retroperitoneal, intra-articular or pericardial, or intramuscular with compartment syndrome Bleeding causing a fall in hemoglobin level of 20 g L^{-1} (1.24 mmol L^{-1}) or more, or leading to transfusion of two or more units of whole blood or red cells *Clinically relevant nonmajor* Requiring medical intervention by a healthcare professional Leading to hospitalization or increased level of care Prompting a face to face (i.e., not just a telephone or electronic communication) evaluation *Minor* Overt (bleeding visible to the eye or detectable on an imaging study) bleed that does not meet criteria for the above criteria
TIMI (Thrombolysis in Myocardial Infarction)	*Non-CABG-related bleeding* *Major* Any intracranial bleeding (excluding microhemorrhages <10 mm evident only on gradient-echo MRI) Clinically overt signs of hemorrhage associated with a drop in hemoglobin of ≥5 g/dL Fatal bleeding (bleeding that directly results in death within 7 d) *Minor* Clinically overt (including imaging), resulting in hemoglobin drop of 3 to <5 g/dL or ≥10% decrease in hematocrit No observed blood loss: ≥4 g/dL decrease in the hemoglobin concentration or ≥12% decrease in hematocrit Any overt sign of hemorrhage that meets one of the following criteria and does not meet criteria for a major or minor bleeding event, as defined above:
	Requiring intervention (medical practitioner-guided medical or surgical treatment to stop or treat bleeding, including temporarily or permanently discontinuing or changing the dose of a medication or study drug) Leading to or prolonging hospitalization Prompting evaluation (leading to an unscheduled visit to a healthcare professional and diagnostic testing, either laboratory or imaging) *Minimal* Any overt bleeding event that does not meet the criteria above *Bleeding in the setting of CABG* Fatal bleeding (bleeding that directly results in death) Perioperative intracranial bleeding Reoperation after closure of the sternotomy incision for the purpose of controlling bleeding Transfusion of ≥5 U PRBCs or whole blood within a 48-h period; cell saver transfusion will not be counted in calculations of blood products Chest tube output >2 L within a 24-h period

(continued)

Table 3.1 (continued)

Classification	Bleeding definition
GUSTO (Global use of strategies to open occluded arteries)	*Severe or life-threatening* Intracerebral hemorrhage Resulting in substantial hemodynamic compromise requiring treatment *Moderate* Requiring blood transfusion but not resulting in hemodynamic compromise *Mild* Bleeding that does not meet above criteria
PARAGON-B (Platelet IIb/IIIa antagonist for the reduction of acute coronary syndrome events in a global organization network)	*Major or life-threatening* Any intracranial hemorrhage or bleeding that led to hemodynamic compromise that required intervention *Intermediate* Bleeding that required transfusion or a decrease in hemoglobin of ≥5 g/dl (or a decrease ≥15% in hematocrit when hemoglobin was unavailable)
CURE	*Major bleeding* Life-threatening (fatal, intracranial, requiring surgical intervention, results in substantial hypotension requiring the use of intravenous inotropic agents) Hemoglobin decrease ≥5 g/dL or required ≥4 U of blood *Other major bleeding* Transfusion of 2–3 U, intraocular *Minor* Led to discontinuation of study drug
ACUITY (acute catheterization and urgent intervention triage strategy), HORIZONS AMI (harmonizing outcomes with revascularization and stents in acute myocardial infarction)	*Major* Intracranial or intraocular hemorrhage Access-site hemorrhage requiring intervention ≥5-cm hematoma Retroperitoneal Reduction in hemoglobin concentration of ≥4 g/dL without an overt source of bleeding Reduction in hemoglobin concentration of ≥3 g/dL with an overt source of bleeding Reoperation for bleeding Use of any blood product transfusion
CURRENT-OASIS 7	*Severe* Requiring transfusion ≥4 U of PRBCs or equivalent whole blood Resulting in hemoglobin drop ≥5 g/dL Leading to hypotension that requires inotropes Requiring surgery Symptomatic intracranial hemorrhage Fatal *Other major* Requiring transfusion of 2–3 U Significantly disabling, intraocular bleeding leading to significant loss of vision *Minor* Other bleeding that leads to modification of drug regimen *Other* Bleeding not meeting criteria for major or minor
STEEPLE	*Major bleeding* Fatal bleeding Retroperitoneal, intracranial, or intraocular bleeding Bleeding that causes hemodynamic compromise requiring specific treatment Bleeding that requires intervention (surgical or endoscopic) or decompression of a closed space to stop or control the event Clinically overt bleeding, requiring any transfusion of ≥1 U PRBC or whole blood Clinically overt bleeding, causing a decrease in hemoglobin of ≥3 g/dL (or, if hemoglobin level is not available, a decrease in hematocrit of ≥10%) *Minor* Gross hematuria not associated with trauma (e.g., from instrumentation) Epistaxis that is prolonged, is repeated, or requires plugging or intervention Gastrointestinal hemorrhage Hemoptysis Subconjunctival hemorrhage Hematoma >5 cm or leading to prolonged or new hospitalization Clinically overt bleeding, causing a decrease in hemoglobin of 2–3 g/dL Uncontrolled bleeding requiring protamine sulfate administration

(continued)

Table 3.1 (continued)

Classification	Bleeding definition
PLATO (platelet inhibition and patient outcomes trial)	*Major life-threatening* Fatal Intracranial Intrapericardial with cardiac tamponade Resulting in hypovolemic shock or severe hypotension that requires pressors or surgery Clinically overt or apparent bleeding associated with decrease in hemoglobin >5 g/dL Requiring transfusion of ≥4 U whole blood or PRBCs *Other major* Significantly disabling (e.g., intraocular with permanent vision loss) Associated drop in hemoglobin of 3–5 g/dL Requiring transfusion of 2–3 U whole blood or PRBCs *Any major* Any one of the above criteria *Minor* Requiring medical intervention to stop or treat bleeding (e.g., epistaxis requiring visit to medical facility for packing) *Minimal* All others (e.g., bruising, bleeding gums, oozing from injection sites) not requiring intervention or treatment
GRACE	*Major* Requiring a transfusion of ≥2 U PRBCs Resulting in a decrease in hematocrit b of ≥10% Occurring intracerebrally Resulting in stroke or death
REPLACE-2/ ISAR-REACT 3	*Major* Intracranial, intraocular, or retroperitoneal Overt blood loss with hemoglobin decrease >3 g/dL Any hemoglobin decrease >4 g/dL Transfusion of ≥2 U blood products *Minor* Overt bleeding not meeting criteria for major bleeding
ESSENCE	*Major* Clinically overt bleeding that was fatal (bleeding reported to cause death) Symptomatic intracranial hemorrhage Retroperitoneal hemorrhage Intraocular hemorrhage leading to significant vision loss Decrease in hemoglobin of at least 3.0 g/dL (with each blood transfusion unit counting for 1.0 g/dL hemoglobin) Bleeding requiring transfusion of ≥2 U RBCs or equivalent of whole blood *Minor* All other clinically significant bleeding not meeting the definition for major bleeding and that led to interruption of the study drug for at least 24 h, surgical intervention, or transfusion of ≤1 U blood
Amlani et al.	*Major* Hemoglobin drop ≥5 g/dL Intracranial hemorrhage Bleeding requiring surgery Blood transfusion of at least 2 U

TIMI indicates Thrombolysis in Myocardial Infarction, *CABG* coronary artery bypass graft, *MRI* magnetic resonance imaging, *PRBC* packed red blood cell, *GUSTO* Global Use of Strategies to Open Occluded Arteries, *CURE* Clopidogrel in Unstable Angina to Prevent Recurrent Events, *ACUITY* Acute Catheterization and Urgent Intervention Triage Strategy, *HORIZONS* Harmonizing Outcomes With Revascularization and Stents, *CURRENT-OASIS 7* Clopidogrel optimal loading Dose Usage to Reduce Recurrent Events/Optimal Antiplatelet Strategy for Interventions, *STEEPLE* Safety and Efficacy of Enoxaparin in PCI Patients, an International Randomized Evaluation, *PLATO* Platelet Inhibition and Patient Outcomes, *GRACE* Global Registry of Acute Coronary Events, *REPLACE-2* Randomized Evaluation in PCI Linking Angiomax to Reduced Clinical Events, *ISAR-REACT* Intracoronary Stenting and Antithrombotic Regimen: Rapid Early Action for Coronary Treatment, and *ESSENCE* Efficacy and Safety of Subcutaneous Enoxaparin in Non-Q-Wave Coronary Events risks of death and/or MI [25]. The lack of objective components however may result in variations in event rates across practices, and lower event rates when compared to more contemporary definitions. Thus, trials applying the GUSTO definition may require additional attention, re-evaluation, and event adjudication to ensure consistently captured outcomes.

Thrombolysis in Myocardial Infarction (TIMI) bleeding criteria were also developed in the IVT era and have been the most popular criteria for 40 years. The original TIMI definition relied predominantly on drops in hemoglobin or hematocrit level and was therefore affected by laboratory follow-up protocols [26]. The definitions have now been updated to capture a broader range of bleeding events, detected clinically or via imaging [13, 14, 27–30]. The current TIMI criteria and its components are shown in Tables 3.1 and 3.2, respectively.

The TIMI criteria however are still limited by the legacy of its development in the IVT era. A TIMI "minor" bleeding, such as an upper gastrointestinal (GI) bleeding requiring a transfusion, holds greater clinical significance than that implied by the term "minor." Moreover, the timing of hemoglobin assessment may not reflect the actual timing of the bleeding. Notably, the TIMI criteria were the first to classify bleeding in patients revascularized by coronary artery bypass graft (CABG) surgery and to emphasize the importance of this: approximately two-thirds of all major bleeding events in the TRACER trial occurred in patients undergoing CABG, necessitating specific attention for risk assessment and decision guidance [31]. Finally, the TIMI classification was the first to introduce different types of death in relation to bleeding events, which with modification has been adopted by the BARC definitions.

The ISTH (International Society on Thrombosis and Haemostasis) bleeding criteria were designed to monitor bleeding events following long-term anticoagulation therapy; thus, they also apply to venous thromboembolisms and patients with atrial fibrillation. It has undergone several updates. As bleeding criteria for long-term medication, the ISTH definition emphasizes the clinical relevance of the bleeding, wherein it has the lowest threshold for drops in hemoglobin (2 g/dl) compared to the bleeding criteria (drop ≥3 g/dl) used in interventional cardiology trials. In addition, ISTH doesn't differentiate between major or fatal bleeding, as both result in drug discontinuation. Notably, the current ISTH definitions were developed after the BARC definition and thus could be harmonized with other bleeding definitions (Fig. 3.2) [32].

Given the imperfections of the TIMI and GUSTO definitions, trialists in the POBA and early stent era merged elements from both criteria to leverage their strengths and overcome the limitations; however, as stated above, this created variations and confusion. The ASSENT-3 and the COMMIT trials incorporated elements from both the TIMI and GUSTO definitions [33]. Some trials have introduced their own bleeding definitions such as the Clopidogrel in Unstable Angina to Prevent Recurrent Events (CURE), Acute Catheterization and Urgent Intervention Triage Strategy (ACUITY), Organization for the Assessment of Strategies for Ischemic Syndromes (OASIS), Safety and Efficacy of Enoxaparin in PCI Patients, an International Randomized Evaluation (STEEPLE), and Platelet Inhibition and Patient Outcomes (PLATO) trials (Table 3.2) [19, 34–37]. For example, the more recent PLATO trial classifies bleeding as major (life-threatening or not), minor or minimal.

The *BARC definition* was developed in 2011 by a consortium of experts across the Atlantic, joined by FDA and industry representatives, to satisfy the need for future trials and to capture and stratify better clinically significant bleeding events. The BARC utilized an ordinal system with multiple subcategories ranging from Type 1 to Type 5, allowing for better granularity and risk stratification. Importantly, the BARC definition adopted the most comprehensive criteria, allowing detailed recording of minor bleeding, bleeding-related death, and bleeding in CABG patients.

Table 3.2 Components of bleeding classifications used across clinical trials in interventional cardiology

Classification/trial	Levels	Special criteria for CABG	Target population	Year of publication	Hemoglobin/hematocrit	Transfusion	require surgery/intervention	Hemodynamic unstable	Intracranial of close space bleeding	Fatal bleeding	Discontinue medication	Imaging
BARC	4	Yes	Coronary stent trials	2011	+	+	+	+	+	+	+	(+)
ISTH	3	No	Evaluation of antithrombotic agents	2005; updated 2014	+	+	+	–	+	+	–	(–)
TIMI	3	Yes	AMI treated with thrombolysis	1987; updated 2009	+	+	+	–	+	+	+	(+)
GUSTO	3	No	AMI treated with thrombolysis	1993	–	+	–	+	+	–	–	(–)
PARAGON-B	2	No	ACS treated with IIb/IIIa inhibitors	2002	+	+	+	+	+	–	–	(–)
CURE	2	No	AMI treated with clopidogrel	2001	+	+	+	+	+	–	+	(–)
ACUITY, HORIZONS	1	No	ACS treated with bivalirudin	2006	+	+	+	–	+	+	–	(–)
CURRENT-OASIS 7	4	No	ACS treated with clopidogrel	2010	+	+	+	+	+	+	+	(–)
STEEPLE	2	No	Elective PCI, enoxaparin	2006	+	+	+	+	+	+	+	(–)
PLATO	4	No	ACS treated with ticagrelor	2009	+	+	+	+	+	+	–	(–)
GRACE	1	No	ACS	2003	+	+	–	–	+	+	–	(–)
REPLACE-2/ISAR-REACT 3	2	No	Urgent or elective PCI, bivalirudin	2003	+	+	–	–	+	–	–	(–)
ESSENCE	2	No	Non-Q wave MI, unstable angina, enoxaparin	1997	+	+	+	–	+	–	–	(–)
Amlani et al.	1	No	AMI	2010	+	+	+	–	+	–	–	(–)

AMI acute myocardial infarction

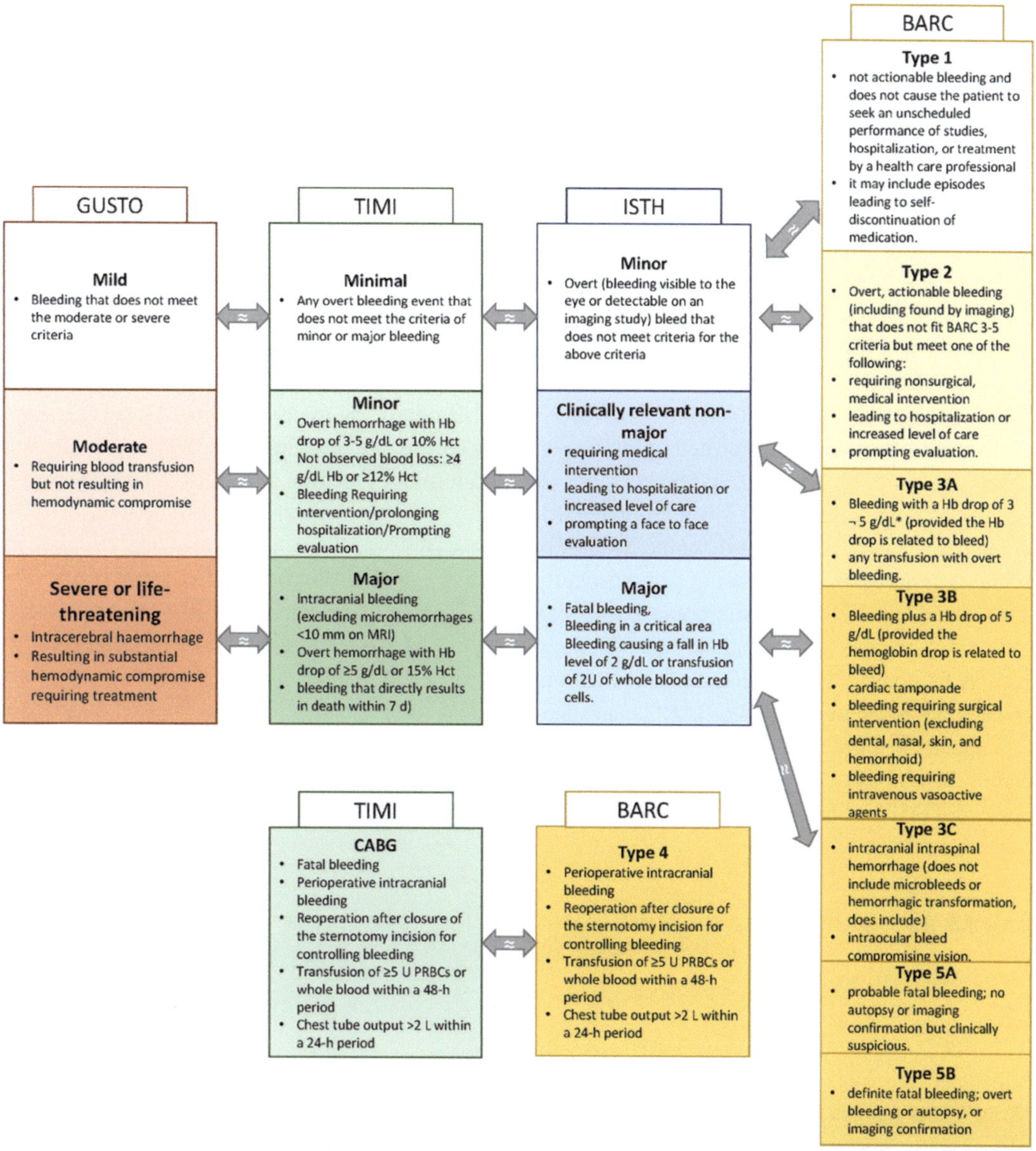

Fig. 3.2 Comparison of the most used bleeding classifications. ISTH classifies bleeding according to clinical relevance. TIMI, GUSTO, and BARC represent the most used bleeding classifications. ISTH, TIMI, and GUSTO are divided into three levels of severity, while BARC is divided into five, numerically graded, levels. Prognostically, a bleed classified as "mild" by GUSTO corresponds to a "minimal" bleed by TIMI and to a "1" or "2" bleed by BARC. A bleed classified as "moderate" according to GUSTO corresponds to a "minor" bleed by TIMI and to a "3a" bleed according to BARC. Finally, a bleed classified as "severe" according to GUSTO corresponds to a "major" bleed according to TIMI and to a "3b," "3c," "4," or "5" bleed according to BARC. Abbreviations: ISTH International Society on Thrombosis and Haemostasi, BARC Bleeding Academic Research Consortium, GUSTO Global Use of Strategies to Open Occluded Coronary Arteries, TIMI Thrombolysis in Myocardial Infarction

3.4 Comparison of Different Bleeding Risk Classifications

The components of each bleeding definition are shown in Table 3.2. Intracranial hemorrhage, often with severe sequelae, is classified as severe in all definitions; however, the TIMI classification excludes microhemorrhages measuring ≤10 mm and does not provide subcategorization for intracranial hemorrhage, potentially missing nuances in severity, while other definitions, such as the STEEPLE, ESSENCE, BARC, and ISTH, have recognized intraocular bleeding as severe.

The need for transfusion or hemoglobin drop is also unanimously recognized; however, not all definitions request additional information regarding interventions or put hemodynamic instability in the criteria despite both being prognostically important [38]. Hemodynamic compromise can stem from various factors other than bleeding, such as hemodilution, sedation, and medication, and can be transient. Thus, the BARC classification specified the need for vasoactive agents to define hemodynamic disturbance. Lastly, the updated TIMI and BARC classifications include imaging findings, which are critical to identify asymptomatic bleeding.

Generally, the early definitions capture fewer events, classify events as less severe, and are also more susceptible to variations in local practices, imaging utilization, and blood bank resources (Table 3.3). Nevertheless, the bleeding definitions can still be roughly interpreted as interchangeably (Fig. 3.2). In modern clinical trials, clinical bleeding events are frequently classified as BARC 3 and BARC 5, (BARC 4 if CABG is involved) which, respectively, corresponds to TIMI minor and major bleeding, GUSTO moderate and severe bleeding, and ISTH clinically relevant minor bleeding and major bleeding.

3.5 Validation and Comparison of the Different Bleeding Classifications in Prospective Cohorts

The BARC classification was developed by updating previous classifications without a source database, such as the Framingham risk score;

Table 3.3 The incidence of bleeding event defined by different bleeding classification across trials

			GUSTO		TIMI		BARC	
Trial	Population	Medication	Severe	Moderate	Major	Minor	3 or 5	2
CURE	ACS	DAPT	2.2	1.2	3.7	5.1	NR	NR
TRACER	NSTEMI	Vorapaxar	4.0		3.7		15.4	
ENGAGE AF-TIMI 48 trial	AF	Edoxaban vs. warfarin	1.6	NR	2.5	NR	1.3	NR
Pooled data from: PURSUIT and PARAGON B	ACS	IIb/IIIa	1.2	11.4	8.2	8.4	NR	NR
PRODIGY	All comer	DAPT	3.1		2.5		7.1	
Kikkert et al.	STEMI	DAPT	2.7	6.3	5.0	7.9	14.5	4.4
ISAR trials	STEMI	Abciximab	NR	NR	0.9	2.1	3.48	1.7

AF atrial fibrillation, *IIb/IIIa* platelet IIb/IIIa antagonism, *ACS* acute coronary syndrome, *NR* no reports, *PRODIGY* (Prolonging Dual anti-platelet treatment after Grading stent-induced Intimal hyperplasia study) trial, *TRACER* Thrombin Receptor Antagonist for Clinical Event Reduction in Acute Coronary Syndrome https://doi.org/10.1016/j.jacc.2016.02.056, *ENGAGE AF* (Effective Anticoagulation With Factor Xa Next Generation in Atrial Fibrillation)-TIMI 48 trial (NCT00781391) https://doi.org/10.1161/CIRCULATIONAHA.119.041346, Intracoronary Stenting and Antithrombotic Regimen (ISAR) clinical trials https://doi.org/10.1161/CIRCULATIONAHA.111.060871, *PURSUIT* Inhibition of Platelet Glycoprotein IIb/IIIa with Eptifibatide in Patients with Acute Coronary Syndromes; https://doi.org/10.1056/NEJM199808133390704, *PARAGON* Platelet IIb/IIIa Antagonism for the Reduction of Acute Coronary Syndrome Events in a Global Organization Network trial

Table 3.4 Validation of the BARC bleeding score [42]

	Ndreppa et al. (*N* = 12,499)	Kikkert et al. (*N* = 2002)	Vranckx et al. (*N* = 2013)	Yoon et al. (*N* = 6166)	Vranckx et al. (*N* = 12,944)
Study design	Six pooled clinical trials	Single-center registry	Multicenter clinical trial	Multicenter registry	Multicenter clinical trial
Study population	PCI for angina or NSTEACS	PCI for STEMI	PCI, all comers	PCI, all comers	PCI for NSTEACS
Timing of bleed	Index hospitalization	Index hospitalization	Any time during study	Index hospitalization	Any time during study
BARC adjudication	Retrospective	Retrospective	Retrospective	Retrospective	Retrospective
Outcome (primary)	Death	Death	Death	MACE	Death
Number of BARC 3 bleeds	492	276	39	207	738
Number of deaths	340	296	163	130	652
Model fit with BARC ≥3 compared with TIMI and GUSTO[a]	Similar	Similar	Similar	Similar (TIMI only)	Similar or better
Bleeding as independent predictor of death					
BARC 3	Yes	No	Yes	N/A	Yes
TIMI minor/major	Yes	No	Yes	N/A	Yes
GUSTO moderate/ severe	Yes	No	Yes	N/A	Yes

BARC Bleeding Academic Research Consortium, *GUSTO* Global Use of Strategies to Open Occluded Arteries, *MACE* major adverse cardiovascular event, *NSTEACS* non-ST-segment elevation acute coronary syndrome, *PCI* percutaneous coronary intervention, *STEMI* ST-segment elevation myocardial infarction, *TIMI* Thrombolysis In Myocardial Infarction
[a]Each bleeding score was included in a multivariate model as a dichotomized binary variable

however, despite this, it has been extensively adopted and validated by clinical trials and has emerged as the most reliable bleeding definition (See Table 3.4).

The first major validation study adjudicated bleeding in 12,459 patients from 6 randomized PCI trials as per the BARC, TIMI, and the REPLACE-2 trial criteria and reported several important findings [39]. First, adjudication using BARC criteria was feasible using the standard data collected in PCI trials. Second, the BARC definition captured significantly more bleeding events with BARC ≥2 bleeding reported in 679 (5.4%) patients, while the corresponding TIMI (major + minor) bleeding was reported in only 374 (3.0%) patients. Third, compared to the TIMI criteria, BARC identified additional patients with clinically relevant bleeding events, and class ≥2 bleeding was associated with a significant increase in 1-year mortality (adjusted hazard ratio 2.72; 95%CI, 2.03–3.63). Lastly, the study showed "a dose-response," with outcomes tracking well with the ordinal BARC classification; however, this study included mainly chronic coronary syndrome patients and applied the BARC classification retrospectively.

The first prospective validation of the BARC definitions occurred in the all-comer PRODIGY trial [40], where they were used alongside the TIMI and GUSTO criteria to adjudicate bleeding events over 2-year follow-up in 2003 patients. The rates of BARC ≥2, TIMI minor or major, and GUSTO moderate or severe bleedings were 7.1%, 5.5%, and 3.1%, respectively, with similar hazard ratio (HRs) for clinical events among all three classifications, and the same "dose-response" phenomenon observed.

The discriminatory power of the multivariable bleeding models to predict 2-year mortality was prospectively assessed by means of external validation, and the performance was described by the Harrell's C statistics. The prediction models with BARC Type 3 (or 5), TIMI (minor or major), or GUSTO (moderate or severe) had similar integrated discrimination improvement suggesting equivalence in prognostic value.

The TRACER trial validated the BARC criteria in 12,994 patients with NSTE-ACS [31], with rates of BARC ≥2, TIMI, and GUSTO bleeding occurring in 15.4%, 3.7%, and 4.0% of patients, respectively [31]. CABG-related bleeding (BARC 4) occurred in 1.2% of patients. Overall the BARC classification consistently identified roughly three times more bleedings with the equivalent predictive power of BARC ≥3 compared to the TIMI or GUSTO criteria.

Like the previous two studies, mortality in patients with BARC [2–4], or bleeding was significantly higher than patients without bleeding (BARC 0 or 1). In addition, a gradual increase in mortality risk with increasing BARC type was observed, where the association between bleeding and mortality appeared to be independent of whether patients experienced bleeding events in-hospital or after discharge.

There are currently no prospective data validating the prognostic importance and comparative ability of BARC in CABG patients. In a retrospective study, BARC 4 bleeding, which occurred in 4.21% of patients having off-pump CABG [41], was shown to be independently associated with an increased risk of in-hospital death and postoperative MI. However, prospective validation of the BARC classification is still warranted to expand the confidence from PCI patients to the CABG population.

3.6 Current Limitations and Future Perspective

With better iterations of bleeding criteria, it is now possible to precisely identify bleeding events in clinical trials and make comparisons. However, despite the BARC classification, there are still contemporary trials using diverse bleeding definitions, suggesting the need for a truly universal bleeding classification [23, 24, 43].

Although extensive validated, the BARC classification still has several limitations. First, BARC was designed to facilitate external CEC adjudication and thus relies heavily on hemoglobin drop. In clinical practice, however, this may (1) not solely rely on bleeding itself (e.g., hemodilution) and (2) be influenced by the response to bleeding (e.g., blood transfusion or medical evaluation). Furthermore, the classification does not guide clinicians in the management of bleeding (e.g., evaluate or intervene). Lastly, no classification considers the individual's susceptibility to bleeding. In clinical trials, the follow-up protocol has a pivotal role in the detection of bleeding events, which aids in risk assessment, guides decision-making, and improves outcome on an individual level, but this might not necessarily reflect daily clinical practice.

It is therefore unknown whether a comprehensive approach to identify bleeding events early in clinical practice could reduce subsequent adverse events. The validation of classifications across specific populations, for example, CABG patients, STEMI patients, patients with structural heart disease, and patients presenting with hemodynamic instability, is still lacking. With the improvement of medical therapy and device technology, the next iteration of bleeding classification facilitating adjudication and accurate prediction of bleeding events will be needed to further guide individualized treatment by optimizing the ischemic and bleeding risk trade-off.

References

1. Grüntzig AR, Senning A, Siegenthaler WE. Nonoperative dilatation of coronary-artery stenosis: percutaneous transluminal coronary angioplasty. N Engl J Med. 1979;301(2):61–8. (In eng). https://doi.org/10.1056/nejm197907123010201.
2. Meier B. The first patient to undergo coronary angioplasty — 23-year follow-up. N Engl J Med. 2001;344(2):144–5. https://doi.org/10.1056/nejm200101113440217.
3. Cao D, Chandiramani R, Chiarito M, Claessen BE, Mehran R. Evolution of antithrombotic therapy in patients undergoing percutaneous coronary intervention: a 40-year journey. Eur Heart J. 2020;42(4):339–51. https://doi.org/10.1093/eurheartj/ehaa824.
4. Iqbal J, Gunn J, Serruys PW. Coronary stents: historical development, current status and future directions. Br Med Bull. 2013;106:193–211. (In eng). https://doi.org/10.1093/bmb/ldt009.

5. Miyazaki Y, Suwannasom P, Sotomi Y, et al. Single or dual antiplatelet therapy after PCI. Nat Rev Cardiol. 2017;14(5):294–303. (In eng). https://doi.org/10.1038/nrcardio.2017.12.
6. Asano T, Ono M, Dai Z, et al. Temporal trends in clinical outcomes after percutaneous coronary intervention: a systematic review of 66,327 patients from 25 all-comers trials. EuroIntervention. 2022;17(16):1318–29. (In eng). https://doi.org/10.4244/eij-d-21-00192.
7. Gruppo Italiano per lo Studio della Sopravvivenza nell'Infarto Miocardico. GISSI-2: a factorial randomised trial of alteplase versus streptokinase and heparin versus no heparin among 12,490 patients with acute myocardial infarction. Lancet. 1990;336(8707):65–71. (In eng)
8. The International Study Group. In-hospital mortality and clinical course of 20,891 patients with suspected acute myocardial infarction randomised between alteplase and streptokinase with or without heparin. Lancet. 1990;336(8707):71–5. (In eng)
9. ISIS-3 (Third International Study of Infarct Survival) Collaborative Group. ISIS-3: a randomised comparison of streptokinase vs tissue plasminogen activator vs anistreplase and of aspirin plus heparin vs aspirin alone among 41,299 cases of suspected acute myocardial infarction. Lancet. 1992;339(8796):753–70. (In eng)
10. Gusto Investigators. An international randomized trial comparing four thrombolytic strategies for acute myocardial infarction. N Engl J Med. 1993;329(10):673–82. https://doi.org/10.1056/nejm199309023291001.
11. Granger CB. The global utilization of streptokinase and tissue plasminogen activator for occluded coronary arteries (GUSTO) pilot study: combined streptokinase and t-PA (abstract). Circulation. 1991;84:II-573. https://cir.nii.ac.jp/crid/1573387449301660288
12. Rao SV, O'Grady K, Pieper KS, et al. Impact of bleeding severity on clinical outcomes among patients with acute coronary syndromes. Am J Cardiol. 2005;96(9):1200–6. (In eng). https://doi.org/10.1016/j.amjcard.2005.06.056.
13. Bovill EG, Terrin ML, Stump DC, et al. Hemorrhagic events during therapy with recombinant tissue-type plasminogen activator, heparin, and aspirin for acute myocardial infarction. Results of the thrombolysis in myocardial infarction (TIMI), phase II trial. Ann Intern Med. 1991;115(4):256–65. (In eng). https://doi.org/10.7326/0003-4819-115-4-256.
14. Wiviott SD, Braunwald E, McCabe CH, et al. Prasugrel versus clopidogrel in patients with acute coronary syndromes. N Engl J Med. 2007;357(20):2001–15. (In eng). https://doi.org/10.1056/NEJMoa0706482.
15. Sabatine MS, Morrow DA, Giugliano RP, et al. Association of hemoglobin levels with clinical outcomes in acute coronary syndromes. Circulation. 2005;111(16):2042–9. https://doi.org/10.1161/01.CIR.0000162477.70955.5F.
16. Secemsky EA, Matteau A, Yeh RW, et al. Comparison of short- and long-term cardiac mortality in early versus late stent thrombosis (from pooled PROTECT trials). Am J Cardiol. 2015;115(12):1678–84. (In eng). https://doi.org/10.1016/j.amjcard.2015.03.010.
17. Thornton MA, Gruentzig AR, Hollman J, King SB 3rd, Douglas JS. Coumadin and aspirin in prevention of recurrence after transluminal coronary angioplasty: a randomized study. Circulation. 1984;69(4):721–7. (In eng). https://doi.org/10.1161/01.cir.69.4.721.
18. Schömig A, Neumann FJ, Kastrati A, et al. A randomized comparison of antiplatelet and anticoagulant therapy after the placement of coronary-artery stents. N Engl J Med. 1996;334(17):1084–9. (In eng). https://doi.org/10.1056/nejm199604253341702.
19. Effects of clopidogrel in addition to aspirin in patients with acute coronary syndromes without ST-segment elevation. N Engl J Med. 2001;345(7):494–502. https://doi.org/10.1056/NEJMoa010746.
20. Camenzind E. Do drug-eluting stent increase death. Barcelona: ESC Congress News; 2006.
21. Mehran R, Rao SV, Bhatt DL, et al. Standardized bleeding definitions for cardiovascular clinical trials. Circulation. 2011;123(23):2736–47. https://doi.org/10.1161/CIRCULATIONAHA.110.009449.
22. Investigators ST. Enoxaparin vs unfractionated heparin in high-risk patients with non–ST-segment elevation acute coronary syndromes managed with an intended early invasive strategy primary results of the SYNERGY randomized trial. JAMA. 2004;292(1):45–54. https://doi.org/10.1001/jama.292.1.45.
23. Wang Y, Meng X, Wang A, et al. Ticagrelor versus clopidogrel in CYP2C19 loss-of-function carriers with stroke or TIA. N Engl J Med. 2021;385(27):2520–30. https://doi.org/10.1056/NEJMoa2111749.
24. Kim BK, Hong SJ, Cho YH, et al. Effect of ticagrelor monotherapy vs ticagrelor with aspirin on major bleeding and cardiovascular events in patients with acute coronary syndrome: the TICO randomized clinical trial. JAMA. 2020;323(23):2407–16. (In eng). https://doi.org/10.1001/jama.2020.7580.
25. Rao SV, O'Grady K, Pieper KS, et al. A comparison of the clinical impact of bleeding measured by two different classifications among patients with acute coronary syndromes. J Am Coll Cardiol. 2006;47(4):809–16. https://doi.org/10.1016/j.jacc.2005.09.060.
26. Chesebro JH, Knatterud G, Roberts R, et al. Thrombolysis in myocardial infarction (TIMI) trial, phase I: a comparison between intravenous tissue plasminogen activator and intravenous streptokinase. Clinical findings through hospital discharge. Circulation. 1987;76(1):142–54. https://doi.org/10.1161/01.CIR.76.1.142.
27. Fuchs J, Cannon CP. Hirulog in the treatment of unstable angina. Circulation. 1995;92(4):727–33. https://doi.org/10.1161/01.CIR.92.4.727.
28. Antman EM, McCabe CH, Gurfinkel EP, et al. Enoxaparin prevents death and cardiac ischemic events in unstable angina/non–Q-wave myocardial

infarction. Circulation. 1999;100(15):1593–601. https://doi.org/10.1161/01.CIR.100.15.1593.
29. Antman EM, McCabe CH, Braunwald E. Bivalirudin as a replacement for unfractionated heparin in unstable angina/non-ST-elevation myocardial infarction: observations from the TIMI 8 trial. Am Heart J. 2002;143(2):229–34. https://doi.org/10.1067/mhj.2002.120405.
30. Mega JL, Braunwald E, Mohanavelu S, et al. Rivaroxaban versus placebo in patients with acute coronary syndromes (ATLAS ACS-TIMI 46): a randomised, double-blind, phase II trial. Lancet. 2009;374(9683):29–38. (In eng). https://doi.org/10.1016/s0140-6736(09)60738-8.
31. Vranckx P, White HD, Huang Z, et al. Validation of BARC bleeding criteria in patients with acute coronary syndromes: the TRACER trial. J Am Coll Cardiol. 2016;67(18):2135–44. (In eng). https://doi.org/10.1016/j.jacc.2016.02.056.
32. Kaatz S, Ahmad D, Spyropoulos AC, Schulman S. Definition of clinically relevant non-major bleeding in studies of anticoagulants in atrial fibrillation and venous thromboembolic disease in non-surgical patients: communication from the SSC of the ISTH. J Thromb Haemost. 2015;13(11):2119–26. https://doi.org/10.1111/jth.13140.
33. Efficacy and safety of tenecteplase in combination with enoxaparin, abciximab, or unfractionated heparin: the ASSENT-3 randomised trial in acute myocardial infarction. Lancet. 2001;358(9282):605–13. https://doi.org/10.1016/S0140-6736(01)05775-0.
34. Stone GW, Bertrand M, Colombo A, et al. Acute Catheterization and Urgent Intervention Triage strategY (ACUITY) trial: study design and rationale. Am Heart J. 2004;148(5):764–75. (In eng). https://doi.org/10.1016/j.ahj.2004.04.036.
35. Piegas LS, Flather M, Pogue J, et al. The Organization to Assess Strategies for Ischemic Syndromes (OASIS) registry in patients with unstable angina. Am J Cardiol. 1999;84(5a):7m–12m. (In eng). https://doi.org/10.1016/s0002-9149(99)00551-2.
36. Montalescot G, Gallo R, White HD, et al. Enoxaparin versus unfractionated heparin in elective percutaneous coronary intervention 1-year results from the STEEPLE (SafeTy and efficacy of enoxaparin in percutaneous coronary intervention patients, an international randomized evaluation) trial. JACC Cardiovasc Interv. 2009;2(11):1083–91. (In eng). https://doi.org/10.1016/j.jcin.2009.08.016.
37. Wallentin L, Becker RC, Budaj A, et al. Ticagrelor versus clopidogrel in patients with acute coronary syndromes. N Engl J Med. 2009;361(11):1045–57. https://doi.org/10.1056/NEJMoa0904327.
38. Matic DM, Milasinovic DG, Asanin MR, et al. Prognostic implications of bleeding measured by Bleeding Academic Research Consortium (BARC) categorisation in patients undergoing primary percutaneous coronary intervention. Heart. 2014;100(2):146–52. (In eng). https://doi.org/10.1136/heartjnl-2013-304564.
39. Ndrepepa G, Schuster T, Hadamitzky M, et al. Validation of the Bleeding Academic Research Consortium definition of bleeding in patients with coronary artery disease undergoing percutaneous coronary intervention. Circulation. 2012;125(11):1424–31. (In eng). https://doi.org/10.1161/circulationaha.111.060871.
40. Vranckx P, Leonardi S, Tebaldi M, et al. Prospective validation of the Bleeding Academic Research Consortium classification in the all-comer PRODIGY trial. Eur Heart J. 2014;35(37):2524–9. (In eng). https://doi.org/10.1093/eurheartj/ehu161.
41. Xi Z, Gao Y, Yan Z, Zhou Y-J, Liu W. The prognostic significance of different bleeding classifications in off-pump coronary artery bypass grafting. BMC Cardiovasc Disord. 2020;20(1):3. https://doi.org/10.1186/s12872-019-01315-0.
42. Ben-Yehuda O, Redfors B. Validation of the bleeding academic research consortium bleeding definition. J Am Coll Cardiol. 2016;67(18):2145–7. https://doi.org/10.1016/j.jacc.2016.03.505.
43. van der Sangen NMR, Küçük IT, Sivanesan S, et al. Less bleeding by omitting aspirin in non-ST-segment elevation acute coronary syndrome patients: rationale and design of the LEGACY study. Am Heart J. 2023;265:114–20. (In eng). https://doi.org/10.1016/j.ahj.2023.07.011.

The Conundrum Between HBR and HTR

Managing High Bleeding and Thrombotic Risks in Patients Undergoing Coronary Intervention

Gabriel Tensol Rodrigues Pereira,
Bernardo Cortese, and Luis Augusto Palma Dallan

4.1 Introduction

In recent years, there has been a significant focus on finding the optimal medical treatments and their duration for patients undergoing coronary interventions, especially percutaneous coronary intervention (PCI). The goal is to achieve a delicate balance between preventing stent or vessel thrombosis while minimizing the risk of bleeding. A particular challenge arises in managing patients who are at high risk for both bleeding (HBR) and thrombosis (HTR), requiring a sophisticated approach to their treatment and care (Fig. 4.1). This chapter will explore the concepts of HBR and HTR, methods for identifying at-risk patients, and the intricate strategies involved in managing these risks effectively.

G. Tensol Rodrigues Pereira · L. A. Palma Dallan (✉)
University Hospitals Cleveland Medical Center, Cleveland, OH, USA

Case Western Research University School of Medicine, Cleveland, OH, USA
e-mail: gabriel.tensolrodriguespereira@uhhospitals.org

B. Cortese
University Hospitals Harrington Heart & Vascular Institute, Cleveland, OH, USA

Fondazione Ricerca e Innovazione Cardiovascolare, Milan, Italy

DCB Academy, Milan, Italy

B. Cortese, S. Rigattieri (eds.), *High Bleeding Risk Patients in Interventional Cardiology*,
https://doi.org/10.1007/978-3-031-87302-7_4

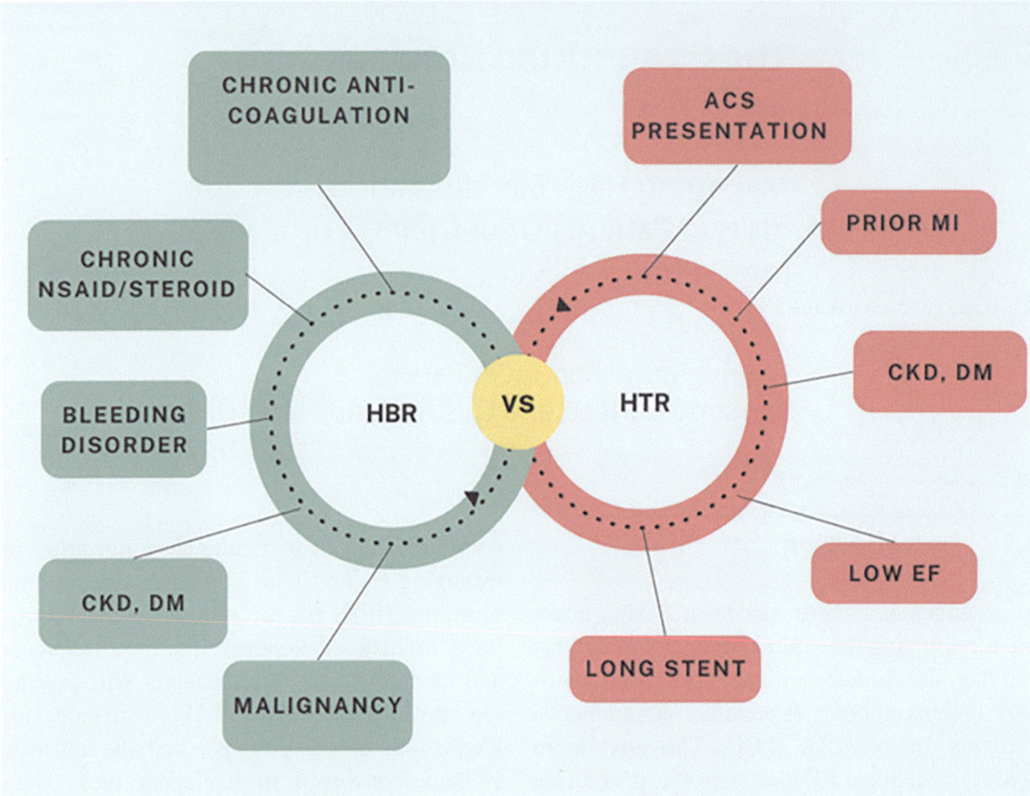

Fig. 4.1 Several aspects that interplay when evaluation HBR and HTR patients. *ACS* Acute Coronary Syndrome, *CKD* Chronic Kidney Disease, *DM* Diabetes Melitus, *NSAID* Non-steroidal anti-inflamatory drug

4.2 High Bleeding Risk (HBR) in Coronary Intervention

High bleeding risk for patients undergoing coronary intervention was an ill-defined entity, up until 2011, when the Academic Research Consortium (ARC) created the Bleeding ARC (BARC), providing bleeding end-point definitions for clinical trials, which, in turn, lead to the establishment of ARC-HRB in 2018. After the creation of the ARC-HRB, a consensus definition of patients at HBR were created, representing the very first systematic approach to those patients. Prior to the creation of the ARC-HRB, HBR was loosely defined as patients with a high propensity for bleeding complications post-PCI, with several proposed scores such as the PRECISE-DAPT or BleeMACS score.

The ARC-HRB (Academic Research Consortium-High Bleeding Risk) bleeding risk classification is based on the BARC (Bleeding Academic Research Consortium) 3–5 bleeding events. These events range from major bleeds causing a drop in hemoglobin levels of at least 3 g/dL to potentially fatal bleeding events. The annual risk of such bleeding events, including the risk of intracranial hemorrhage within a year, is used to identify high bleeding risks. A risk of 4% or more per annum is classified as a major criterion for being considered at high bleeding risk (HBR), while any risk under 4% annually is deemed a minor criterion. Patients are identified as being at HBR if they meet at least one major criterion or two minor criteria, as per defined below (Table 4.1).

The Academic Research Consortium for High Bleeding Risk (ARC-HBR) identifies certain

Table 4.1 Criteria for bleeding risk. Legends: bAVM indicates brain arteriovenous malformation

Major	Minor
Age ≥ 75	
Anticipated use of long-term oral anticoagulation*	
Severe or end-stage CKD (eGFR <30 mL/min)	Moderate CKD (eGFR 30–59 mL/ min)
Hemoglobin <11 g/dL	Hemoglobin 11–12.9 g/dL for men and 11–11.9 g/dL for women
Spontaneous bleeding requiring hospitalization or transfusion in the past 6 months or at any time, if recurrent	Spontaneous bleeding requiring hospitalization or transfusion within the past 12 months not meeting the major criterion
Moderate or severe baseline thrombocytopenia (platelet count <100 × 109/L)	
Chronic bleeding diathesis	
Liver cirrhosis with portal hypertension	
	Long-term use of oral NSAIDs or steroids
Active malignancy‡ (excluding non-melanoma skin cancer) within the past 12 months	
Previous spontaneous ICH (at any time); previous traumatic ICH within the past 12 months; presence of a bAVM; moderate or severe ischemic stroke§ within the past 6 months	Any ischemic stroke at any time not meeting the major criterion
Nondeferrable major surgery on DAPT	
Recent major surgery or major trauma within 30-day before PCI	

CKD chronic kidney disease, *DAPT* dual antiplatelet therapy, *eGFR* estimated glomerular filtration rate, *HBR* high bleeding risk, *ICH* intracranial hemorrhage, *NSAID* nonsteroidal anti-inflammatory drug and *PCI* percutaneous coronary intervention

*This excludes vascular protection doses.42 †Baseline thrombocytopenia is defined as thrombocytopenia before PCI. ‡Active malignancy is defined as diagnosis within 12 months and/or ongoing requirement for treatment (including surgery, chemotherapy, or radiotherapy). §National Institutes of Health Stroke Scale score ≥ 5

conditions that, while not included in the official scoring system, should nevertheless be considered when evaluating a patient's bleeding risk. These conditions include frailty, presentation with acute coronary syndrome (ACS), and medication nonadherence. Despite their significance, there is a lack of consensus on defining frailty and medication nonadherence, making it challenging to gather reliable data for inclusion in current guidelines. On the other hand, in the case of ACS, it can be difficult to discern whether increased bleeding risks are directly due to the condition itself or the result of more aggressive dual antiplatelet therapy (DAPT). However, evidence tends to indicate that the latter—more aggressive DAPT—is a contributing factor, thus, ACS not being included.

The binary nature of current bleeding risk scoring systems, such as the ARC-HRB, presents a significant limitation in capturing the nuanced realities of patient conditions. For example, consider two patients, both above 75 years old with moderate chronic kidney disease (CKD). One patient leads an active lifestyle, exercises regularly, and has no history of recurrent falls, indicating a relatively lower risk profile despite their age and CKD. In contrast, the other patient is chronically frail, has the same age and CKD severity, but with a history of multiple falls in recent months, clearly presenting a higher risk. The binary scoring system categorizes both patients similarly, failing to account for the considerable differences in their health status, activity levels, and overall risk of bleeding. This lack of granularity can lead to oversimplified risk assessments, potentially impacting the tailored management and care these individuals require.

4.3 High Thrombotic Risk (HTR) in Coronary Intervention

Patients categorized as having a high thrombotic risk (HTR) face a greater likelihood of experiencing severe, potentially catastrophic outcomes such as stent thrombosis and myocardial infarction after undergoing percutaneous coronary intervention (PCI). The risk of such events was particularly notable during the shift from bare-metal stents to first-generation drug-eluting stents (DES). The potent antiproliferative drugs coated on these early DES led to inadequate endothelialization, resulting in an increased incidence of late and very late stent thrombosis. However, advancements in DES technology have significantly mitigated these risks in subsequent generations.

Research has delved into the factors that predict the likelihood of thrombosis, revealing the complexity and nuanced nature of these predictors. Clinical factors such as diabetes, multivessel disease, whether the patient presented with acute coronary syndrome (ACS) or not, chronic kidney disease (CKD), malignancy, cocaine use, and left ventricular function have all been shown to influence thrombosis risk. Nonclinical determinants, including procedural aspects like side-branch stenting, the length and type of stent (bare metal vs. DES), post-procedure blood flow (TIMI flow), the use of overlapping stents, and the degree of stent expansion, also play critical roles in assessing thrombosis risk.

Stent thrombosis can occur at various times postimplantation, categorized as early (within 1 month), late (from 1 month to 1 year), or very late (after 1 year). The majority of cases are early thromboses, often tied to the discontinuation or absence of dual antiplatelet therapy (DAPT) at the time of the event. This highlights the importance of timing in relation to PCI and suggests that thrombosis risk decreases as time elapses from the initial procedure.

The complex interaction of various factors means there is no single, universally agreed-upon method to accurately gauge a patient's high thrombotic risk (HTR). Despite this, several scoring systems like the CREDO-Kyoto and ACE-Syntax scores have been introduced to aid clinicians in identifying individuals at an increased risk of thrombosis. To truly comprehend the thrombotic risk faced by a patient, it's essential to combine insights from clinical determinants with anatomical and procedural data. This holistic approach is vital for a more accurate assessment of thrombotic risk.

4.4 Balancing HBR and HTR: Recommendations and Strategies

Navigating the complex interplay between high bleeding risk (HBR) and high thrombotic risk (HTR) necessitates innovative approaches for patient assessment and management. A pivotal contribution to this field is the ARC-HBR trade-off model, which meticulously identifies and quantifies baseline or procedural characteristics associated with an increased risk of myocardial infarction (MI), stent thrombosis (ST), or major bleeding (defined as BARC types 3–5 bleeding). This model's findings highlight key factors such as anemia, kidney insufficiency, current smoking, and complex PCI procedures as significantly elevating the risk for both thrombotic events and major bleeding. Distinct variables have also been pinpointed that specifically heighten the risk for either thrombosis (e.g., prior MI, diabetes, acute MI presentation, and use of bare metal stents) or bleeding (e.g., age $\geq$ 65 years, chronic obstructive pulmonary disease, certain comorbidities, and planned oral anticoagulation post-PCI).

The ARC-HBR model offers a nuanced understanding of risk, distinguishing between factors that universally increase vulnerability to adverse outcomes and those that predominate in either bleeding or thrombotic scenarios. Its dual prediction models for MI/ST and BARC types 3–5 bleeding demonstrate moderate discrimination, underscoring the complexity of accurately forecasting patient-specific risks. The alignment of observed and predicted rates across quintiles of risk further validates the model's utility in stratifying patients according to their individual risk profiles.

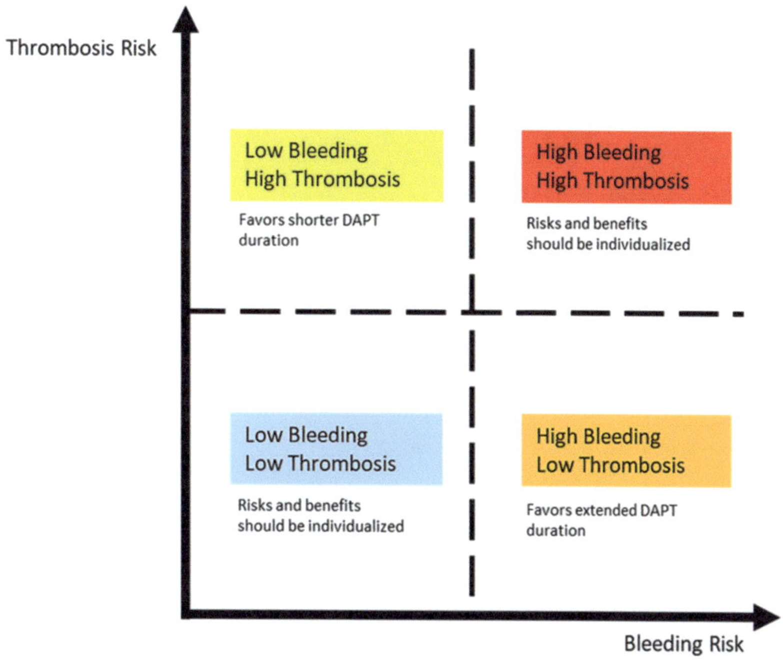

Fig. 4.2 Adaptation of the ARC-HBR trade-off model, in which both a bleeding and thrombotic risks are calculated from several clinical and demographic information, ultimately guiding physicians to what should be favored. The red and blue section are the "white zone" on the model in which an individualized approach is necessary given the balanced risks on those situations

Crucially, the ARC-HBR trade-off model visualizes the predicted risks of MI/ST and major bleeding for patients, allowing for a comparative risk analysis that incorporates the associated mortality of these events. This comparison reveals a significant stratification among patients, with a notable proportion presenting a higher predicted risk for either bleeding or thrombotic events. Moreover, a "white zone" is identified, encapsulating patients whose risks of bleeding and thrombotic complications are comparably balanced, indicating a critical need for personalized treatment strategies that carefully weigh the benefits and risks of interventions (Fig. 4.2).

Parallel to the ARC-HBR model, the DAPT score offers a framework for assessing the benefits and risks associated with prolonged dual antiplatelet therapy, targeting the reduction of thrombotic events post-PCI. By evaluating clinical variables and procedural characteristics, the DAPT score aids clinicians in making informed decisions about the duration of antiplatelet therapy, balancing the prevention of stent thrombosis against the increased risk of bleeding.

Other relevant studies in the field further underscore the complexity of managing patients with concurrent HBR and HTR. These studies advocate for a multidimensional approach to risk assessment, integrating both clinical judgment and evidence-based scores. They suggest that the management of such patients should not rely solely on binary classifications but rather on a comprehensive evaluation that includes patient lifestyle, disease presentation, and procedural specifics.

In light of these considerations, recommendations for balancing HBR and HTR include the following:

1. **Individualized assessment**: Utilize the ARC-HBR trade-off model and DAPT score as part of a broader, individualized risk assessment strategy, taking into account the unique aspects of each patient's clinical presentation and lifestyle.
2. **Integrated decision-making**: Engage in multidisciplinary decision-making, incorporating input from cardiologists, surgeons, and primary care providers to ensure a holistic understanding of the patient's health status and risk factors.
3. **Evidence-based management**: Follow guidelines informed by the latest evidence, adjusting treatment plans as new data emerges and as patient conditions evolve.

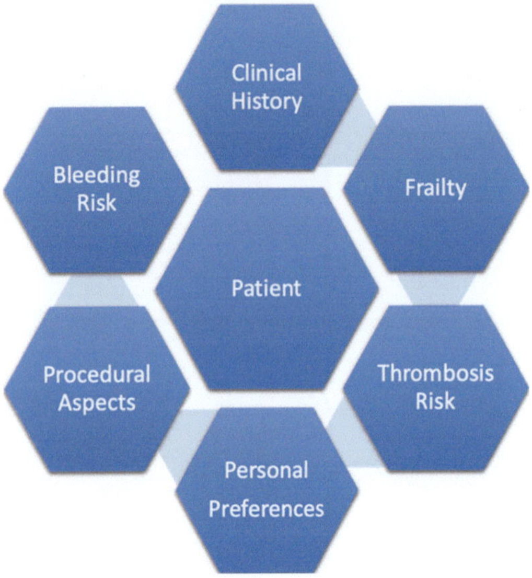

Fig. 4.3 A representation of a patient centered approach, in which multiple aspects are taken into account, including patient preferences

4. **Patient-centered care**: Prioritize patient education and involvement in treatment decisions, ensuring patients understand the risks and benefits of various treatment strategies and are active participants in their care (Fig. 4.3).
5. **Continued research and innovation:** Support ongoing research into the development of more nuanced risk assessment tools and treatment strategies that can accommodate the complexities of balancing HBR and HTR in PCI patients.

By adopting these recommendations and strategies, clinicians can more effectively manage the delicate balance between preventing thrombotic events and minimizing bleeding risk, ultimately improving outcomes for patients undergoing coronary interventions.

Suggested Reading

Urban P, Mehran R, Colleran R, Angiolillo DJ, Byrne RA, Capodanno D, Cuisset T, Cutlip D, Eerdmans P, Eikelboom J, Farb A, Gibson CM, Gregson J, Haude M, James SK, Kim HS, Kimura T, Konishi A, Laschinger J, Leon MB, Magee PFA, Mitsutake Y, Mylotte D, Pocock S, Price MJ, Rao SV, Spitzer E, Stockbridge N, Valgimigli M, Varenne O, Windhoevel U, Yeh RW, Krucoff MW, Morice MC. Defining high bleeding risk in patients undergoing percutaneous coronary intervention: a consensus document from the academic research consortium for high bleeding risk. Eur Heart J. 2019 Aug 14;40(31):2632–2653. https://doi.org/10.1093/eurheartj/ehz372. PMID: 31116395; PMCID: PMC6736433.

Mehran R, Rao SV, Bhatt DL, Gibson CM, Caixeta A, Eikelboom J, Kaul S, Wiviott SD, Menon V, Nikolsky E, Serebruany V, Valgimigli M, Vranckx P, Taggart D, Sabik JF, Cutlip DE, Krucoff MW, Ohman EM, Steg PG, White H. Standardized bleeding definitions for cardiovascular clinical trials: a consensus report from the bleeding academic research consortium. Circulation. 2011;123(23):2736–47. https://doi.org/10.1161/CIRCULATIONAHA.110.009449.

Costa F, van Klaveren D, James S, Heg D, Räber L, Feres F, Pilgrim T, Hong MK, Kim HS, Colombo A, Steg PG, Zanchin T, Palmerini T, Wallentin L, Bhatt DL, Stone GW, Windecker S, Steyerberg EW, Valgimigli M, PRECISE-DAPT Study Investigators. Derivation and validation of the predicting bleeding complications in patients undergoing stent implantation and subsequent dual antiplatelet therapy (PRECISE-DAPT) score: a pooled analysis of individual-patient datasets from clinical trials. Lancet. 2017;389(10073):1025–34. https://doi.org/10.1016/S0140-6736(17)30397-5.

Lyu SQ, Zhu J, Wang J, Wu S, Zhang H, Shao XH, Yang YM. Performance of the REACH, PARIS, BleeMACS, and PRECISE-DAPT scores for predicting 1-year bleeding events in patients undergoing coronary drug-eluting stent implantation. Platelets. 2022 July 4;33(5):719–726. https://doi.org/10.1080/09537104.2021.1981847. Epub 2021 Oct 11.

Natsuaki M, Morimoto T, Yamaji K, Watanabe H, Yoshikawa Y, Shiomi H, Nakagawa Y, Furukawa Y, Kadota K, Ando K, Akasaka T, Hanaoka KI, Kozuma K, Tanabe K, Morino Y, Muramatsu T, Kimura T; CREDO-Kyoto PCI/CABG Registry Cohort 2, RESET, and NEXT trial investigators. Prediction of thrombotic and bleeding events after percutaneous coronary intervention: CREDO-Kyoto Thrombotic and Bleeding Risk Scores. J Am Heart Assoc. 2018 May 22;7(11):e008708. https://doi.org/10.1161/JAHA.118.008708. PMID: 29789335; PMCID: PMC6015347.

Urban P, Gregson J, Owen R, Mehran R, Windecker S, Valgimigli M, Varenne O, Krucoff M, Saito S, Baber U, Chevalier B, Capodanno D, Morice MC, Pocock S. Assessing the risks of bleeding vs thrombotic events in patients at high bleeding risk after coronary stent implantation: the ARC-high bleeding risk trade-off model. JAMA Cardiol. 2021 Apr 1;6(4):410–419. https://doi.org/10.1001/jamacardio.2020.6814. PMID: 33404627; PMCID: PMC7788509.

Part II

Revascularization Strategies in HBR Patients

5 Percutaneous Coronary Intervention in the Elderly

Sergio Barrera and Jose M. de la Torre Hernandez

5.1 Introduction

Ischemic heart disease continues to be the main cause of morbidity and mortality in elderly patients. The proportion of older people has increased significantly in recent years, and this trend will continue. Decision-making in older patients can be challenging for cardiologists, and population aging is a reality we face every day in the catheterization laboratory. In addition, older people has been observed to have lower cardiac catheterization requests despite the fact that reduced mortality after percutaneous coronary intervention (PCI) has been observed, especially in the setting of acute coronary syndromes.

Aging leads to a higher prevalence of ischemic heart disease. Nonetheless, elderly patients are underrepresented in most clinical trials, and therefore there is a paucity of evidence regarding therapeutic strategies. The complexity of coronary intervention is the greatest challenge in percutaneous revascularization of the elderly, not only because of concomitant multiple comorbidities but also for anatomical and functional aspects in these patients. However, it has been shown that elderly patients with acute coronary syndrome (ACS) may experience similar or even greater benefit than other age groups when the procedure is performed on time [1].

In elderly patients, the risk of mortality remains high both during and after the procedure, particularly in patients with long and complex procedures. The development of new techniques and the implementation of new technology in PCI has allowed complex coronary procedures to be performed in elderly patients and in very-high-risk patients increasing their quality of life. To establish the greatest benefit from percutaneous revascularization, it is important to identify the patients most likely to obtain it, so a comprehensive evaluation of the patient is essential.

There are different tools available to establish risk stratification in patients with ACS to guide decision-making on the type of revascularization, potential complications, and adjunctive medication. This assessment takes on an important role essentially in elderly patients, since they are at higher risk of ischemic and hemorrhagic events (Fig. 5.1).

S. Barrera · J. M. de la Torre Hernandez (✉)
Hospital Universitario Marques de Valdecilla, Servicio de Cardiología, Unidad de Cardiología Intervencionista, IDIVAL, Santander, Spain

B. Cortese, S. Rigattieri (eds.), *High Bleeding Risk Patients in Interventional Cardiology*,
https://doi.org/10.1007/978-3-031-87302-7_5

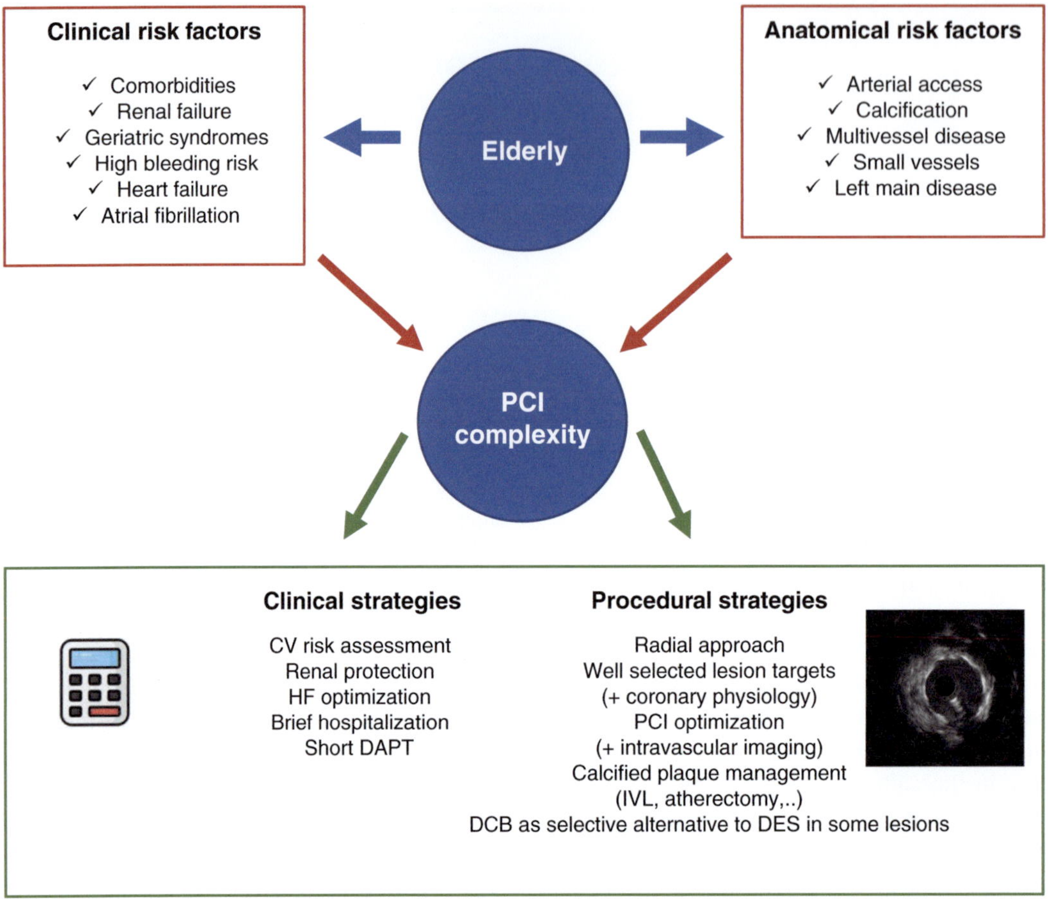

Fig. 5.1 Factors defining PCI complexity and practical implications of this condition. *CV* cardiovascular, *DCB* drug-coated balloon, *DES* drug-eluting stent, *HF* heart failure, *IVL* intravascular lithotripsy

5.2 Risk Assessment in the Elderly

Risk assessment allows cardiologists to identify patients who receive greater benefit than others for percutaneous revascularization. There are many tools that stratify risk according to patient characteristics, and this assessment by different scores should be done routinely in all patients who might undergo invasive treatment as part of the decision to revascularize and to anticipate any possible complications. Subjective patient assessment is also important; however, it can be prone to bias. Early recognition of high-risk older adults may facilitate the administration of appropriate and necessary therapies more likely to provide benefit and plays an important role in complex decision-making.

A large number of risk stratification scores for PCI exist with excellent performance in the general population, but these models have not been validated in adults older than 75 years or have failed to incorporate the contributions of geriatric-specific risk factors. While older age is an independent risk variable in general, several other contributors are present in these patients. Conventional risk approach identifies periprocedural risk from three perspectives; assessment of cardiovascular risk based on demographic, clinical and presenting characteristics, and anatomic and procedural considerations. However, the conventional approach does not incorporate geriatric syndromes [1–3].

5.3 Cardiovascular Risk Assessment Tools

Several scores for estimation of prognosis, thrombotic risk, and bleeding risk are nowadays available. Conventional risk scores can quantify the risk of all-cause mortality, bleeding, and readmission risk [4].

5.3.1 GRACE Score

A score derived from an international, multicenter registry in patients with ACS with and without ST-segment elevation to stratify the risk of infarction and death at 1 month and 6 months. The GRACE risk score uses eight factors: age, heart rate, systolic blood pressure, renal function, congestive heart failure, ST-segment deviation, cardiac arrest, and elevated biomarkers. The GRACE score has been tested for accuracy in predicting in-hospital mortality in very elderly persons with acute coronary syndromes and has been shown to be accurate in predicting in-hospital mortality from ACS, similar to younger patients [5].

5.3.2 TIMI Score

It was designed based on two interventional studies in non-ST-elevation ACS: TIMI 11B11 and ESSENCE. The Thrombolysis in Myocardial Infarction (TIMI) score is considered a tool for early risk stratification. Seven factors help to assess the risk of mortality and the risk of other adverse cardiac events: age 65 years or older, presence of at least three risk factors for coronary artery disease (i.e., diabetes mellitus, hypertension, hyperlipidemia, smoking, and family history), history of coronary stenosis of 50% or more, presence of greater than or equal to two episodes of angina 24 hours prior to presentation, aspirin use within the past 7 days, ST-segment deviations greater than or equal to 0.05 mV on initial ECG on admission, and elevated serum cardiac markers of necrosis. This tool has been validated in elderly women; greater adverse outcomes were observed with a higher TIMI risk score for in-hospital and post-discharge follow-up [6].

5.3.3 CRUSADE

It is a predictive model of eight variables associated with an increased likelihood of bleeding in patients with non-ST-segment elevation ACS. The variables evaluated are low hematocrit, high creatinine clearance, elevated heart rate, female sex, presence of heart failure on admission, previous known vascular disease, and end-tidal blood pressures. Both this bleeding predictive tool, as well as others, have shown a lower performance in elderly patients [7].

The EPIC05-Sierra75 trial investigated outcomes in elderly patients treated with antithrombotic strategy guided by bleeding and ischemic risks (clinical presentation, PCI complexity, and PRECISE DAPT score) after revascularization with latest-generation everolimus-eluting stent [8]. It was concluded that the application of this risk-adjusted antithrombotic protocol after revascularization with latest-generation everolimus-eluting stents seems to be associated with a better prognosis in terms of ischemic and bleeding outcomes.

5.4 Defining High Bleeding Risk in the Elderly

Factors related to bleeding risk have been identified, most of them are related to age, the older the age, and the higher the risk of bleeding. Having said this, it is important to remark that age per se is not a high bleeding risk factor. Female sex and some comorbidity such as hypertension, diabetes mellitus, peripheral artery disease, stroke, peripheral artery disease, and history of bleeding have also been identified as bleeding risk predictors [9, 10]. In trials that have evaluated short antiplatelet therapy in PCI patients at high risk of bleeding, the most common risk factors are advanced age, use of anticoagulants, and impaired renal function. High bleeding risk is defined according to

Table 5.1 Bleeding scores for patients undergoing PCI

Scores	PRECISE DAPT	DAPT score	ARC-HBR
Year of publication	2017	2016	2019
Validating data set	PLATO Bern PCI Registry	PROTECT	Bern PCI Registry CREDO Registry Mount Sinai Registry
Criteria for HBR	≥25	<2	≥1 major or ≥2 minor ARC-HBR criteria

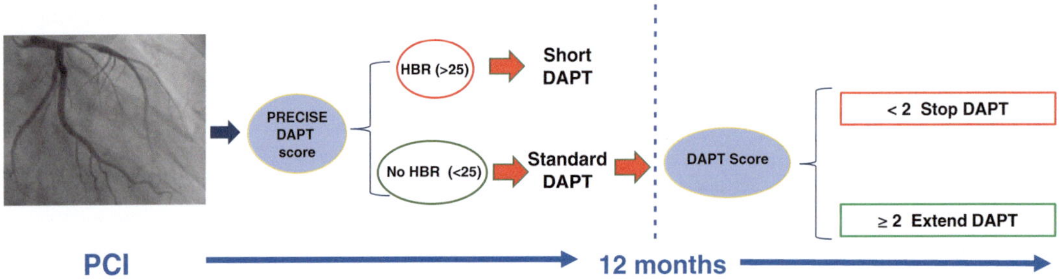

Fig. 5.2 Application of bleeding scores in the time course after PCI

Academic Research Consortium as a BARC 3 or 5 bleeding risk of ≥4% per year or an intracranial hemorrhage (ICH) risk of ≥1% per year [11].

Several scores such as the PRECISE-DAPT and DAPT score have been validated to guide antiplatelet therapy after PCI (Table 5.1 and Fig. 5.2).

5.5 Impact of Geriatric Syndromes

Geriatric syndromes refer to clinical conditions that do not fall into the category of a disease and share multiple risk factors including cognitive as well as functional impairment. Geriatric syndromes complicate decision-making in elderly patients, delays patient care, and increases procedural risk in catheterization laboratory [12].

5.5.1 Frailty

A state of increased vulnerability to stressors due to decreased physiological reserve. Frailty is measured as greater than or equal to three abnormal domains of the following: weight loss, weakness, poor stamina and energy, sluggishness, and low level of physical activity.

Frailty is independently associated with an increased risk of developing cardiovascular disease, morbidity, and mortality. Compared with non-frail subjects, frail older patients had a higher incidence of major adverse cardiac events, including mortality, during a 6-year follow-up period.

Frailty is associated with greater susceptibility to stressful events, and they have a higher prevalence of coronary heart disease. One study showed that one-fifth of patients older than 65 years are frail at the time of catheterization, and frailty is associated with greater comorbidities, higher burden of coronary artery disease, and worse functional status. Frail older adults presenting NSTEMI have more challenging angiographic findings regardless of age, as these patients have severe calcification of the culprit lesion, higher SYNTAX score, and high-risk lesions.

The FRAIL scale [13]: It was proposed by the geriatric advisory panel of the International Academy of Nutrition and Aging; it is an easy-to-use self-questionnaire and seeks to measure frailty in the clinical setting. For each affirmative answer, one point is indicated, with a score of 3 or more being considered frail and a score of 1 or 2 being considered pre-frail.

F = fatigue: Are you fatigued?
R = resistance: Unable to climb one flight of stairs?
A = aerobic: Unable to walk a block?
I = Illnesses- disease: Do you have more than five diseases?
L = loss of weight—weight loss: Have you lost more than 5% of your weight in the last 6 months?

5.5.2 Cognitive Impairment

Decreasing ability to care for oneself and to complete activities of daily living, loss of independence, and reduced quality of life. The prevalence of cognitive impairment increases with age and CVD further worsens cognitive function.

Atrial fibrillation was associated with an excess risk of developing dementia when subjects were followed for several years. Patients with heart failure have high prevalence of cognitive impairment and proposed mechanisms include risk factors shared with CVD and dementia that may lead to neurodegeneration, CVD leading to clinical or subclinical strokes causing cognitive impairment, or CVD that decreases cerebral perfusion.

Cognitive assessment before and after cardiac procedures is an important marker of quality of life and marker of mortality. Cognitive impairment can lead to decreased medication adherence and therefore influences treatment goals. Higher incidence of delirium leads to longer duration of hospitalization, greater cognitive impairment, rehospitalization, and death.

5.5.3 Falls

This is perhaps the greatest concern in elderly patients undergoing PCI, since it is associated with high morbidity and mortality. The use of sedative medication, analgesics, and prolonged procedures predisposes to falls, and the use of antiplatelet and anticoagulant drugs further increases the risk. Falls can cause impaired function, morbidity, mortality, and poor quality of life in the elderly.

Many cardiovascular medications, including vasoactive medications and atrioventricular node blockers, can contribute to falls. These geriatric patients with CVD are frequently prescribed multiple medications as a result of their comorbidities, which can further accentuate the negative effects of some cardiovascular medications, resulting in falls.

Falls present with a risk of bleeding resulting in challenges in weighing the risks and benefits of anticoagulation or prolonged antiplatelet therapy in older adults undergoing complex coronary or structural heart disease interventions. Falls risk and polypharmacy should be assessed before prescribing most cardiovascular medications.

5.5.4 Sarcopenia

Sarcopenia is defined as progressive loss of skeletal muscle mass, quality, and function with associated weakness. It can be diagnosed by a combination of instruments that measure muscle strength, muscle mass, and physical performance. Cardiovascular disease is a risk factor for the accelerated development of sarcopenia, with a prevalence of 30% in older adults.

Biochemical markers of sarcopenia (sarcopenia index: ratio of serum creatinine to cystatin C) have been associated with poorer quality of life. Furthermore, sarcopenia predicts atherosclerotic cardiovascular disease and is an independent predictor of adverse cardiovascular events. Elderly patients with sarcopenia undergoing PCI information is limited; however, sarcopenia has been shown to predict mortality in TAVR.

5.6 Anatomical and Procedural Risk Factors in the Elderly

In elderly patients, certain factors should be considered prior PCI. This initial evaluation should consider the cardiovascular aging process which among other things is characterized by increased stiffness of the aorta and large central arteries, LV concentric hypertrophy, elevated LV end-diastolic pressure, calcification, etc. In advanced age, many patients have undergone multiple surgical interventions during their lifetime, which could modify the normal anatomy of the cardiovascular system. In addition, certain neurological diseases predispose to limb stiffness making it difficult to adopt a neutral position and, in some patients, predisposes to abnormal movements.

Regarding coronary angiography, these patients present high-risk anatomical lesions, such as left main coronary artery disease, ostial lesions, severe calcification, long lesions (>60 mm), or in-stent restenosis. We should not forget that in previous years coronary revascularization surgery was more common, so catheterization is more frequently requested in previously operated patients, which is important when choosing the arterial access.

Complex high-risk indicated percutaneous coronary intervention (CHIP-PCI) is a poorly defined concept, which has not been validated in an older population before. Our group conducted a study aimed to evaluate the predictive value of the CHIP-PCI score in a large cohort of elderly patients and to identify potential further risk factors [14]. A total of 2725 patients were included in the study. Of the 12 investigated original CHIP-PCI score variables, 5 were independent predictors: previous myocardial infarction, left ventricular ejection fraction <30%, chronic kidney disease, left main coronary artery percutaneous coronary intervention, and non-radial access. Furthermore, diabetes mellitus, anemia, and severe calcification showed to be significant predictors of MACCEs. The additional variables improved the discriminatory value of the CHIP-PCI score for 1-year MACCEs (modified CHIP-PCI score: area under the curve (AUC) 0.647 vs original CHIP-PCI score: AUC 0.598, $p = 0.02$) and in-hospital MACCEs (AUC 0.729 vs 0.657, $p = 0.003$, respectively). In conclusion, the CHIP-PCI score retains its prognostic value in older patients for in-hospital MACCEs; however, it is of limited value at 1-year follow-up. The modified CHIP-PCI score, including the five patient-related and three procedure-related factors, significantly improved its discriminatory potential.

5.6.1 Arterial Access

Arterial access is essential in PCI in the elderly. The correct choice of arterial access ensures a shorter procedure, with sufficient catheter support and lower complications. In addition, it allows the procedure to be performed in comfort for the patient and for the physician. However, this is not always possible, as elderly patients have a high prevalence of peripheral vascular disease, especially those with a history of smoking and diabetes. Nevertheless, it is always recommended to choose an access that allows working comfortably, as coronary lesions are often complex.

Radial access is the first choice. Previous studies have shown that radial access reduces the risk of vascular complications and bleeding associated with PCI. It is important to know that radial access becomes more difficult in elderly patients due to anatomical alterations. Advanced age, female sex, and hypertension have been described as clinical predictors of failure of right radial access for coronary angiography. In a study in patients older than 70 years, those who underwent a radial approach had a lower mortality rate and a lower rate of major bleeding compared to those who underwent a femoral approach [15]. In another study it was observed that, in elderly patients with suspected coronary artery disease, the rate of bleeding requiring surgery or blood transfusion was 0% in the radial approach and 3.2% in the femoral approach [16].

Although radial access is becoming increasingly common for PCI, femoral access remains a common access. When choosing femoral access, whether right or left, ultrasound guidance of the puncture is recommended to avoid complications. A recent trial showed that routine use of ultrasound during femoral puncture did not reduce major complications or increased bleeding in patients undergoing cardiac intervention; however, it did reduce the risk of venous puncture and the number of attempts [17].

Although hemostasis after femoral sheath removal is traditionally achieved by manual compression, vascular closure devices have been developed as an alternative strategy. These devices have been developed with the goal of achieving rapid hemostasis and early ambulation. Contemporary randomized trials demonstrated that femoral closure devices decrease the risk of access site complications after coronary angiography, mainly due to lower rates of hematoma ≥5 mm, but not of major bleeding or other no hemorrhage-related complications. We currently have femoral arterial closure devices with sheath sizes between 5 Fr and 8 Fr such as Angio-Seal device (Angio-Seal VIP; Terumo), Perclose device (Perclose A-T or Perclose ProGlide; Abbott), or using a Mynx device (Mynx ACE or MYNXGRIP; Cordis).

A trial demonstrated, in patients older than 60 years, that the use of a vascular closure device does not significantly reduce access-site bleeding and the risk of hematoma compared with manual arterial compression alone for patients undergoing diagnostic catheterization alone. In contrast, patients who underwent PCI and therefore generally require larger sheath sizes and periprocedural anticoagulation demonstrated a significant reduction in access site bleeding, risk of hematoma, and a lower risk of vascular complications with the use of a closure device [18].

Hemostasis in radial access has traditionally been done with radial band; some common complications of this access is hematoma and radial artery occlusion. The ideal duration for the removal of the band has been evaluated in a meta-analysis, and it has been observed that a duration of at least 2 h is effective for the prevention of radial occlusion and hematoma prevention.

5.6.2 Drug-Eluting Stents and Drug-Coated Balloons

Some studies have used older age as a factor in deciding the type of stent to implant in PCI. Factors associated with the use of DESs in patients undergoing primary PCI for STEMI showed that older age was associated with a decrease in the use of DESs compared to bare metal stents (BMS).

The XIMA (Xience or Vision Stents for the Management of Angina in the Elderly) trial comparing DES with BMS showed that octogenarians have similar procedural success as younger patients; the rate of all-cause mortality, myocardial infarction (4.3% vs 8.7%; $p = 0.01$), and revascularization of the treated vessel (2.0% vs 7%; $p = 0.001$) was significantly lower in the DES group than in the BMS group. Remarkably, the incidence of major bleeding events did not increase despite the longer use of dual antiplatelet therapy in the DES group versus the BMS group [19].

Outcomes have also been studied in patients >75 years with DES or BMS implantation for stable angina, silent ischemia, or ACS. In the SENIOR trial [20], the primary outcome of major adverse cardiac and cerebrovascular events (composite of all-cause mortality, myocardial infarction, stroke, or ischemia-directed revascularization) was compared between the DES and BMS group in an intention-to-treat population at 30 days, 180 days, and 1 year. The primary outcome occurred in 12% of patients in the DES group and 16% of patients in the BMS group (relative risk, 0.71; 95% CI, 0.52–0.94; $p = 0.02$).

On current limited data, among elderly patients with PCI, a DES, and a short duration of dual antiplatelet therapy, have been shown to be better than BMS and a short duration of dual antiplatelet therapy with respect to all-cause mortality, myocardial infarction, stroke, and ischemia-driven target lesion revascularization. But there are not only DES; there is also the alternative of drug-coated balloons. These have been shown to be equally effective and safe regardless of age and reduce or even obviate the need for DAPT [21]. There are already registries with monotherapy after treatment with DCB that suggest safety [22].

5.7 Coronary Calcification

Coronary calcification is associated with high rates of immediate procedural failure and adverse clinical outcomes and is common in elderly patients. Coronary calcification induces a difficult advancement of devices (coronary guidewires, stents, coronary balloons) and stents expansion. Therefore, it may lead to PCI-related complications such as vessel dissection, perforation, or mechanical problems of stent (under expansion, distortion, detachment, or loss of the stent). The presence of moderate-severe calcification in coronary angiography has been associated with older age, greater coronary artery complexity, lower final minimum luminal diameter, higher residual stenosis, and higher periprocedural complication rates [23].

Recent advances in intracoronary imaging and adjunctive technologies now allow the operator to select the most appropriate strategy in patients with severe calcium treated percutaneously and with greater success.

In intracoronary imaging, characterization of calcium is important in pre-PCI planning to choose the appropriate approach. The circumferential arc angle, longitudinal extent, and axial thickness of calcium deposits have been shown to determine the outcome of PCI and therefore may help to select the use of adjunctive intracoronary devices.

5.7.1 Balloons (Scoring, Cutting, and Super High Pressure)

Scoring balloons AngioSculpt (AngioScore, California, USA), Scoreflex (OrbusNeich Medical, B.V. Hoevelaken, the Netherlands), and cutting balloons such as Flextome and Wolverine (Boston Scientific, Natick, Massachusetts, USA).

These are modified coronary balloon which create incisions within the lesion to increase balloon expansion during inflation. Cutting balloons have multiple microscopic blades attached longitudinally to a semiflexible balloon to create tracts that maximize balloon expansion.

Scoring balloons are semiflexible balloons with a helical nylon scoring rim that can allow dilation of the lesion while potentially preventing slippage. Scoring balloons are potentially more effective than cutting balloons, but there are limited data on their use in calcified arteries.

Super-high-pressure balloons such as OPN NC (SIS Medical AG, Winterthur, Switzerland) have a nominal burst pressure of 35 atm and may be beneficial for calcified plaque preparation.

5.7.2 Ablative Atherectomy Techniques

The two most commonly used ablative atherectomy techniques are rotational and orbital atherectomy. Rotational atherectomy (Boston Scientific, Boston, Massachusetts, USA) is an intracoronary device consisting of a diamond-encrusted elliptical burr passed over a 0.009″ custom guidewire with a 0.014″ tip (RotaWire) that rotates at speeds of ~150,000 rpm and advances with a helical drive shaft. To facilitate forward ablation and non-ablative removal of the rotating bur, only the front half of the bur is diamond inlaid. The device is 6 or 7 Fr. Currently, the optimal technique recommends sizing the burr:artery ratio to 50%, using a pecking motion (to avoid embolization of macroparticles), restricting ablations to <20 s and avoiding decelerations >5000 rpm during ablation to avoid complications.

The orbital atherectomy device (Diamondback 360) is 6 Fr compatible and mounted on a dedicated wire: 0.0012″ ViperWire Advance. It consists of a drive shaft with an eccentrically mounted diamond-coated crown that rotates and orbits within the artery, thus applying centrifugal force on the calcification. As with rotational, the goal of the treatment is to modify vessel stiffness, thus allowing stent placement. However, the main difference with RA is that in orbital atherectomy the ablation area increases with rotational speed, becoming substantially larger than the cross-sectional area of the rotating element.

5.7.3 Laser Atherectomy (Spectranetics, Colorado Springs, Colorado, USA)

LA uses xenon chloride gas as a medium to generate ultrasound violet pulses at 308 nm. These pulses exert a photochemical effect where the pulses destroy carbon bonds in the vascular material, a photothermal effect where intracellular water is heated and causes cell destruction and also a photomechanical effect, where bubbles formed at the catheter tip burst and modify the obstructing material. The benefit of the 308-nm laser range is that it exhibits less tissue penetration (<30 microM), less heat production, and overall less tissue damage than higher laser ranges, while maintaining adequate modification of coronary calcification. The device is compatible with any 0.014″ coronary guidewire and is available in four diameters: 0.9, 1.4 mm (6 Fr. compatible) and 1.7, 2.0 mm (7 Fr. compatible).

5.7.4 Intravascular Lithotripsy (Shockwave Medical, Fremont, California, USA)

It delivers acoustic pulse waves circumferentially to break superficial and deep calcification. The system is composed of a 0.014″ monorail system dilatable balloon catheter that is prepared in a conventional manner. It has a dual port hub, one of which is connected to the balloon inflator and the other to a connector cable, which is attached to the pulse generator console.

Pulses are delivered by activating a button on the connector cable for 10 s (one pulse/s). The system is compatible with all conventional 0.014″ coronary guidewires and is compatible with 6 Fr. A major potential advantage compared to RA and OA is that intravascular lithotripsy can be performed on lesions located at the bifurcations while keeping the side branch coronary guidewires in place.

5.8 Left Main Coronary Artery Disease

Left main coronary artery (LM) disease is found in 4% of all diagnostic angiographies, and within these it is isolated up to 5–10%. LM disease is associated with significant morbidity and mortality, even more so in an older population. Currently there is no standard revascularization strategy for all types of LM lesions; both surgical and percutaneous revascularization are valid strategies. Elderly patients are often more frail than younger patients, and, consequently, physicians may be reluctant to recommend an invasive surgical strategy to treat LM.

In a prespecified subgroup analysis of the SYNTAXES trial (Synergy Between PCI with Taxus and Cardiac Surgery Extended Survival) [24], the impact of revascularization modality on all-cause death and 10-year life expectancy was investigated, as well as on major adverse cardiac or cerebrovascular event (MACE) rates and quality of life up to 5 years between elderly and non-elderly patients with LM and three-vessel disease; it was observed that there was no significant difference in the risk of all-cause death between PCI and CABG in elderly patients at 5 years and 10 years.

LM is evaluated by conventional coronary angiography. The evaluation should be careful if LM disease is suspected, avoiding excessive intubation with the catheter, monitoring the aortic pressure curve (flattening or ventricularization), and performing angiographic projections that allow us to evaluate the three segments of the LM. Revascularization is indicated if angiographic stenosis is >50% and evidence of myocardial ischemia. The pressure guidewire is another tool that provides valuable information when assessing LM disease; obtaining measurements from LAD and LCX provides a better assessment of the LM.

There are other tools for LM evaluation such as intracoronary imaging; IVUS allows us to obtain more information about the structure and anatomy of the LM, as well as the presence of plaque, composition, and calcification, but above all it allows us to evaluate the extension of plaque to proximal LAD or LCX. IVUS allows us to assess revascularization by measuring the minimum luminal area and has proven its usefulness and performance in deferring revascularization after 6 mm^2. In addition, IVUS is very useful after percutaneous angioplasty for stent optimization in LM [25].

In IVUS optimization, adequate stent expansion and apposition as well as the proximal and distal border should be evaluated. After stent implantation, deformation with the guide catheter at the proximal edge is common in ostial lesions. When treating the distal trunk, in the case of using the provisional stent technique, plaque burden and optimization can be assessed after stent recrossing. If we use the two-stent technique, we can assess the expansion and distal edge of the stent in both branches.

5.9 Multivessel Disease

Older adults with ischemic heart disease often present with multivessel coronary artery disease which makes the procedure difficult due to the complex anatomy and extent of coronary disease.

In fact, patients with multivessel disease show more major adverse cardiac events (heart failure, reinfarction, stroke, hospitalization for cardiovascular disease, unscheduled revascularization, and all-cause mortality). A critical step is to decide on the most appropriate strategy for revascularization by PCI. Whereas complete revascularization treats all hemodynamically significant coronary artery lesions, incomplete revascularization treats the culprit lesion only when multivessel disease is present, leaving any lesion untreated [26].

The benefit of complete revascularization in patients older than 75 years with myocardial infarction and multivessel disease was recently studied. In this study, elderly patients undergoing PCI were randomized to complete physiology-guided revascularization of non-culprit lesions or to receive no further revascularization except for the culprit lesion. A composite of death, myocardial infarction, stroke, or any revascularization at 1 year was studied. It was concluded that patients aged 75 years or older with myocardial infarction and multivessel disease and those who underwent complete revascularization had less risk of the composite of death, myocardial infarction, stroke, and revascularization at 1 year compared with those who only had the culprit lesion revascularized. Physiologic evaluation and PCI of non-culprit lesions were performed during the index procedure or in a staged in-hospital procedure [27].

5.10 Results of PCI in Acute Settings

5.10.1 Non-ST-Segment Elevation Myocardial Infarction

Currently, randomized studies that have investigated the invasive strategy in elderly patients with NSTEMI most have found no benefit compared with conservative management. However, one of these studies, the largest in population, demonstrated that invasive strategy reduced recurrent myocardial infarction and repeated urgent revascularization. The Italian Elderly ACS trial [28] assigned patients to early invasive versus conservative strategy; patients in the conservative strategy had higher rates of ischemic events during hospitalization, which led to urgent angiography; although it led to a 20% reduction in the rate of death, disability rate, stroke, or rehospitalization, this was not statistically significant. It is important to note that geriatric syndromes were not evaluated in these trials. In the MOSCA-Frail trial [29], if frailty was evaluated, it did not show any benefit from the invasive strategy. If we consider observational and randomized studies, as well as systematic reviews and even meta-analyses, the invasive strategy has shown some reduction in myocardial infarction and recurrent revascularization, but no survival benefit.

5.10.2 ST-Segment Elevation Myocardial Infarction

Older patients present atypical symptoms when they suffer STEMI, which can cause delay in reperfusion treatment and therefore greater risk of complications (death, mechanical complications). It is estimated that about 20% of patients >85 years with STEMI are admitted with a diagnosis other than an ACS [30].

The superiority of primary PCI over fibrinolysis seems to extend to elderly patients, although the findings are limited in very elderly patients and there is no evaluation of the role of geriatric syndromes. The low inclusion or noninclusion of older adults in most clinical trials limits decision-making in this group of patients, but it seems that the trend indicates a greater number of primary PCIs in octogenarians; perhaps this increase reflects a greater toolbox for PCI and therefore greater comfort in performing complex angioplasties. In a meta-analysis of elderly patients, 70 to 80 years of age who were randomized to primary PCI, a reduction in all causes of mortality, reinfarction, and stroke was observed. Elderly patients should not be denied revascularization solely because of their age.

In Spain we conducted a nationwide registry of consecutive patients older than 75 years treated with primary angioplasty (ESTROFA MI + 75) [31]. The study included 3576 patients (39.3% women, 48.5% with renal failure, 11.5% in Killip III or IV, and 29.8% with >6 h of chest pain). Radial access was used in 56.4%, bivalirudin in 11.8%, thromboaspiration in 55.9%, and drug-eluting stents in 26.6%. The 1-month and 2-year incidences of cardiovascular death were 10.1% and 14.7%, respectively. The 2-year rates of definite or probable thrombosis, repeat revascularization, and BARC bleeding >2 were 3.1%, 2.3%, and 4.2%, respectively. Predictive factors were diabetes mellitus, renal failure, atrial fibrillation, delay to reperfusion >6 h, ejection fraction <45%, Killip class III–IV, radial access, bivalirudin, drug-eluting stents, final TIMI flow of III, and incomplete revascularization at discharge.

In a subgroup-analysis of this nationwide registry of primary angioplasty in the elderly (ESTROFA MI + 75) patients with multivessel disease were analyzed to describe treatment approaches and 2-year outcomes. Of 1830 patients, 847 (46%) underwent multivessel PCI either in acute (51%), staged (44%), or both procedures (5%). Multivessel PCI was independent predictor of cardiac death and infarction with the best prognosis corresponding to those undergoing staged procedures [32].

5.10.3 Cardiogenic Shock

In the setting of cardiogenic shock and cardiac arrest, age is an independent predictor of death after PCI. Furthermore, the value of mechanical circulatory support in these cases, e.g., with intra-aortic balloon pump or Impella, is uncertain. Therefore, careful selection of patients most likely to benefit from PCI is required.

There are few studies reporting clinical outcomes in elderly patients with cardiogenic shock. In the SHOCK (Should We Emergently Revascularize Occluded Coronaries for Cardiogenic Shock) trial [33], patients aged ≥75 years did not benefit from early revascularization and may have been harmed; their 30-day mortality rate was 75%. However, the low representation of older adults in this trial (<20%) limits the applicability of this analysis. In the CULPRIT-SHOCK (Culprit Lesion Only PCI Versus Multivessel Percutaneous Coronary Intervention in Cardiogenic Shock) trial [34], in which the mean age of the study population was 70 years and 31% were >75 years of age, no interaction between age and treatment was observed regarding benefit in favor of culprit vessel PCI alone compared with multivessel PCI during the index procedure.

Currently there are insufficient trials to determine the best selection of elderly patients who might benefit from an invasive strategy after myocardial infarction with or without cardiogenic shock; however, although there is higher mortality in older patients, this should not discourage the strategy of emergency revascularization.

An additional analysis of the previously mentioned nationwide registry of primary angioplasty in the elderly was aimed to depict the characteristics and outcomes of the 332 patients in cardiogenic shock in order to derive a baseline risk prediction score for 1-year mortality [35]. Baseline independent predictors of mortality were anterior myocardial infarction (HR 2.8, 95%CI, 1.4–6.0; $p = 0.005$), ejection fraction<40% (HR 2.3, 95%CI, 1.14–4.50; $p = 0.018$), and time from symptom onset to angioplasty >6 h (HR 3.2, 95%CI, 1.6–7.5; $p = 0.001$). A score was designed that included these predictive factors (score "6-ANT-40"). Survival at 1 year was 54.5% for patients with score 0, 32.3% for score 1, 27.4% for score 2, and 17% for score 3 ($p = 0.004$, c-statistic 0.70). The score was validated in an independent cohort of 124 patients.

5.11 In Summary

Society is aging, life expectancy is increasing, and more patients are surviving acute cardiac events, so chronic comorbidities are common. The incidence of ischemic heart disease is high and so is the need for PCI procedures. Older patients are at greater risk for these procedures, mainly because of comorbidities and frailty rather than because of age itself. Several scores are available to estimate the risk of PCI in these contexts. It is also important to estimate bleeding risk. In general, patients cannot be ruled out for PCI procedures due to age, even in the setting of infarction or shock, but individualization is necessary. We have multiple techniques to help optimize PCI and make it safer, and we must adjust antithrombotic therapies according to the balance of bleeding and ischemic risks. Initiatives such as this book are very relevant to help to better manage these complex but highly valuable patients.

Conflicts of Interest Jose M de la Torre Hernandez: Receipt of grants/research supports: Boston Scientific, Abbott Vascular, Biotronik. Receipt of honoraria or consultation fees: Boston Scientific, Medtronic, Biotronik, Abbott.

References

1. Nanna MG, Sutton NR, Kochar A, et al. Assessment and management of older adults undergoing PCI, Part 1: A JACC: Advances Expert Panel. JACC Adv. 2023;2(4):100389.
2. Nanna MG, Sutton NR, Kochar A, et al. A geriatric approach to percutaneous coronary interventions in older adults, Part II: A JACC: Advances Expert Panel. JACC Adv. 2023;2(5):100421.
3. Damluji AA, Forman DE, Wang TY, et al. Management of acute coronary syndrome in the older adult population: a scientific statement from the American Heart Association. Circulation. 2023;147(3):e32–62.
4. Shanmugam VB, Harper R, Meredith I, Malaiapan Y, Psaltis PJ. An overview of PCI in the very elderly. J Geriatr Cardiol. 2015;12(2):174–84.
5. Eagle KA, Lim MJ, Dabbous OH, Pieper KS, Goldberg RJ, van de Werf F, et al. A validated prediction model for all forms of acute coronary syndrome: estimating the risk of 6-month postdischarge death in an international registry. GRACE Investigat JAMA. 2004;291:2727–33.
6. Antman EM, Cohen M, Bernink PJ, McCabe CH, Horacek T, Papuchis G, Mautner B, Corbalan R, Radley D, Braunwald E. The TIMI risk score for unstable angina/non-ST elevation MI: a method for prognostication and therapeutic decision making. JAMA. 2000;284(7):835–42.
7. Alexander KP, Chen AY, Newby LK, et al. Sex differences in major bleeding with glycoprotein IIb/IIIa inhibitors: results from the CRUSADE (Can Rapid risk stratification of Unstable angina patients Suppress ADverse outcomes with Early implementation of the ACC/AHA guidelines) initiative. Circulation. 2006;114(13):1380–7.
8. De la Torre Hernandez JM, Palop RL, Jimenez Mazuecos JM, et al. Prospective application of a bleeding and ischemic risks-adjusted antithrombotic protocol in elderly patients revascularized with everolimus-eluting stents: EPIC05-Sierra75 study. J Geriatr Cardiol. 2022;19(5):354–66.
9. Ariza-Solé A, Formiga F, Lorente V, et al. Efficacy of bleeding risk scores in elderly patients with acute coronary syndromes. Rev Esp Cardiol (Engl Ed). 2014;67(6):463–70.
10. Riobóo-Lestón L, Raposeiras-Roubin S, Abu-Assi E, Iñiguez-Romo A. Bleeding risk assessment in elderly patients with acute coronary syndrome. J Geriatr Cardiol. 2019;16(2):145–50.
11. Urban P, Mehran R, Colleran R, et al. Defining high bleeding risk in patients undergoing percutaneous coronary intervention: a consensus document from the Academic Research Consortium for High Bleeding Risk. Eur Heart J. 2019;40(31):2632–53.
12. Aïdoud A, Gana W, Poitau F, et al. High prevalence of geriatric conditions among older adults with cardiovascular disease. J Am Heart Assoc. 2023;12(2):e026850.
13. Morley JE, Malmstrom TK, Miller DK. A simple frailty questionnaire (FRAIL) predicts outcomes in middle aged African Americans. J Nutr Health Aging. 2012;16(7):601–8.
14. Marschall A, Martí Sánchez D, Ferreiro JL, et al. Outcomes prediction in complex high-risk indicated percutaneous coronary interventions in the older patients. Am J Cardiol. 2023;205:465–72.
15. Cantor WJ, Mehta SR, Yuan F, et al. Radial versus femoral access for elderly patients with acute coronary syndrome undergoing coronary angiography and intervention: insights from the RIVAL trial. Am Heart J. 2015;170(5):880–6.
16. Achenbach S, Ropers D, Kallert L, et al. Transradial versus transfemoral approach for coronary angiography and intervention in patients above 75 years of age. Catheter Cardiovasc Interv. 2008;72(5):629–35.
17. Jolly SS, AlRashidi S, d'Entremont MA, et al. Routine ultrasonography guidance for femoral vascular access for cardiac procedures: The UNIVERSAL Randomized Clinical Trial. JAMA Cardiol. 2022;7(11):1110–8.
18. Kreutz RP, Phookan S, et al. Femoral artery closure devices vs manual compression during cardiac catheterization and percutaneous coronary intervention. J Soc Cardiovasc Angiogr Intervent. 2022;1(5):100370.
19. De Belder A, de la Torre Hernandez JM, Lopez-Palop R, et al. A prospective randomized trial of everolimus-

eluting stents versus bare-metal stents in octogenarians: the XIMA Trial (Xience or Vision Stents for the Management of Angina in the Elderly). J Am Coll Cardiol. 2014;63(14):1371–5.
20. Varenne O, Cook S, Sideris G, et al. Drug-eluting stents in elderly patients with coronary artery disease (SENIOR): a randomised single-blind trial. Lancet. 2018;391(10115):41–50.
21. Sella G, Gandelman G, Tuvali O, et al. Utilization of drug-coated balloons for the treatment of coronary lesions in the elderly population. J Clin Med. 2022;11(9):2616.
22. Cortese B, Serruys PW. Single-antiplatelet treatment after coronary angioplasty with drug-coated balloon. J Am Heart Assoc. 2023;12(6):e028413.
23. Hennessey B, Pareek N, Macaya F, et al. Contemporary percutaneous management of coronary calcification: current status and future directions. Open Heart. 2023;10(1):e002182.
24. Takahashi K, Serruys PW, Gao C, et al. Ten-year all-cause death according to completeness of revascularization in patients with three-vessel disease or left main coronary artery disease: insights from the SYNTAX extended survival study. Circulation. 2021;144(2):96–109.
25. De la Torre Hernandez JM, Garcia Camarero T, Baz Alonso JA, et al. Outcomes of predefined optimisation criteria for intravascular ultrasound guidance of left main stenting. EuroIntervention. 2020;16(3):210–7.
26. Carmona-Segovia ADM, Doncel-Abad MV, Becerra-Muñoz VM, et al. Prognostic stratification of older patients with multivessel coronary artery disease treated with percutaneous transluminal coronary angioplasty based on clinical and biochemical measures: protocol for a prospective cohort study. BMJ Open. 2022;12(2):e058042.
27. Biscaglia S, Guiducci V, Escaned J, et al. Complete or culprit-only PCI in older patients with myocardial infarction. N Engl J Med. 2023;389(10):889–98.
28. Savonitto S, Cavallini C, Petronio AS, et al. Early aggressive versus initially conservative treatment in elderly patients with non-ST-segment elevation acute coronary syndrome: a randomized controlled trial. JACC Cardiovasc Interv. 2012;5(9):906–16.
29. Sanchis J, Bueno H, Miñana G, et al. Effect of routine invasive vs conservative strategy in older adults with frailty and non-ST-segment elevation acute myocardial infarction: a randomized clinical trial. JAMA Intern Med. 2023;183(5):407–15.
30. Kumar S, McDaniel M, Samady H, Forouzandeh F. Contemporary revascularization dilemmas in older adults. J Am Heart Assoc. 2020;9(3):e014477.
31. De la Torre Hernández JM, Brugaletta S, Gómez Hospital JA, et al. Primary angioplasty in patients older than 75 years. Profile of patients and procedures, outcomes, and predictors of prognosis in the ESTROFA IM+75 Registry. Rev Esp Cardiol (Engl Ed). 2017;70(2):81–7.
32. De La Torre Hernandez JM, Gomez Hospital JA, Baz JA, et al. Multivessel disease in patients over 75 years old with ST elevated myocardial infarction. Current management strategies and related clinical outcomes in the ESTROFA MI+75 nation-wide registry. Cardiovasc Revasc Med. 2018;19(5 Pt B):580–8.
33. Hochman JS, Sleeper LA, Godfrey E, et al. SHould we emergently revascularize Occluded Coronaries for cardiogenic shocK: an international randomized trial of emergency PTCA/CABG-trial design. The SHOCK Trial Study Group. Am Heart J. 1999;137(2):313–21.
34. Thiele H, Akin I, Sandri M, et al. PCI strategies in patients with acute myocardial infarction and cardiogenic shock. N Engl J Med. 2017;377(25):2419–32.
35. De la Torre Hernández JM, Brugaletta S, Gómez Hospital JA, et al. Baseline risk stratification of patients older than 75 years with infarction and cardiogenic shock undergoing primary angioplasty. Rev Esp Cardiol (Engl Ed). 2019;72(12):1005–11.

Revascularisation Strategies in Frail Patients

6

Gregory B. Mills, Graziella Pompei, Francesca Rubino, and Vijay Kunadian

6.1 Frailty and Cardiovascular Disease

Discrete from chronological age, frailty is 'a state of increased vulnerability to poor resolution of homeostasis following stress' [1]. Frailty is common in the community population of older people (~13%) but is much more prevalent in those with cardiovascular disease [2, 3]. Moreover, frailty is significantly less frequent in men than in women in NSTEACS patients aged 80 years and older [4]. The evaluation of frailty and comorbidity in older patients with acute coronary syndromes (ACS) is emphasised by scientific guidelines from the European Society of Cardiology (ESC) and the American Heart Association (AHA) [5, 6]. Information on frailty is crucial to guide the treatment choice and improves the discriminating ability of risk scores based on cardiovascular parameters [7].

Despite numerous frailty assessment scales—relying on either a phenotype definition or physician-judged cumulative deficit models—there remains no consensus on the optimal evaluation of frailty in older patients with cardiovascular disease [2, 8, 9]. The relationship between frailty and cardiovascular disease is bidirectional—they share common risk factors and biochemical mechanisms such as low-grade inflammation [10]. Frailty and pre-frailty have been associated with a greater chance of suffering from cardiovascular disease. In particular, frailty resulted to be associated with an increased risk of ischaemic heart disease (IHD), heart failure (HF) and risk of cardiovascular mortality, whereas prefrailty carried a higher risk of HF and cardiovascular mortality [11]. Patients living with cardiovascular disease and frailty may also present with other 'geriatric syndromes' such as multimorbidity, cognitive impairment, polypharmacy and decline in functional status as measured by health-related quality of life or needing assistance with activi-

G. B. Mills · V. Kunadian (✉)
Translational and Clinical Research Institute, Faculty of Medical Sciences, Newcastle University, Newcastle upon Tyne, UK

Cardiothoracic Centre, Royal Victoria Infirmary/Freeman Hospital, Newcastle upon Tyne Hospitals NHS Foundation Trust, Newcastle upon Tyne, UK
e-mail: vijay.kunadian@newcastle.ac.uk

G. Pompei
Translational and Clinical Research Institute, Faculty of Medical Sciences, Newcastle University, Newcastle upon Tyne, UK

Cardiovascular Institute, Azienda Ospedaliero-Universitaria di Ferrara, Cona, FE, Italy

F. Rubino
Translational and Clinical Research Institute, Faculty of Medical Sciences, Newcastle University, Newcastle upon Tyne, UK

Division of Cardiology, Department of Medicine, University of Verona, Verona, Italy

B. Cortese, S. Rigattieri (eds.), *High Bleeding Risk Patients in Interventional Cardiology*,
https://doi.org/10.1007/978-3-031-87302-7_6

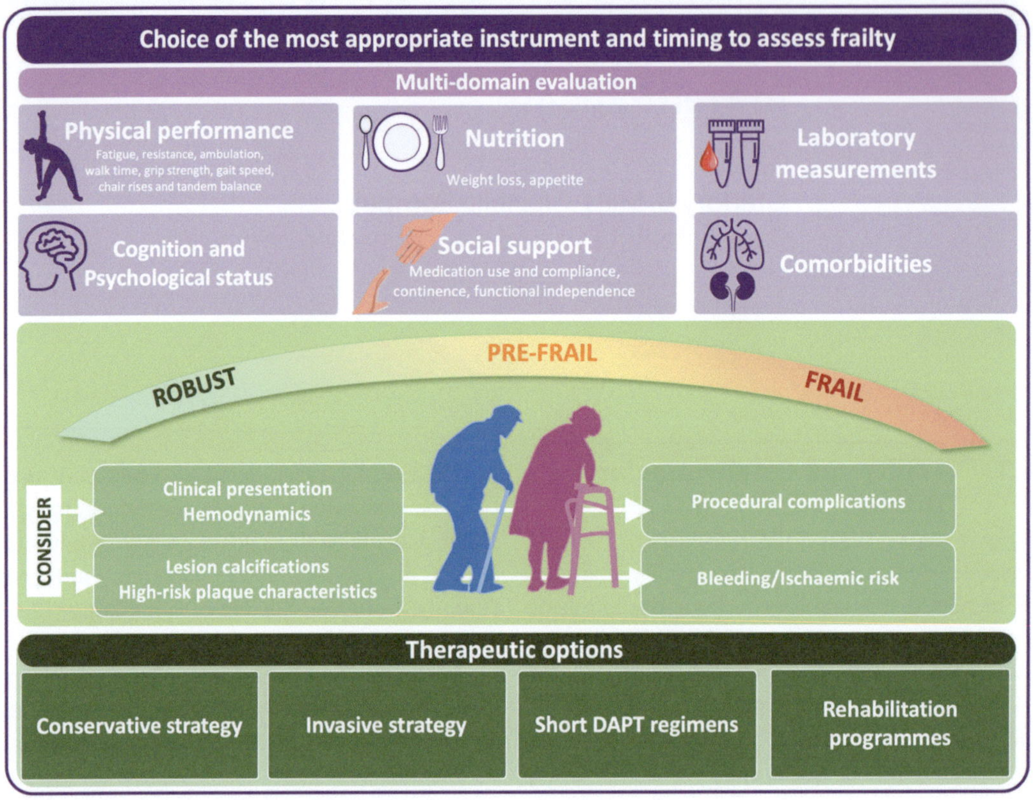

Fig. 6.1 A tailored and integrated (multispecialty and multidisciplinary) approach in frail older patients living with cardiovascular disease is crucial for decision-making regarding optimising management plans

ties of daily living [12]. This complexity requires both an individualised and integrated (multispecialty and multidisciplinary) approach to decision-making regarding optimising management plans (Fig. 6.1).

6.2 Frailty and Acute Coronary Syndrome

Older patients are more likely to present with either non-ST-elevation myocardial infarction (NSTEMI) or unstable angina—grouped as non-ST-elevation acute coronary syndrome (NSTEACS)—than ST-elevation myocardial infarction (STEMI) [13]. The clinical characteristics of this patient group are heterogenous, such that frailty may be a better prognostic indicator of adverse outcomes after ACS compared to chronological age [14, 15]. Frailty score assessment at the time of myocardial infarction (MI) predicts mortality and hospitalisations over subsequent years of follow-up. Re-evaluating frailty over time has been demonstrated to be a reliable tool providing the possibility to define a frailty trajectory, a superior predictor of mortality compared to baseline frailty and with a high discriminatory power in predicting death beyond classic predictors [16]. Frail patients are less likely to receive evidence-based medications and coronary angiography too [17, 18].

Frailty is associated with a greater risk of mortality and ischaemic events (reinfarction or stroke) after ACS [19–21]. This specifically includes in-hospital mortality and all-cause death at 1 year after STEMI [22, 23]. The risk of a composite of major adverse cardiovascular events (MACE) is greatest in frail older patients with NSTEACS, driven by higher rates of all-cause mortality and reinfarction. The study to Improve Clinical

Outcomes in high-risk patients with ACS (ICON-1) is a multicentre, observational, prospective cohort study providing evidence regarding risk stratification factors in older frail ACS patients undergoing invasive care. An analysis performed by Batty et al. led to the development of a novel risk score based on a significant association between the Fried frailty classification, age, systolic blood pressure and raised Killip class on admission, history of peripheral vascular disease and problems dressing self with 1-year primary outcome (a composite of all-cause mortality, MI, stroke, unplanned revascularisation and major bleeding), outperforming the GRACE 2 score [24]. The association between frailty and the abovementioned composite outcomes persisted for at least 5 years after the index event even after adjustment for age and sex, demonstrating that biological age has a more relevant influence on prognosis for older people with NSTEACS than chronological age alone [25]. Given the impact of frailty on adverse outcomes after ACS, the assessment of frailty can support benefit-risk decision-making in older patients. Studies reporting association between frailty assessment in older ACS patients and clinical outcomes are listed in Table 6.1.

Table 6.1 Studies reporting correlation between frailty and clinical outcomes in ACS patients

Study	Patients (*n*)	Age (years)	Frailty score	Results
Ekerstad et al. (2011) [74]	307	≥75	CSHA	Frailty strongly and independently associated with the following:
			CFS	Primary composite EP (death from any cause, MI, revascularisation due to ischemia, hospitalisation for any cause, major bleeding, stroke/TIA and the need for dialysis up to 1 month after inclusion) (OR, 2.2; 95% CI, 1.3–3.7)
				In-hospital mortality (OR, 4.6; 95% CI, 1.3–16.8)
				1-month mortality (OR, 4.7; 95% CI, 1.7–13.0)
Myers et al. (2014) [16]	1521	≤65	Rockwood Frailty Index	Baseline frailty positively associated with mortality
		Re-assessed		Unadjusted HR for mortality = 4.14 (95% CI 3.07–5.59) for the frailest compared to the least frail group
		10–13 years after MI		The frailest patients more than twice as likely to be hospitalised during follow-up compared to the least frail (adjusted rate ratio 2.14, 95% CI 1.63–2.81)
Sanchis et al. (2014) [75]	342	≥65	Fried criteria	Frailty using the Green score had the strongest discriminative accuracy (area under the receiver operating characteristic curve 0.76 for mortality)
			Green score	A Green score ≥5 points was the strongest mortality predictor
				The incremental predictive information was greater over the GRACE score
Alonso Salinas et al. (2016) [76]	190	≥75	SHARE-FI	Frailty predicted major bleeding during 30-day follow-up
				Frailty showed a trend to correlation, not statistically significant, with mortality, reinfarction or stroke rates on univariate analysis
Alegre et al. (2017) [20]	532	≥80	FRAIL scale	Higher all-cause mortality rate for both pre-frailty and frailty groups at 6 months compared with patients without frailty criteria ($p < 0.001$)
				Higher incidence of mortality or readmission at 6 months in prefrail and frail patients ($p < 0.001$)
Blanco et al. (2017) [77]	236	≥80	EFS	Frailty significantly and independently associated with a significant increase in the risk of all-cause death
				EFS score of 4–6 ➔ HR 1.59 (95% CI, 0.78–3.26; P 1/4 0.20)
				EFS score ≥7 ➔ HR 4.03 (95% CI, 2.02–8.04; $p < 0.001$)

(continued)

Table 6.1 (continued)

Study	Patients (n)	Age (years)	Frailty score	Results
Ekerstad et al. (2018) [7]	307	≥75	CSHA CFS	Higher long-term all-cause mortality (median 6.7 years) amongst frail patients than non-frail patients ($p < 0.001$)
				In Cox regression analysis, frailty independently associated with mortality from the index hospital admission to the end of follow-up (HR 2.06, 95%CI 1.51–2.81; $p < 0.001$) together with age ($p < 0.001$), EF (P 1/4 0.012) and Charlson comorbidity index (P 1/4 0.018)
Batty et al. (2019) [24]	279	≥75	Fried criteria	Significant difference in the primary EP (composite of all-cause mortality, MI, stroke, unplanned revascularisation and major bleeding) at 1 year in the three frailty groups (robust 18.0%, pre-frail 27.5% and frail 39%; $p = 0.03$; HR for frail vs robust: 2.79, 95% CI 1.28–6.08)
Gu et al. (2019) [49]	90	≥75	Fried criteria	Compared to robust patients, significantly greater presence of high-risk lesions (VH TCFA ($p = 0.011$), MLA ≤ 4 mm² ($p = 0.016$), TCFA + MLA ≤ 4 mm² ($p = 0.005$), TCFA + PB ≥ 70% ($p = 0.005$) and TCFA + PB ≥ 70% + MLA ≤ 4 mm² ($p = 0.003$)) in pre-frail group
				By age- and sex-adjusted logistic regression analysis, frailty strongly and independently associated with the presence of TCFA (OR 2.81, 95% CI:1.06–7.48, $p = 0.039$)
Ratcovich et al. (2022) [25]	263	≥75	CSHA CFS	Higher composite EP (all-cause mortality, unplanned revascularisation, MI, stroke, bleeding) at 5 y amongst frail patients according to CFS (frail: 22, 66.7%; pre-frail: 81, 53.3%; robust: 27, 34.6%, $p = 0.003$)
			Fried criteria	Similar trend with Fried criteria (frail: 55.7%; pre-frail: 49.0%; robust: 34.8%, $p = 0.085$)
				Frailty measured with both criteria associated with the primary EP (age and sex-adjusted HR) compared with robust groups. CFS: 2.22, 95% CI 1.23–4.02, $p = 0.008$; Fried: HR 1.81, 95% CI 1.00–3.27, $p = 0.048$
Beska et al. (2023) [50]	271	≥75	Fried criteria	Compared with robust patients, more severe CL calcification in frail patients (OR 5.40; 95% CI (1.75–16.8); $p = 0.03$)
				Smaller mean improvement in post-PCI CL stenosis in frail patients (50.6%; 95% CI (45.7–55.6)) than robust patients (58.6%; 95% CI (53.5–63.7); $p = 0.042$)

Abbreviations: *CSHA CFS* Canadian Study of Health and Aging Clinical Frailty Scale, *EP* endpoint, *MI* myocardial infarction, *TIA* transient ischemic attack, *OR* odds ratio, *CI* confidence interval, *SHARE-FI* Survey of Health, Ageing and Retirement in Europe—Frailty Index, *EFS* Edmonton Frail scale, *HR* hazard ratio, *HF* ejection fraction, *CL* culprit lesion, *PCI* percutaneous coronary intervention

6.3 Instruments to Measure Frailty in Acute Coronary Syndromes

Frailty is influenced by several variables, and its definition encompasses multiple domains of human functioning. This reflects the mutability of frailty over time and emphasizes that physical, psychological and social factors are part of a complex dynamic system. There is ample availability of frailty risk scores developed in recent years and taking into account several factors, such as nutritional status, physical activity mobility, energy, strength, psychological aspect, social relations/support and cognition. Table 6.2 provides a list of the main available frailty scales to assess older ACS patients. The choice of a particular instrument is dependent on the set-

Table 6.2 Frailty scales in ACS patients

Instrument	Brief description	Score assessment	Physical performance assessment
FRAIL scale	Interview-based tool evaluating five items (fatigue, resistance, ambulation, concomitant diseases, weight loss)	Pre-frailty (<3 criteria) Frailty (≥3 criteria)	No
Rockwood Frailty Index or Deficit Accumulation Index (DAI)	Evaluation based on 32 different variables about symptoms, signs, disabilities, diseases and laboratory measurements	Final point with a threshold of 0.25 defining frailty	No
Clinical Frailty Scale	A judgement-based frailty tool evaluating specific domains including comorbidity, function and cognition	Nine frailty levels ranging from 1 (very fit) to 9 (terminally ill)	No
Fried criteria	Five criteria: unintentional weight loss>4.5 kg in the past year, exhaustion, physical activity, walk time and grip strength	Frailty is defined by the presence of three or more criteria	Yes
SHARE- FI	Standardised questionnaire addressing exhaustion, appetite, physical activity, ambulation, resistance and grip strength	Score results in a continuous measure, and accordingly, patients are classified in three groups: frail, pre-frail and non-frail	Yes
Edmonton Frail Scale	Questions and tasks about nutrition, symptoms, mood and physical performance	It ranges from 0 (not frail) to 17 (very frail)	Yes
Reported Edmonton Frail Scale	Self-reported questionnaire including nine domains: cognition, general health status, functional independence, social support, medication use, nutrition, mood, continence and functional performance	Frailty is identified by a score of at least 8	No
Green score	Scale of four items (physical activity, serum albumin, gait speed, grip strength)	Ranging from 0 to 12	Yes
Tilburg Frailty Indicator	Questionnaire consisting of two parts Part A: 10 questions on frailty determinants (age, sex, marital status, education level, social circumstances, lifestyle) Part B: 15 frailty elements across 3 domains: physical, psychological and social	Each item in Part B scores 1 point. Patients are considered frail if they score at least 5 of a possible 15	No
SPPB	Three timed physical performance tests, including gait speed, chair rises and tandem balance	Each test is scored from 0 to 4, with a total score ≤5 (of a possible 12) indicating frailty	Yes

Abbreviations: *SHARE-FI* Survey of Health, Ageing and Retirement in Europe—Frailty Index, *SPPB* short physical performance battery

ting, the aim of the measurement, the qualities of the person who administers the instrument, and available time [26]. Some of them can be calculated at the hospital admission. Conversely, other tests and scales can be performed only after mobilisation due to the necessity of objectivation of the physical performance. Therefore, these are ideal to assess patients before the discharge [27].

The physical frailty phenotype, also called Fried's frailty scale, is the most frequently used instrument. Fried's scale accurately predicts mortality in patients with CVD and, according to a systematic review, it seems to be the most suitable instrument to be used as an evaluative outcome measure in frailty research [26]. However, Fried criteria are not readily measurable in acute clinical situations because they encompass a walking test, grip strength measurement and a detailed quality of life questionnaire [9]. Therefore, the clinimetric properties of this and other indexes need to be explored far more extensively.

6.3.1 The Impact of Physical Performance

A limitation in physical functioning alone seems to be associated with important clinical outcomes. Newman et al. used an extended walking test (400 m) to evaluate frailty in 3075 community-dwelling adults. Compared with the quartile with the fastest walk time, the quartile with the slowest walk time had a significantly higher adjusted risk of mortality (HR 3.23; 95%CI (2.11–4.94)) and cardiovascular disease (HR 1.61; 95% CI (1.05–2.45)) [28]. Similarly, cardiovascular events in STEMI patients undergoing percutaneous coronary intervention (PCI) can be predicted using gait speed (HR for 0.1 m/s increase in gait speed: 0.71). This shows the variety of available frailty tools that can be administered to predict worse outcomes in ACS patients and those undergoing invasive interventions [29]. The Short Physical Performance Battery (SPPB) is an instrument measuring three timed physical performance tests, and it is relatively simple, cheap and takes a few minutes to complete. However, in acute settings, it may be difficult to assess it. Recent evidence showed that SPPB test before hospital discharge increases the ability to predict adverse events in older ACS patients. Therefore, it may be useful in the clinical decision-making process [9]. Campo et al. measured the risk of major adverse cardiovascular and cerebrovascular events (MACCE) and all-cause mortality at 1 year in a comparison study of seven frailty scales for patients admitted for ACS (33% STEMI, 45% NSTEMI, 22% unstable angina). The SPPB, Edmonton Frail Scale (EFS) and Fried criteria were associated with all-cause mortality, but the SPPB resulted to be the best predictor for MACCE (ΔC-statistic: 0.043) and all-cause mortality (ΔC-statistic: 0.063). The addition of SPPB scale on top of TIMI or GRACE risk scores led to a considerable improvement in MACCE and all-cause mortality prediction (about 15% and 20%, respectively) [30]. The choice of the correct timing to evaluate frailty or physical performance is still debatable in an acute scenario. Both approaches (before an acute event or at the time of hospital discharge) show advantages and drawbacks, and there is lack of evidence reporting a direct comparison.

6.4 Frailty and Bleeding

Older patients with ACS are at increased risk of both thrombotic and bleeding events [31, 32]. However, in the era of contemporary clinical practice following procedural and pharmacological advances—such as radial access, modern dual antiplatelet therapy strategies and drug-eluting stents—bleeding risk is reduced in older patients [33–35]. Current bleeding risk scores account for chronological age but do not consider the heterogeneity in the older patient population such as frailty status. Frail patients with ACS have higher rates of bleeding independent of age and despite less frequent use of antiplatelet therapy [36]. Furthermore, major bleeding events are associated with all-cause mortality.

Small registries enrolling older patients with NSTEACS undergoing coronary angiography have demonstrated no association between frailty status and bleeding events up to 5 years post-discharge [24, 25]. Likewise, data from the randomised TRILOGY trial has shown no association between frailty status and bleeding events in patients with NSTEACS receiving medical management only [37].

However, large-scale studies have established more robust findings. A registry including over 7 million patients with ACS found significantly higher rates of bleeding events in frail patients irrespective of management strategy, whilst the risk of in-hospital bleeding complications, in comparison to patients without frailty, was at least doubled [38]. This finding has been replicated in other meta-analyses and recent retrospective studies enrolling older patients with ACS undergoing coronary angiography [19, 39].

Interestingly, frailty as measured by high Clinical Frailty Scale (CFS) score is associated with major bleeding up to 1 year after PCI, irrespective of patients fulfilling the criteria of numerous 'High Bleeding Risk' definitions [40].

6.5 Frailty and Revascularisation

Older patients living with frailty are less likely to receive coronary angiography, PCI or coronary artery bypass (CABG) surgery following acute myocardial infarction (AMI) [18]. Revascularisation is most often percutaneous in older patients, given the anaesthetic requirement, invasive nature and greater risk profile of major cardiac surgery. The risk of procedural complications such as contrast-induced nephropathy is greater in older patients due to the prevalence of comorbidities like chronic kidney disease (CKD) [41]. However, contemporary data shows that coronary angiography and PCI can be performed safely in this patient group, with very low rates of bleeding events [42]. There is no difference in rates of procedural complications or in-hospital adverse outcomes between frail and robust patients with NSTEACS.

6.5.1 Angiographic Features

Left anterior descending (LAD) artery involvement and multi-vessel coronary artery disease (CAD) are more common with increasing age [43]. Older patients also have more severe coronary artery calcification [44]. This is associated with common comorbidities in this patient group, such as diabetes and CKD [45, 46]. Patients with more severe coronary artery calcification experience significantly higher 10-year rates of all-cause mortality, reinfarction and target lesion revascularisation (TLR) independent of age or the type of stent deployed [47]. Given these characteristics, high-risk lesions are frequently encountered in clinical practice when older patients with ACS undergo coronary angiography.

Optical coherence tomography (OCT) shows that frail patients undergoing PCI have vulnerable plaque characteristics such as more lipid-rich plaque and thin-cap fibroatheroma (TCFA), in comparison to robust patients, despite lower body mass index and serum lipid/triglyceride levels [48]. A previously published analysis of the ICON1 study cohort had already shown a greater presence of high-risk lesions phenotypes—including TCFA and significant plaque burden—detected by virtual histology intravascular ultrasound (VH-IVUS) imaging in non-robust NSTEACS patients regardless of age [49]. Compared to robust patients, older frail patients with NSTEACS have significantly higher baseline SYNTAX scores—indicating more complex CAD—associated with adverse outcomes at 5 years, and are five times more likely to have severe culprit lesion calcification, independent of age [50].

6.5.2 Coronary Revascularisation Guided by Functional Assessment

Myocardial revascularisation of intermediate coronary stenosis based on fractional flow reserve (FFR) and instantaneous wave-free-ratio (iFR) is strongly recommended by the international guidelines [51, 52]. Large randomised controlled trials demonstrated the superiority of FFR-guided PCI versus the standard angiography-based approach and the non-inferiority of iFR over FFR. However, older patients were underrepresented in these trials and growing results suggested that the findings obtained in the young population were not totally applicable to the older one. Regarding the coronary functional assessment in the frailty patients, there is a total gap in the evidence.

A sub-study of the Fractional Flow Reserve Versus Angiography for Multivessel Evaluation (FAME) trial highlighted that older patients tended to have a higher mean value of FFR than younger patients considering the same angiographical stenosis category [53]. Indeed, increasing age correlated positively with FFR, but not with iFR [54].

FFR is defined as the ratio between the mean distal pressure (Pd) of a stenosis and the aortic pressure (Pa) during maximal hyperaemia inducted by vasodilating agents. iFR is defined as the trans-stenotic pressure ratio (Pd/Pa) during the wave-free period of the diastole when microvascular resistance in minimal. Non-adequate achievement of the maximal hyperaemia status might explain the minor proportion of functional significant stenosis (FFR $\leq$ 0.80) found in the older population compared to the younger one [53]. The aging process induces structural and functional changes in the vascular wall of the whole coronary circulation leading to endothelial dysfunction which reduces the hyperaemic response in older patients [55].

The coronary flow reserve (CFR) describes the capacity of increasing blood flow to the heart under physical or pharmacological stress. It considers the blood flow in the epicardial and microvascular circulation, and a CFR value $\geq$2 is defined as normal. It was demonstrated that CFR decreases with advancing age [56, 57]. On the other hand, the index of hyperaemic coronary microcirculatory resistance (IMR), which measures the resistance of microvascular circulation, increases with the age (normal value <25) [57]. A high value of IMR might explain the vasodilatory incompetence of the older patients.

These results suggest a possible overestimation of the FFR values and question the safety of deferring revascularisation based on FFR in older patients. However, the FAME trial sub-study did not find significant difference in the death, myocardial infarction and repeat revascularisation between patients older or younger than 65 years old who underwent FFR-guided PCI [53]. Analysing only the older patients deferred based on FFR, the findings of impaired CFR and iFR have been associated with adverse outcome compared to those with normal CFR and iFR [54, 57, 58].

Another mechanism influencing the FFR-iFR discordance might be the pattern of atherosclerotic disease [59]. Older adults tend to show diffuse disease and vessel calcification rather than focal lesions, which are associated with a larger trans-lesion pressure gradient during hyperaemia with abnormal FFR [54, 59, 60].

Therefore, in older patients, undergoing coronary physiology assessment might be useful to measure both FFR and iFR, performed easily with the same intracoronary pressure wire guide. A careful evaluation of the atherosclerotic pattern is fundamental to plan the appropriate management of CAD. In addition, evaluating the CFR in older patients, especially with normal value of FFR, might add an important prognostic value.

In the case of discordant values of FFR and iFR, the revascularisation strategy might be based on the iFR if abnormal (iFR < 0.90). Nevertheless, further evidence needed to support the hypothesis that non-hyperaemic index, as iFR, could guide the revascularisation strategy in this population. Additional studies are expected to improve the benefits of physiology-guided revascularisation in older patients particularly in frailty patients.

6.5.3 Percutaneous Coronary Intervention

Evidence is lacking regarding frailty status, characteristics from revascularisation and clinical outcomes. There is very limited data on the use of contemporary calcium-debulking techniques in older frail patients. One registry of older patients with NSTEACS has shown that regardless of more complex CAD and smaller mean improvements in culprit stenosis after PCI, compared to robust patients, there is no association between frailty status and achievement of complete revascularisation [50]. In an exploratory analysis, both baseline and post-PCI SYNTAX scores were associated with long-term MACE. Larger trials are needed to confirm that PCI is equally successful in robust and frail patients with ACS.

Given the prevalence of multi-vessel CAD and high-risk lesions in older patients with ACS, it has been hypothesised that a strategy of incomplete revascularisation targeting a single-culprit lesion may produce greater clinical benefits than an approach of complete revascularisation. In one study, although mortality rates were non-significantly higher in patients receiving incomplete revascularisation, there was no difference in long-term adverse outcomes between the two approaches [61]. However, a meta-analysis of registry data has demonstrated conflicting results, with complete revascularisation associated with lower rates of cardiac mortality and reinfarction in older patients [62]. Although these studies consistently demonstrate similar safety profiles and bleeding rates between culprit-only and complete revascularisation, the optimal approach to PCI in patients with frailty is yet to be investigated [63].

6.5.4 Clinical Benefit of Revascularisation

International treatment guidelines recognise the lack of consensus regarding the safety and effectiveness of invasive or conservative management strategies in frail older patients with ACS [5]. Given this paucity of evidence and recommendations [64], it is suggested that 'management decisions are based on the risks of procedural complications and clinical outcomes' (Fig. 6.2).

Of the few studies published, they suggest that the presence or absence of frailty affects any clinical benefit derived from an invasive approach. Robust data from randomised controlled trials often informs guideline recommendations, but such studies have historically had strict eligibility such that the frailest older patients were excluded. Registries better-reflect the heterogenous older population encountered in clinical practice today but can be limited by selection bias whereby the frailest patients are not referred for coronary angiography or PCI.

An observational study evaluated the occurrence of frailty and its association with quality of life (QoL) and clinical outcomes at a mean follow-up of 107 days in a population of older patients with CAD referred to hospital and undergoing different treatments strategy: PCI, CABG and medical therapy. The QoL score by Short Form-12 was divided into a physical composite score and a mental composite score. Although cardiovascular symptoms status and the mental composite score of QoL significantly improved (52.7 ± 11.5 at baseline vs 55.1 ± 10.6 at follow-up, $p = 0.04$), the overall frailty status did not significantly change, nor the physical health composite score of QoL (37.2 ± 11.0 at baseline vs 38.5 ± 11.3 at follow-up, $p = 0.27$) [65].

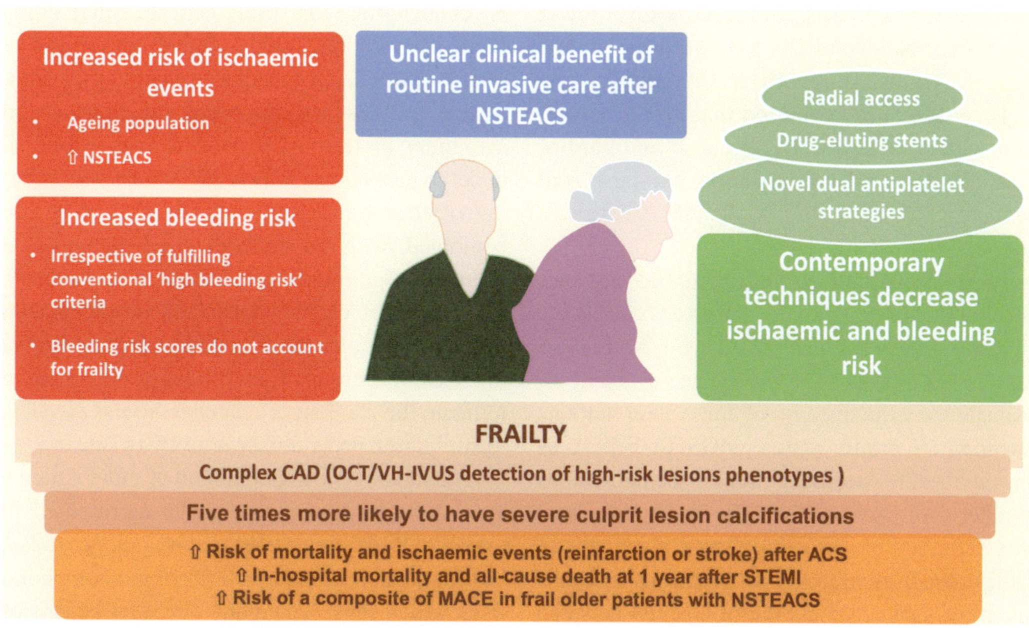

Fig. 6.2 Considerations in the revascularisation of older patients with acute coronary syndrome and frailty include baseline bleeding risk increased beyond chronological age and conventional 'high bleeding risk' criteria, the lack of clear clinical benefit of a routine invasive approach in this patient group and the application of contemporary interventional techniques which have decreased bleeding rates in older patients

Preliminary results from the *Impact of Frailty and Functional Status on Outcomes in Elderly Patients with ST-Segment Elevation Myocardial Infarction Undergoing Primary Angioplasty* (IFFANIAM) registry of older patients with STEMI managed by primary PCI have shown that the rate of in-hospital mortality is nearly four times higher in frail patients [66].

Based on registry data, the clinical benefit of PCI in frail older patients with NSTEACS is unclear and inconclusive. One observational study has demonstrated that the risk of a composite of adverse ischaemic events (cardiac death, reinfarction or urgent revascularisation) is reduced in non-frail patients managed by coronary angiography and PCI as opposed to conservative medical management [67]. However no such benefit was observed in frail patients, and the differential impact of frailty status on bleeding events was not assessed. Large-scale patient-level analysis has shown that frail patients still receive, albeit slightly reduced, reductions in in-hospital survival rates following PCI compared to medical management [18]. In another retrospective study, invasive management was associated with a lower mortality risk beyond 18 months irrespective of baseline frailty status [68]. Conversely, one registry study has suggested that PCI is associated with a reduction in all-cause and cardiovascular-cause rehospitalisation amongst frail patients, whilst no similar benefit is seen in non-frail patients [69].

Previous randomised controlled trials comparing a routine invasive strategy with a conservative medical strategy in older patients with NSTEACS have failed to assess the prevalence of frailty or evaluate the effectiveness of these interventions according to frailty status. MOSCA-FRAIL is the only trial to specifically report such outcomes in older frail patients [70]. There was no difference in the risk of ischaemic events (composite of cardiac death, reinfarction or urgent revascularisation) or days alive and out of hospital between the management strategies. Bleeding rates were higher in invasively managed patients, although this endpoint lacked statistical power and there were likely differences in adherence to dual-antiplatelet therapy between the groups. The results suggest an initially conservative approach may be appropriate in this patient group.

6.5.5 Measuring Benefits of Revascularisation

Studies enrolling older patients still evaluate endpoints with a predominantly clinical focus, such as mortality rates. Arguably, in patients with reduced life expectancy, frailty and multimorbidity, outcomes which better reflect patients' priorities and health goals may be more appropriate. Examples include health-related QoL, functional status and 'days alive and out of hospital'. It is frail patients with NSTEACS who have the proportionally largest improvements in health-related quality of life 1 year after PCI [71]. If replicated in larger-scale studies, as well as being significant for patients individually, this could have important implications for cost-effective evaluations.

Recovering from cardiovascular disease and adapting to changes in life after hospital discharge is challenging for frail patients undergoing PCI. The HULK study found a significant improvement in QoL indices (including psychological profiles and improved functional/social activities) in frail ACS patients randomised to undergo an exercise intervention strategy consisting of four supervised sessions after discharge combined with an individualised home-based exercise programme. Furthermore, the cumulative occurrence of cardiac death and hospitalisation for cardiovascular cause was significantly higher in the control group. These findings might help to mitigate the challenges related to access physical rehabilitation programmes after PCI [72].

The heterogenous population of older patients with ACS are historically under-represented in research. Reflecting contemporary practice today, frail patients have many elevated and competing risks which may negate any potential benefit of revascularisation—including the higher risk of adverse ischaemic events, higher risk of procedural complications and bleeding and higher risk of non-cardiovascular death related to other comorbidities. The benefits of revascularisation have typically been observed in patients with greatest baseline cardiovascular risk—however this is not evident in those with greatest non-cardiac comorbidity burden [73]. The British Heart Foundation SENIOR-RITA trial (NCT03052036) is comparing routine invasive and conservative medical approaches in older patients with NSTEACS. It is actively enrolling frail patients and will evaluate the impact of frailty status on procedural complications, angiographic analysis and clinical outcomes.

6.6 Summary

- Frail patients are at increased risk of death, ischaemic events and bleeding complications following acute coronary syndrome.
- Older patients with frailty are less likely to receive evidence-based medications, coronary angiography or revascularisation.
- Frailty is associated with high-risk angiographic characteristics.
- Robust trial data investigating interventional strategies in older patients with frailty is lacking. Hence there is a paucity of international guidelines for the optimal management of patients with acute coronary syndrome and frailty.

References

1. Clegg A, Young J, Iliffe S, Rikkert MO, Rockwood K. Frailty in elderly people. Lancet. 2013;381:752–62. https://doi.org/10.1016/s0140-6736(12)62167-9.
2. Fried LP, Tangen CM, Walston J, Newman AB, Hirsch C, Gottdiener J, Seeman T, Tracy R, Kop WJ, Burke G, et al. Frailty in older adults: evidence for a phenotype. J Gerontol A Biol Sci Med Sci. 2001;56:M146–56. https://doi.org/10.1093/gerona/56.3.m146.
3. Walker DM, Gale CP, Lip G, Martin-Sanchez FJ, McIntyre HF, Mueller C, Price S, Sanchis J, Vidan MT, Wilkinson C, et al. Editor's choice – frailty and the management of patients with acute cardiovascular disease: a position paper from the acute cardiovascular care association. Eur Heart J Acute Cardiovasc Care. 2018;7:176–93. https://doi.org/10.1177/2048872618758931.
4. Vicent L, Ariza-Sole A, Alegre O, Sanchis J, Lopez-Palop R, Formiga F, Gonzalez-Salvado V, Bueno H, Vidan MT, Diez-Villanueva P, et al. Octogenarian women with acute coronary syndrome present frailty and readmissions more frequently than men. Eur Heart J Acute Cardiovasc Care. 2019;8:252–63. https://doi.org/10.1177/2048872618798226.
5. Collet JP, Thiele H, Barbato E, Barthelemy O, Bauersachs J, Bhatt DL, Dendale P, Dorobantu M, Edvardsen T, Folliguet T, et al. 2020 ESC Guidelines for the management of acute coronary syndromes in patients presenting without persistent ST-segment elevation. Eur Heart J. 2021;42:1289–367. https://doi.org/10.1093/eurheartj/ehaa575.
6. Amsterdam EA, Wenger NK, Brindis RG, Casey DE Jr, Ganiats TG, Holmes DR Jr, Jaffe AS, Jneid H, Kelly RF, Kontos MC, et al. 2014 AHA/ACC guideline for the management of patients with non-ST-elevation acute coronary syndromes: a report of the American College of Cardiology/American Heart Association Task Force on Practice Guidelines. J Am Coll Cardiol. 2014;64:e139–228. https://doi.org/10.1016/j.jacc.2014.09.017.
7. Ekerstad N, Pettersson S, Alexander K, Andersson D, Eriksson S, Janzon M, Lindenberger M, Swahn E, Alfredsson J. Frailty as an instrument for evaluation of elderly patients with non-ST-segment elevation myocardial infarction: a follow-up after more than 5 years. Eur J Prev Cardiol. 2018;25:1813–21. https://doi.org/10.1177/2047487318799438.
8. Rockwood K, Song X, MacKnight C, Bergman H, Hogan DB, McDowell I, Mitnitski A. A global clinical measure of fitness and frailty in elderly people. CMAJ. 2005;173:489–95. https://doi.org/10.1503/cmaj.050051.
9. Chung K, Wilkinson C, Veerasamy M, Kunadian V. Frailty scores and their utility in older patients with cardiovascular disease. Interv Cardiol. 2021;16:e05. https://doi.org/10.15420/icr.2020.18.
10. Afilalo J. Frailty in patients with cardiovascular disease: why, when, and how to measure. Curr Cardiovasc Risk Rep. 2011;5:467–72. https://doi.org/10.1007/s12170-011-0186-0.
11. Veronese N, Cereda E, Stubbs B, Solmi M, Luchini C, Manzato E, Sergi G, Manu P, Harris T, Fontana L, et al. Risk of cardiovascular disease morbidity and mortality in frail and pre-frail older adults: results from a meta-analysis and exploratory meta-regression analysis. Ageing Res Rev. 2017;35:63–73. https://doi.org/10.1016/j.arr.2017.01.003.
12. Aïdoud A, Gana W, Poitau F, Debacq C, Leroy V, Nkodo JA, Poupin P, Angoulvant D, Fougère B. High prevalence of geriatric conditions among older adults with cardiovascular disease. J Am Heart Assoc. 2023;12:e026850. https://doi.org/10.1161/jaha.122.026850.
13. Gale CP, Cattle BA, Woolston A, Baxter PD, West TH, Simms AD, Blaxill J, Greenwood DC, Fox KA, West RM. Resolving inequalities in care? Reduced mortality in the elderly after acute coronary syndromes.

The Myocardial Ischaemia National Audit Project 2003–2010. Eur Heart J. 2012;33:630–9. https://doi.org/10.1093/eurheartj/ehr381.
14. Murali-Krishnan R, Iqbal J, Rowe R, Hatem E, Parviz Y, Richardson J, Sultan A, Gunn J. Impact of frailty on outcomes after percutaneous coronary intervention: a prospective cohort study. Open Heart. 2015;2:e000294. https://doi.org/10.1136/openhrt-2015-000294.
15. Sanchis J, Ruiz V, Bonanad C, Valero E, Ruescas-Nicolau MA, Ezzatvar Y, Sastre C, García-Blas S, Mollar A, Bertomeu-González V, et al. Prognostic value of geriatric conditions beyond age after acute coronary syndrome. Mayo Clin Proc. 2017;92:934–9. https://doi.org/10.1016/j.mayocp.2017.01.018.
16. Myers V, Drory Y, Gerber Y, Israel Study Group on First Acute Myocardial I. Clinical relevance of frailty trajectory post myocardial infarction. Eur J Prev Cardiol. 2014;21:758–66. https://doi.org/10.1177/2047487312462828.
17. Bebb O, Smith FG, Clegg A, Hall M, Gale CP. Frailty and acute coronary syndrome: A structured literature review. Eur Heart J Acute Cardiovasc Care. 2018;7:166–75. https://doi.org/10.1177/2048872617700873.
18. Damluji AA, Huang J, Bandeen-Roche K, Forman DE, Gerstenblith G, Moscucci M, Resar JR, Varadhan R, Walston JD, Segal JB. Frailty among older adults with acute myocardial infarction and outcomes from percutaneous coronary interventions. J Am Heart Assoc. 2019;8:e013686. https://doi.org/10.1161/jaha.119.013686.
19. Dou Q, Wang W, Wang H, Ma Y, Hai S, Lin X, Liu Y, Zhang X, Wu J, Dong B. Prognostic value of frailty in elderly patients with acute coronary syndrome: a systematic review and meta-analysis. BMC Geriatr. 2019;19:222. https://doi.org/10.1186/s12877-019-1242-8.
20. Alegre O, Formiga F, Lopez-Palop R, Marin F, Vidan MT, Martinez-Selles M, Carol A, Sionis A, Diez-Villanueva P, Aboal J, et al. An easy assessment of frailty at baseline independently predicts prognosis in very elderly patients with acute coronary syndromes. J Am Med Dir Assoc. 2018;19:296–303. https://doi.org/10.1016/j.jamda.2017.10.007.
21. Graham MM, Galbraith PD, O'Neill D, Rolfson DB, Dando C, Norris CM. Frailty and outcome in elderly patients with acute coronary syndrome. Can J Cardiol. 2013;29:1610–5. https://doi.org/10.1016/j.cjca.2013.08.016.
22. Calvo E, Teruel L, Rosenfeld L, Guerrero C, Romero M, Romaguera R, Izquierdo S, Asensio S, Andreu-Periz L, Gómez-Hospital JA, et al. Frailty in elderly patients undergoing primary percutaneous coronary intervention. Eur J Cardiovasc Nurs. 2019;18:132–9. https://doi.org/10.1177/1474515118796836.
23. Yoshioka N, Takagi K, Morita Y, Yoshida R, Nagai H, Kanzaki Y, Furui K, Yamauchi R, Komeyama S, Sugiyama H, et al. Impact of the clinical frailty scale on mid-term mortality in patients with ST-elevated myocardial infarction. Int J Cardiol Heart Vasc. 2019;22:192–8. https://doi.org/10.1016/j.ijcha.2019.02.014.
24. Batty J, Qiu W, Gu S, Sinclair H, Veerasamy M, Beska B, Neely D, Ford G, Kunadian V. One-year clinical outcomes in older patients with non-ST elevation acute coronary syndrome undergoing coronary angiography: an analysis of the ICON1 study. Int J Cardiol. 2019;274:45–51. https://doi.org/10.1016/j.ijcard.2018.09.086.
25. Ratcovich H, Beska B, Mills G, Holmvang L, Adams-Hall J, Stevenson H, Veerasamy M, Wilkinson C, Kunadian V. Five-year clinical outcomes in patients with frailty aged ≥75 years with non-ST elevation acute coronary syndrome undergoing invasive management. Eur Heart J Open. 2022;2:oeac035. https://doi.org/10.1093/ehjopen/oeac035.
26. de Vries NM, Staal JB, van Ravensberg CD, Hobbelen JS, Olde Rikkert MG, Nijhuis-van der Sanden MW. Outcome instruments to measure frailty: a systematic review. Ageing Res Rev. 2011;10:104–14. https://doi.org/10.1016/j.arr.2010.09.001.
27. Tonet E, Pavasini R, Biscaglia S, Campo G. Frailty in patients admitted to hospital for acute coronary syndrome: when, how and why? J Geriatr Cardiol. 2019;16:129–37. https://doi.org/10.11909/j.issn.1671-5411.2019.02.005.
28. Newman AB, Simonsick EM, Naydeck BL, Boudreau RM, Kritchevsky SB, Nevitt MC, Pahor M, Satterfield S, Brach JS, Studenski SA, et al. Association of long-distance corridor walk performance with mortality, cardiovascular disease, mobility limitation, and disability. JAMA. 2006;295:2018–26. https://doi.org/10.1001/jama.295.17.2018.
29. Matsuzawa Y, Konishi M, Akiyama E, Suzuki H, Nakayama N, Kiyokuni M, Sumita S, Ebina T, Kosuge M, Hibi K, et al. Association between gait speed as a measure of frailty and risk of cardiovascular events after myocardial infarction. J Am Coll Cardiol. 2013;61:1964–72. https://doi.org/10.1016/j.jacc.2013.02.020.
30. Campo G, Maietti E, Tonet E, Biscaglia S, Ariza-Sole A, Pavasini R, Tebaldi M, Cimaglia P, Bugani G, Serenelli M, et al. The assessment of scales of frailty and physical performance improves prediction of major adverse cardiac events in older adults with acute coronary syndrome. J Gerontol A Biol Sci Med Sci. 2020;75:1113–9. https://doi.org/10.1093/gerona/glz123.
31. Gharacholou SM, Becker RC. Hemostasis and thrombosis in older adults. J Thromb Thrombolysis. 2009;27:249–51. https://doi.org/10.1007/s11239-009-0308-4.
32. Hernández B, Fuentes E, Palomo I, Alarcón M. Increased platelet function during frailty. Exp Hematol. 2019;77:12–25.e12. https://doi.org/10.1016/j.exphem.2019.08.006.
33. Varenne O, Cook S, Sideris G, Kedev S, Cuisset T, Carrié D, Hovasse T, Garot P, El Mahmoud R, Spaulding C, et al. Drug-eluting stents in elderly

patients with coronary artery disease (SENIOR): a randomised single-blind trial. Lancet. 2018;391:41–50. https://doi.org/10.1016/s0140-6736(17)32713-7.
34. Valgimigli M, Gagnor A, Calabró P, Frigoli E, Leonardi S, Zaro T, Rubartelli P, Briguori C, Andò G, Repetto A, et al. Radial versus femoral access in patients with acute coronary syndromes undergoing invasive management: a randomised multicentre trial. Lancet. 2015;385:2465–76. https://doi.org/10.1016/s0140-6736(15)60292-6.
35. Valgimigli M, Frigoli E, Heg D, Tijssen J, Jüni P, Vranckx P, Ozaki Y, Morice MC, Chevalier B, Onuma Y, et al. Dual antiplatelet therapy after PCI in patients at high bleeding risk. N Engl J Med. 2021;385:1643–55. https://doi.org/10.1056/NEJMoa2108749.
36. Alonso Salinas GL, Sanmartín Fernández M, Pascual Izco M, Marco del Castillo Á, Rincón Díaz LM, Lozano Granero C, Valverde Gómez M, Pastor Pueyo P, del Val MD, Pardo Sanz A, et al. Frailty predicts major bleeding within 30days in elderly patients with Acute Coronary Syndrome. Int J Cardiol. 2016;222:590–3. https://doi.org/10.1016/j.ijcard.2016.07.268.
37. White HD, Westerhout CM, Alexander KP, Roe MT, Winters KJ, Cyr DD, Fox KA, Prabhakaran D, Hochman JS, Armstrong PW, et al. Frailty is associated with worse outcomes in non-ST-segment elevation acute coronary syndromes: insights from the TaRgeted platelet Inhibition to cLarify the Optimal strateGy to medicallY manage Acute Coronary Syndromes (TRILOGY ACS) trial. Eur Heart J Acute Cardiovasc Care. 2016;5:231–42. https://doi.org/10.1177/2048872615581502.
38. Kwok CS, Lundberg G, Al-Faleh H, Sirker A, Van Spall HGC, Michos ED, Rashid M, Mohamed M, Bagur R, Mamas MA. Relation of frailty to outcomes in patients with acute coronary syndromes. Am J Cardiol. 2019;124:1002–11. https://doi.org/10.1016/j.amjcard.2019.07.003.
39. Dodson JA, Hochman JS, Roe MT, Chen AY, Chaudhry SI, Katz S, Zhong H, Radford MJ, Udell JA, Bagai A, et al. The association of frailty with in-hospital bleeding among older adults with acute myocardial infarction: insights from the ACTION Registry. JACC Cardiovasc Interv. 2018;11:2287–96. https://doi.org/10.1016/j.jcin.2018.08.028.
40. Kanenawa K, Yamaji K, Tashiro H, Morimoto T, Hiromasa T, Hayashi M, Hiramori S, Tomoi Y, Kuramitsu S, Domei T, et al. Frailty and bleeding after percutaneous coronary intervention. Am J Cardiol. 2021;148:22–9. https://doi.org/10.1016/j.amjcard.2021.02.041.
41. Madhavan MV, Gersh BJ, Alexander KP, Granger CB, Stone GW. Coronary artery disease in patients ≥80 years of age. J Am Coll Cardiol. 2018;71:2015–40. https://doi.org/10.1016/j.jacc.2017.12.068.
42. Tegn N, Eek C, Abdelnoor M, Aaberge L, Endresen K, Skårdal R, Berg ES, Gullestad L, Bendz B. Patients aged 80 years or older with non-ST-elevation myocardial infarction or unstable angina pectoris randomised to an invasive versus conservative strategy: angiographic and procedural results from the After Eighty study. Open Heart. 2020;7:7. https://doi.org/10.1136/openhrt-2020-001256.
43. Mahjoob MP, Sadeghi S, Khanaman HF, Naderian M, Khaheshi I. Comparison of coronary risk factors and angiographic findings in younger and older patients with significant coronary artery disease. Rom J Intern Med. 2018;56:90–5. https://doi.org/10.1515/rjim-2017-0048.
44. Généreux P, Madhavan MV, Mintz GS, Maehara A, Palmerini T, Lasalle L, Xu K, McAndrew T, Kirtane A, Lansky AJ, et al. Ischemic outcomes after coronary intervention of calcified vessels in acute coronary syndromes. Pooled analysis from the HORIZONS-AMI (Harmonizing Outcomes With Revascularization and Stents in Acute Myocardial Infarction) and ACUITY (Acute Catheterization and Urgent Intervention Triage Strategy) TRIALS. J Am Coll Cardiol. 2014;63:1845–54. https://doi.org/10.1016/j.jacc.2014.01.034.
45. Schurgin S, Rich S, Mazzone T. Increased prevalence of significant coronary artery calcification in patients with diabetes. Diabetes Care. 2001;24:335–8. https://doi.org/10.2337/diacare.24.2.335.
46. Wang XR, Zhang JJ, Xu XX, Wu YG. Prevalence of coronary artery calcification and its association with mortality, cardiovascular events in patients with chronic kidney disease: a systematic review and meta-analysis. Ren Fail. 2019;41:244–56. https://doi.org/10.1080/0886022x.2019.1595646.
47. Rheude T, Koch T, Joner M, Lenz T, Xhepa E, Wiebe J, Coughlan JJ, Aytekin A, Cassese S, Laugwitz KL, et al. Ten-year clinical outcomes of drug-eluting stents with different polymer coating strategies by degree of coronary calcification: a pooled analysis of the ISAR-TEST 4 and 5 randomised trials. EuroIntervention. 2023;18:1188–96. https://doi.org/10.4244/eij-d-22-00781.
48. Amano H, Noike R, Yabe T, Watanabe I, Okubo R, Koizumi M, Toda M, Ikeda T. Frailty and coronary plaque characteristics on optical coherence tomography. Heart Vessel. 2020;35:750–61. https://doi.org/10.1007/s00380-019-01547-2.
49. Gu SZ, Qiu W, Batty JA, Sinclair H, Veerasamy M, Brugaletta S, Neely D, Ford G, Calvert PA, Mintz GS, et al. Coronary artery lesion phenotype in frail older patients with non-ST-elevation acute coronary syndrome undergoing invasive care. EuroIntervention. 2019;15:e261–8. https://doi.org/10.4244/EIJ-D-18-00848.
50. Beska B, Ratcovich H, Bagnall A, Burrell A, Edwards R, Egred M, Jordan R, Khan A, Mills GB, Morrison E, et al. Angiographic and procedural characteristics in frail older patients with non-ST elevation acute coronary syndrome. Interv Cardiol. 2023;18(e04):2023. https://doi.org/10.15420/icr.2022.20.
51. Neumann FJ, Sousa-Uva M, Ahlsson A, Alfonso F, Banning AP, Benedetto U, Byrne RA, Collet JP, Falk V, Head SJ, et al. 2018 ESC/EACTS guidelines on myocardial revascularization. Kardiol

Pol. 2018;76:1585–664. https://doi.org/10.5603/KP.2018.0228.

52. Lawton JS, Tamis-Holland JE, Bangalore S, Bates ER, Beckie TM, Bischoff JM, Bittl JA, Cohen MG, DiMaio JM, Don CW, et al. 2021 ACC/AHA/SCAI guideline for coronary artery revascularization: a report of the American College of Cardiology/American Heart Association Joint Committee on Clinical Practice Guidelines. J Am Coll Cardiol. 2022;79:e21–e129. https://doi.org/10.1016/j.jacc.2021.09.006.
53. Lim HS, Tonino PA, De Bruyne B, Yong AS, Lee BK, Pijls NH, Fearon WF. The impact of age on fractional flow reserve-guided percutaneous coronary intervention: a FAME (Fractional Flow Reserve versus Angiography for Multivessel Evaluation) trial substudy. Int J Cardiol. 2014;177:66–70. https://doi.org/10.1016/j.ijcard.2014.09.010.
54. Faria DC, Lee JM, van der Hoef T, Mejía-Rentería H, Echavarría-Pinto M, Baptista SB, Cerrato E, Garcia-Garcia HM, Davies J, Onuma Y, et al. Age and functional relevance of coronary stenosis: a post hoc analysis of the ADVISE II trial. EuroIntervention. 2021;17:757–64. https://doi.org/10.4244/EIJ-D-20-01163.
55. van de Hoef TP, Echavarria-Pinto M, Meuwissen M, Stegehuis VE, Escaned J, Piek JJ. Contribution of age-related microvascular dysfunction to abnormal coronary: hemodynamics in patients with ischemic heart disease. JACC Cardiovasc Interv. 2020;13:20–9. https://doi.org/10.1016/j.jcin.2019.08.052.
56. van de Hoef TP, van Lavieren MA, Damman P, Delewi R, Piek MA, Chamuleau SA, Voskuil M, Henriques JP, Koch KT, de Winter RJ, et al. Physiological basis and long-term clinical outcome of discordance between fractional flow reserve and coronary flow velocity reserve in coronary stenoses of intermediate severity. Circ Cardiovasc Interv. 2014;7:301–11. https://doi.org/10.1161/CIRCINTERVENTIONS.113.001049.
57. Mejia-Renteria H, Faria D, Lee JM, Lee SH, Jung JH, Doh JH, Nam CW, Shin ES, Hoshino M, Sugiyama T, et al. Association between patient age, microcirculation, and coronary stenosis assessment with fractional flow reserve and instantaneous wave-free ratio. Catheter Cardiovasc Interv. 2022;99:1104–14. https://doi.org/10.1002/ccd.30092.
58. Faria D, Mejia-Renteria H, Lee JM, Lee SH, Travieso A, Jung JH, Doh JH, Nam CW, Shin ES, Hoshino M, et al. Age-related changes in the coronary microcirculation influencing the diagnostic performance of invasive pressure-based indices and long-term patient prognosis. Catheter Cardiovasc Interv. 2022;100:1195–205. https://doi.org/10.1002/ccd.30445.
59. Warisawa T, Cook CM, Howard JP, Ahmad Y, Doi S, Nakayama M, Goto S, Yakuta Y, Karube K, Shun-Shin MJ, et al. Physiological pattern of disease assessed by pressure-wire pullback has an influence on fractional flow reserve/instantaneous wave-free ratio discordance. Circ Cardiovasc Interv. 2019;12:e007494. https://doi.org/10.1161/CIRCINTERVENTIONS.118.007494.
60. Araki M, Yonetsu T, Kurihara O, Nakajima A, Lee H, Soeda T, Minami Y, Higuma T, Kimura S, Takano M, et al. Age and phenotype of patients with plaque erosion. J Am Heart Assoc. 2021;10:e020691. https://doi.org/10.1161/JAHA.120.020691.
61. Chen J, Xue Q, Bai J, Gao L, Tian JW, Li K, Xu Q, Li YH, Wang Y. Incomplete revascularization in the drug eluting stent era permits meaningful long-term (12–78 months) outcomes in patients ≥75 years with acute coronary syndrome. J Geriatr Cardiol. 2012;9:336–43. https://doi.org/10.3724/sp.J.1263.2012.05021.
62. Biscaglia S, Erriquez A, Serenelli M, D'Ascenzo F, De Ferrari G, Ariza Sole A, Sanchis J, Giannini F, Gallo F, Scala A, et al. Complete versus culprit-only strategy in older MI patients with multivessel disease. Catheter Cardiovasc Interv. 2022;99:970–8. https://doi.org/10.1002/ccd.30075.
63. Biscaglia S, Guiducci V, Santarelli A, Amat Santos I, Fernandez-Aviles F, Lanzilotti V, Varbella F, Fileti L, Moreno R, Giannini F, et al. Physiology-guided revascularization versus optimal medical therapy of nonculprit lesions in elderly patients with myocardial infarction: Rationale and design of the FIRE trial. Am Heart J. 2020;229:100–9. https://doi.org/10.1016/j.ahj.2020.08.007.
64. van Wyk GW, Berkovsky S, Fraile Navarro D, Coiera E. Comparing health outcomes between coronary interventions in frail patients aged 75 years or older with acute coronary syndrome: a systematic review. Eur Geriatr Med. 2022;13:1057–69. https://doi.org/10.1007/s41999-022-00667-9.
65. Qayyum S, Rossington JA, Chelliah R, John J, Davidson BJ, Oliver RM, Ngaage D, Loubani M, Johnson MJ, Hoye A. Prospective cohort study of elderly patients with coronary artery disease: impact of frailty on quality of life and outcome. Open Heart. 2020;7:7. https://doi.org/10.1136/openhrt-2020-001314.
66. Vila Sala M, Ariza A, Diaz A, Rueda F, Coma N, Aboal J, Vidan MT, Sanchez-Salado JC, Curos A, Garay A. Frailty and prognosis in elderly patients with ST elevation myocardial infarction undergoing primary angioplasty: IFFANIAM study preliminary results [Acute Cardiovascular Care 2014]. Eur Heart J Acute Cardiovasc Care. 2014;3:202. https://doi.org/10.1177/2048872614549721.
67. Llaó I, Ariza-Solé A, Sanchis J, Alegre O, López-Palop R, Formiga F, Marín F, Vidán MT, Martínez-Sellés M, Sionis A, et al. Invasive strategy and frailty in very elderly patients with acute coronary syndromes. EuroIntervention. 2018;14:e336–42. https://doi.org/10.4244/eij-d-18-00099.
68. Fishman B, Sharon A, Itelman E, Tsur AM, Fefer P, Barbash IM, Segev A, Matetzky S, Guetta V, Grossman E, et al. Invasive management in older adults (≥80 Years) with non-ST elevation myocardial infarction. Mayo Clin Proc. 2022;97:1247–56. https://doi.org/10.1016/j.mayocp.2022.03.021.

69. Núñez J, Ruiz V, Bonanad C, Miñana G, García-Blas S, Valero E, Núñez E, Sanchis J. Percutaneous coronary intervention and recurrent hospitalizations in elderly patients with non ST-segment acute coronary syndrome: the role of frailty. Int J Cardiol. 2017;228:456–8. https://doi.org/10.1016/j.ijcard.2016.11.151.
70. Sanchis J, Bueno H, Miñana G, Guerrero C, Martí D, Martínez-Sellés M, Domínguez-Pérez L, Díez-Villanueva P, Barrabés JA, Marín F, et al. Effect of routine invasive vs conservative strategy in older adults with frailty and non-ST-segment elevation acute myocardial infarction: a randomized clinical trial. JAMA Intern Med. 2023;183:407. https://doi.org/10.1001/jamainternmed.2023.0047.
71. Beska B, Coakley D, MacGowan G, Adams-Hall J, Wilkinson C, Kunadian V. Frailty and quality of life after invasive management for non-ST elevation acute coronary syndrome. Heart. 2022;108:203–11. https://doi.org/10.1136/heartjnl-2021-319064.
72. Campo G, Tonet E, Chiaranda G, Sella G, Maietti E, Mazzoni G, Biscaglia S, Pavasini R, Myers J, Grazzi G. Exercise intervention to improve functional capacity in older adults after acute coronary syndrome. J Am Coll Cardiol. 2019;74:2948–50. https://doi.org/10.1016/j.jacc.2019.10.010.
73. Chuang AM, Hancock DG, Halabi A, Horsfall M, Vaile J, De Pasquale C, Sinhal A, Jones D, Brogan R, Chew DP. Invasive management of acute coronary syndrome: interaction with competing risks. Int J Cardiol. 2018;269:13–8. https://doi.org/10.1016/j.ijcard.2018.07.078.
74. Ekerstad N, Swahn E, Janzon M, Alfredsson J, Lofmark R, Lindenberger M, Carlsson P. Frailty is independently associated with short-term outcomes for elderly patients with non-ST-segment elevation myocardial infarction. Circulation. 2011;124:2397–404. https://doi.org/10.1161/CIRCULATIONAHA.111.025452.
75. Sanchis J, Bonanad C, Ruiz V, Fernandez J, Garcia-Blas S, Mainar L, Ventura S, Rodriguez-Borja E, Chorro FJ, Hermenegildo C, et al. Frailty and other geriatric conditions for risk stratification of older patients with acute coronary syndrome. Am Heart J. 2014;168:784–91. https://doi.org/10.1016/j.ahj.2014.07.022.
76. Alonso Salinas GL, Sanmartin Fernandez M, Pascual Izco M, Marco Del Castillo A, Rincon Diaz LM, Lozano Granero C, Valverde Gomez M, Pastor Pueyo P, Del Val MD, Pardo Sanz A, et al. Frailty predicts major bleeding within 30days in elderly patients with acute coronary syndrome. Int J Cardiol. 2016;222:590–3. https://doi.org/10.1016/j.ijcard.2016.07.268.
77. Blanco S, Ferrieres J, Bongard V, Toulza O, Sebai F, Billet S, Biendel C, Lairez O, Lhermusier T, Boudou N, et al. Prognosis impact of frailty assessed by the edmonton frail scale in the setting of acute coronary syndrome in the elderly. Can J Cardiol. 2017;33:933–9. https://doi.org/10.1016/j.cjca.2017.03.026.

Revascularization Strategies in HBR Patients: The Selection of Coronary Stent

7

Angelo Oliva, Mohammad Hashim Mustehsan, Andrea Scotti, Antonio Mangieri, and Azeem Latib

7.1 Introduction

Stent implantation is now considered the standard of care for patients undergoing percutaneous coronary intervention (PCI) for coronary artery disease (CAD) [1]. Historically, bare-metal stents (BMS) were developed with the aim of preventing abrupt vessel closure and flow limiting dissections after plain old balloon angioplasty. Stents were effective for these indications and rapidly gained popularity [2]. However, restenosis and the risk of stent thrombosis emerged as the most undesirable drawbacks of this new technology. For the prevention of stent thrombosis, the implementation of dual antiplatelet therapy (DAPT), consisting in a combination of aspirin and a P2Y12 inhibitor, provided effective protection, with a significantly improved safety profile when compared to anticoagulation—the traditional antithrombotic treatment after PCI [3]. On the other hand, the development of a polymer-based technology for coating an antiproliferative agent to the stent platform targeted the hyperplastic neointimal response to BMS and was effective in reducing the risk of in-stent restenosis and repeat revascularization [2]. However, the first-generation drug-eluting stents (DES) initially showed a worrying rise in the occurrence of stent thrombosis (ST), potentially increasing mortality compared to BMS [4]. These concerns led to significant technology refinements in the key elements of stent design, including strut thickness, drug release kinetics, and polymer biocompatibility that were identified to be crucial for the thrombotic risk. These improvements dramatically enhanced newer generation DES clinical outcomes that progressively outperformed BMS and first-generation DES, in terms of both safety and efficacy. The risk of stent thrombosis was significantly decreased, and this allowed for progressive reduction in the intensity and the length of DAPT, previously maintained for an extended period after DES implantation to ensure adequate ischemic protection, albeit at the expense of increased bleeding complications.

Considerations for stent selection for high-bleeding-risk (HBR) patients undergoing PCI should not be separated from the technological advancements that have progressively shortened DAPT duration. Notably, around 40% of

A. Oliva
The Zena and Michael A. Wiener Cardiovascular Institute, Icahn School of Medicine at Mount Sinai, New York, NY, USA

Department of Biomedical Sciences, Humanitas University, Pieve Emanuele (MI), Italy

M. H. Mustehsan · A. Scotti · A. Latib (✉)
Montefiore-Einstein Center for Heart and Vascular Care, Montefiore Medical Center, Albert Einstein College of Medicine, Bronx, NY, USA

A. Mangieri
Department of Biomedical Sciences, Humanitas University, Pieve Emanuele (MI), Italy

B. Cortese, S. Rigattieri (eds.), *High Bleeding Risk Patients in Interventional Cardiology*,
https://doi.org/10.1007/978-3-031-87302-7_7

patients undergoing PCI are deemed to be at high bleeding risk (HBR) according to criteria provided by the 2019 Academic Research Consortium for HBR (ARC-HBR) [5, 6]. These patients are exposed to a risk of major bleeding ≥4% at 1-year after PCI, which is further increased by prolonged or more intense regimen of DAPT. In this high-risk subgroup of patients, major bleeding complications have been shown to be prognostically equivalent to ischemic events, counteracting the potential benefit of extended DAPT regimen—including in complex coronary disease with higher thrombotic risk [7, 8]. Moreover, patients with HBR had increased mortality at 4-year follow up, with an increase in both bleeding and ischemic complications [9].

Here, we appraise the recent body of evidence concerning the latest generation DES that were tested in HBR populations (Table 7.1).

Table 7.1 Main characteristics of studies comparing new-generation drug-eluting stent in HBR patients

Trial	Design	No. of patients	Stent platform	DAPT duration	Primary endpoint	Results
ZEUS	Randomized, single blinded	1606	Zotarolimus-eluting stent vs BMS	1 month	Death, MI, or TVR at 1 year	Zotarolimus-eluting stent vs BMS: 17.5% vs 22.1% ($p = 0.011$)
LEADERS FREE	Randomized, double blinded	2466	Polymer-free Biolimus A9-eluting stent vs BMS	1 month	Cardiac death, MI, or ST at 1 year	Polymer-free Biolimus A9-eluting stent vs BMS: 9.4% vs 12.9% (p for superiority = 0.005)
LEADERS FREE II	Single-arm, non-inferiority	1203	Polymer-free Biolimus A9-eluting stent	1 month	Cardiac death or MI at 1 year	Polymer-free Biolimus A9-eluting stent vs historical BMS cohort from LEADERS FREE: 7.2% vs 9.2% ($p = 0.0150$)
LEADERS FREE III	Single-arm, non-inferiority (vs stainless steel platform) and superiority (vs BMS)	401	Polymer-free Biolimus A9-eluting stent (cobalt chromium 84–88-μm strut platform)	1 month	Safety endpoint: Cardiac death, MI, or ST at 1 year	Cobalt-chromium vs stainless steel platform
					Efficacy endpoint: TVR at 1 year	Safety: 8% vs 8.9% ($p = 0.001$ for non-inferiority)
						Chromium-cobalt vs BMS
						Safety: 8% vs 9.2% (=0.0007 for non-inferiority)
						Efficacy 4.2% vs 10.6% ($p = 0.007$ for superiority)
SENIOR	Randomized, single-blinded, superiority trial	1200	Biodegradable polymer everolimus-eluting stent vs BMS	1 month (stable presentation) to 6 months (unstable presentation)	Death, nonfatal MI, stroke, or ischemia driven TLR at 1 year	Biodegradable polymer everolimus-eluting stent vs BMS: 12% vs 16% ($p = 0.02$)

(continued)

Table 7.1 (continued)

Trial	Design	No. of patients	Stent platform	DAPT duration	Primary endpoint	Results
EVOLVE SHORT DAPT	Single arm, non-inferiority trial	2009	Bioabsorbable polymer everolimus-eluting stent	3 months vs 12 months	Death or MI and ST between 3 and 15 months	Death or MI 3- vs 12-month: 5.6% vs 5.7% ($p = 0.0016$) Stent thrombosis 3-month DAPT: 0.2% ($p = 0.0005$ vs 1% performance goal)
POEM	Single-arm, prospective, open label	443	Bioresorbable polymer everolimus-eluting stent	1 month	Death, MI, or ST at 1 year	Bioresorbable polymer everolimus-eluting stent vs pre-specified performance criterion: 4.82% vs 9.4% ($p < 0.001$ for non-inferiority)
Onyx ONE	Randomized, single-blinded, non-inferiority	1996	Permanent polymer zotarolimus-eluting stent vs polymer-free Biolimus-eluting stent	1 month	Death, MI, or ST at 1 year	Permanent polymer zotarolimus-eluting stent vs polymer-free biolimus-eluting stent: 17.1% vs 16.9% ($p = 0.01$ for non-inferiority)
Onyx ONE CLEAR	Single-arm	1506	Permanent polymer zotarolimus-eluting stent	1 month	Cardiac death or MI between 1 and 12 months	Permanent polymer zotarolimus-eluting stent vs performance goal: 7% vs 9.7% ($p < 0.001$)
BIOFLOW-DAPT	Randomized, controlled, open-label	1948	Ultrathin bioresorbable sirolimus-eluting stent vs durable polymer zotarolimus-eluting stent	1 month	Cardiac death, MI, or ST at 1 year	Ultrathin bioresorbable sirolimus-eluting stent vs durable polymer zotarolimus-eluting stent: 3.6% vs 3.4% ($p < 0.0001$ for non-inferiority)
COMPARE 60/80 HBR	Randomized controlled trial	732	Ultrathin bioresorbable sirolimus-eluting stent vs thin bioresorbable sirolimus-eluting stent	Per ESC guidelines (median of 30 days)	Death, MI, TVR, stroke, or bleeding at 1 year	Ultrathin bioresorbable sirolimus-eluting stent vs thin bioresorbable sirolimus-eluting stent: 15.4% vs 17.1% ($p = 0.02$ for non-inferiority, $p = 0.55$ for superiority)
XIENCE 28	Single-arm, propensity-stratified non-inferiority (ischemic) and superiority (bleeding)	1605	Durable fluoropolymer everolimus-eluting stent	1-month vs 6-month DAPT	Death or MI (non-inferiority) and bleeding BARC type 3–5 (superiority) from 1- to 6-month follow-up	1-month DAPT vs 6-month DAPT historical cohort: Death or MI: 3.5% vs 4.3% ($p = 0.0005$ for non-inferiority) BARC type 3–5 bleeding: 2.2% vs 4.5% ($p = 0.016$ for superiority)

(continued)

Table 7.1 (continued)

Trial	Design	No. of patients	Stent platform	DAPT duration	Primary endpoint	Results
XIENCE 90	Single-arm, propensity-stratified non-inferiority (ischemic) and superiority (bleeding)	2047	Durable fluoropolymer everolimus-eluting stent	3-month vs 12-month DAPT	Death or MI (non-inferiority) and bleeding BARC type 3–5 (superiority) from 3- to 12-month follow-up	3-month DAPT vs 12-month DAPT historical cohort Death or MI: 5.4% vs 4.4% ($p = 0.0063$ for non-inferiority) BARC type 3–5 bleeding: 2.2% vs 6.3% ($p < 0.0001$ for superiority)
MASTER DAPT	Randomized, multicenter, open-label	4434	Bioresorbable sirolimus-eluting stent	1-month vs prolonged DAPT	Death, MI, stroke, or bleeding at 11 months	1-month vs prolonged DAPT: 7.5% vs 7.7% ($p = <0.001$ for non-inferiority)

DAPT dual antiplatelet therapy, *BMS* bare-metal stent, *MI* myocardial infarction, *TVR* target vessel revascularization, *ST* stent thrombosis, *TVF* target vessel failure, *BARC* Bleeding Academic Research Consortium, *ESC* European Society of Cardiology

7.2 Evidence from Clinical Studies Comparing DES vs BMS

Given the relative safety associated with early DAPT discontinuation in patients receiving BMS, this type of device served as the natural benchmark for testing new-generation DES in HBR populations. Indeed, three large randomized clinical trials compared new DES featuring improved stent platform design and polymer technology against BMS, applying a short DAPT regimen [10–12]. Each trial tested a different DES with different polymer technology with results that were concordant in showing the superiority of DES vs BMS. This led to a paradigm shift in the treatment of HBR patients, establishing these devices as the new standard of care.

Durable Polymer vs BMS In the ZEUS (Zotarolimus-Eluting Versus Bare-Metal Stents in Uncertain Drug-Eluting Stent Candidates) trial, a total of 1606 patients, qualified as uncertain candidates for DES on the basis of thrombotic, bleeding, or restenosis risk criteria, were randomized in a 1:1 fashion to receive the hydrophilic durable polymer-based, second-generation zotarolimus-eluting Endeavor stent (Medtronic, USA) or a BMS, utilizing a 1-month DAPT regimen [10]. The Endeavor stent was shown to reduce the risk of the primary endpoint of major adverse cardiovascular events (MACE) at 1 year (HR 0.76; 95% CI 0.61 to 0.95; $p = 0.011$), and resulted in lower incidence of myocardial infarction (MI), target vessel revascularization (TVR), and definite or probable stent thrombosis (2.0% vs 4.1%; $p = 0.019$). A prespecified analysis of the trial, including 828 (52%) HBR patients, yielded consistent results, with the study device being associated with lower risk of MI, TVR, and ST as compared to BMS [13].

Polymer Free vs BMS The LEADERS FREE (Prospective Randomized Comparison of the BioFreedom Biolimus A9 Drug-Coated Stent versus the Gazelle Bare-Metal Stent in Patients at High Bleeding Risk) was the first study comparing a polymer-free stent with BMS in a total of 2466 HBR randomized patients [11]. The polymer-free biolimusA9-coated stent BioFreedom (Biosensors Europe, Switzerland) followed by 1 month of DAPT significantly reduced the primary safety endpoint, a composite of cardiac death, MI, or ST (HR 0.71; 95% CI, 0.56 to 0.91; p non-inferiority <0.001 and p superiority = 0.005) and the incidence of clinically driven target lesion revascularization (HR 0.50; 95% CI, 0.37 to 0.69; $p < 0.001$). The results were confirmed at 2-year follow-up and in a prespecified sub-analysis including 659 patients presenting with acute coronary syndrome (ACS) [14, 15]. Afterward, the LEADERS FREE II, a single-arm prospective study enrolling an independent cohort of 1203 HBR patients mainly from North-America, yielded consistent results when BioFreedom stent was compared with the historical BMS cohort from LEADERS FREE and provided regulatory basis for US FDA device registration [16]. Finally, BioFreedom Ultra, an updated version with cobalt-chromium and thinner strut platform, was recently shown to be non-inferior to BioFreedom in 401 HBR patients enrolled in the LEADERS FREE III study [17].

Bioresorbable Polymer vs BMS The Synergy everolimus-eluting stent (Boston Scientific, USA) is a thin-strut platinum-chromium metal alloy platform coated with abluminal and bioabsorbable (DL-lactide-co-glycolide) polymer. Everolimus is eluted within 90 days and polymer degradation occurs within 4 months; these design elements were developed to facilitate rapid re-endothelialization and enable shorter durations of DAPT. The SENIOR (Short Duration of Dual Antiplatelet Therapy with Synergy II Stent in Patients Older Than 75 Years Undergoing Percutaneous Coronary Revascularization) trial randomized 1200 elderly patients undergoing PCI to receive either the bioresorbable polymer Synergy stent or a BMS [12]. At 1 year, the primary endpoint—a composite of all-cause death, MI, stroke, or ischemia-driven target lesion revascularization—was significantly reduced in the DES group (RR 0.71, 95% CI 0.52–0.94, $p = 0.02$), compared with BMS. Across enrolled population, most of the patients were classified at intermediate-to-high bleeding risk according to PARIS risk score, and DAPT was recommended for 1 month in stable patients and up to 6 months in patients presenting with ACS. Of note, the Synergy stent platform was subsequently tested in two non-randomized prospective study, conducted in contemporary cohorts of HBR patients. In the EVOLVE Short DAPT study, 1487 HBR patients receiving Synergy stent and 3-month DAPT were matched and compared with a historical cohort of patients receiving DES and 12-month DAPT; non-inferiority with respect to the coprimary endpoint of death or MI was met, and the stent received regulatory approval for HBR patients [18]. The POEM single-arm study prospectively evaluated Synergy stent implantation followed by 1-month DAPT in 443 HBR patients; non-inferiority for cardiac death, MI, or ST was demonstrated with respect to an objective performance criterion [19].

7.3 Evidence from Clinical Studies Comparing Different Types of DES

Once the superiority of new-generation DES over BMS was established, a subsequent series of studies—mostly powered for non-inferiority—gradually expanded the range of devices safely employable with short-term DAPT in HBR patients. In this section and in the following one, the main randomized and non-randomized evidence is summarized, including studies comparing different or same types of DES, and/or different DAPT regimen.

Durable-Polymer vs Polymer-Free Stents Polymer-free BioFreedom stent was used as comparator to evaluate safety and efficacy of the durable-polymer, slow-release zotarolimus-eluting Resolute Onyx stent (Medtronic, USA) among 1996 HBR patients enrolled in the Onyx ONE (Randomized Controlled Trial with Resolute Onyx in One Month Dual Antiplatelet Therapy for High-Bleeding Risk Patients) study [20]. The use of Resolute Onyx, characterized by 81-μm-thick struts and a more biocompatible hydrophilic and hydrophobic polymers blend (BioLinx), resulted in a similar incidence of the primary endpoint, a composite of cardiac death, MI, or stent thrombosis at 1-year compared with BioFreedom (17.1 vs 16.9%; p non-inferiority = 0.011, p superiority = 0.84). Notably, all the patients received a very short DAPT regimen, and nearly half of them presented with ACS. For regulatory purpose, the prospective, nonrandomized Onyx ONE Clear study was designed in parallel with the Onyx ONE trial with the aim to broaden the study population of HBR patients treated with 1-month DAPT and the Resolute Onyx stent in the USA and Japan [21]. By pooling together 1506 patients who were event-free 30 days after PCI, 601 from Onyx ONE US/Japan and 905 from Onyx ONE trial, Onyx ONE Clear provided adequate power to confirm clinical safety and effectiveness of Resolute Onyx with a 1-month DAPT regimen with respect to the composite of cardiac death or MI as compared to performance goal (7.0%, one-sided upper 97.5% CI 8.4%, performance goal of 9.7%; $p < 0.001$). As a result, this stent platform received a specific expanded indication for HBR patients.

Biodegradable Polymer vs Durable Polymer More recently, the Bioflow-DAPT (Biodegradable-Polymer or Durable-Polymer Stents in Patients at High Bleeding Risk: A Randomized, Open-Label Clinical Trial) study was the first randomized trial to actively compare a biodegradable-polymer stent platform with a durable-polymer stent in HBR patients [22]. The Orsiro Mission (Biotronik, Germany) is an ultrathin cobalt-chromium stent coated with a bioabsorbable drug matrix (BIOlute) consisting of sirolimus and polymer poly-l-lactide (PLLA). Efficacy and safety of this stent platform was compared to the durable-polymer zotarolimus-eluting Resolute Onyx stent among 1948 HBR patients undergoing PCI and receiving 1-month DAPT regimen. At 1-year there were no differences between the two platforms with regard to the occurrence of the primary endpoint, a composite of cardiac death, MI or stent thrombosis, and noninferiority was met (3.6% vs 3.4%, p non-inferiority <0.0001).

Ultrathin vs Thin-Strut Stents As mentioned above, alongside with polymer composition, strut thickness may also play a role in ST occurrence [23]. In vivo studies have proved ultrathin (<70 μm) strut stent to be associated with less thrombogenicity, less intimal hyperplasia, and more rapid endothelization [24]. Moreover, when compared with thin-strut second-generation DES, ultrathin strut DES may reduce the risk of long-term target lesion failure and revascularization in all-comer PCI patients [25]. For this reason, the benefit of ultrathin strut stents might be enhanced in high-risk PCI populations such as HBR patients requiring short DAPT.

The aforementioned Bioflow-DAPT trial and an explorative sub-analysis including HBR patients from the BIO-RESORT trial partially try to answer this question [22, 25]. In both studies, an ultrathin biodegradable polymer stent (Synergy or Orsiro) was compared with a thin-strut durable polymer stent (Resolute Onyx or Integrity) in HBR patients undergoing PCI but no significant differences in clinical outcomes were evident. However, more recently, the dedicated COMPARE 60/80 HBR trial was designed to address this issue by comparing the ultrathin-strut (60 μm) biodegradable polymer sirolimus-eluting Supraflex Crux Stent (SMT, India) with the thin-strut (80 μm) biodegradable polymer Ultimaster Tansei (Terumo, Japan) stent in 732 ARC-HBR defined patients included in the study [26]. After a short DAPT treatment (median 30 days), the Supraflex Core Stent met non-inferiority but not superiority with the respect of the primary endpoint of NACE at 1 year, a composite of cardiovascular death, MI, TVR, stroke, or major Bleeding Academic Research Consortium (BARC) Type 3 or 5 bleeding (15.4% vs 17.1%; HR 0.89, 95%CI 0.62–1.28; *p* non-inferiority 0.02; *p*-superiority = 0.55) [27]. Of note, target lesion revascularization and MI were numerically but not significantly lower in the Supraflex Crux arm, although the study was not powered for these secondary endpoints.

7.4 Evidence from Clinical Studies Comparing the Same Type of DES and/or Different DAPT Regimens

Durable Polymer Stent The XIENCE everolimus-eluting stent (Abbott) is a thin-strut (81 μm) cobalt-chromium alloy platform coated with a durable thromboresistant fluoropolymer that has been extensively studied in different clinical scenarios [28]. The XIENCE Short DAPT clinical program was designed to prove safety and efficacy of XIENCE stent in HBR patients undergoing successful PCI followed by a short DAPT regimen of 1 or 3 months [29]. The program included two single-arm prospective studies that compressively enrolled 3652 HBR patients and used propensity-stratified historical cohorts for comparison of the same device with prolonged DAPT, powered for noninferiority on death or myocardial infarction and for superiority on bleeding (BARC Type 2–5). After 1 month (XIENCE 28 study) or 3 months (XIENCE 90 study) of DAPT, propensity-adjusted rates of the primary endpoint of all-cause mortality or myocardial infarction were non-inferior to the 6-month and 12-month DAPT historical controls, respectively (3.5% vs 4.3%, p non-inferiority = 0.0005 and 5.4% vs 5.4%, p non-inferiority = 0.0005, for XIENCE 28 and XIENCE 90, respectively). Major BARC type 3 or 5, but not BARC type 2 to 5 bleedings, were significantly reduced in both experimental groups, and very low rate of stent thrombosis were observed with the experimental device (0.3% and 0.2% for XIENCE 28 or XIENCE 90, respectively). Thus, the XIENCE stent has received labeling for reduced DAPT in HBR patients.

Bioresorbable Polymer Stent The MASTER DAPT (management of high-bleeding-risk patients post bioresorbable polymer-coated stent implantation with an abbreviated versus prolonged DAPT regimen) is the largest multicenter randomized controlled trial on the use of abbreviated DAPT in HBR patients following stenting procedures with thin cobalt-chromium sirolimus-eluting bioresorbable polymer Ultimaster/Ultimaster Tansei (Terumo, Japan) platforms [30]. Among a total of 4434 HBR patients, abbreviated DAPT was noninferior to the continuation of therapy for at least 2 additional months with regard to the occurrence of net adverse clinical events and major adverse cardiac or cerebral events, resulting in a lower incidence of major or clinically relevant nonmajor bleeding. At 1 year, the incidence of all-cause death (3.3% and 3.6%), myocardial infarction (2.7% and 2.2%), and definite or probable stent thrombosis (0.6% and 0.4%) were similar in the abbreviated and the standard-therapy groups, respectively. Moreover, consistent results were reported for subgroups of patients with indication to oral anticoagulation or undergoing complex PCI [31, 32]. To date, Ultimaster/Ultimaster TANSEI stent platforms have received 1-month DAPT CE Mark approval for patients in need of stopping DAPT earlier.

7.5 Clinical Implications

International guidelines have progressively integrated the growing amount of data about the safety and efficacy of new-generation DES, and both European and American guidelines on myocardial revascularization now endorse the use of new-generation DES over BMS for stent implantation in PCI in any clinical setting (class I indication, level of evidence A) [1, 33]. Differently from what was done in the past, guidelines do not provide recommendations for the choice of a specific DES platform in HBR patients; rather more attention is devoted to the implementation of bleeding avoidance strategies and DAPT reduction [34]. Short (1- to 3-month) DAPT is now considered safe and feasible in HBR undergoing PCI, but, as a general rule, the use of DES that have already received regulatory approval for this indication and/or were tested in dedicated clinical studies is recommended. Of note, recent data suggest that HBR patients might benefit from P2Y12 inhibitor monotherapy strategies, consisting in early withdrawal of aspirin after 1 to 3 months of DAPT followed by clopidogrel or ticagrelor alone [35]. With the exception of MASTERDAPT, in which a consistent proportion of patients switched to clopidogrel monotherapy in the abbreviated DAPT arm, aspirin was usually the chronic maintenance drug after short DAPT in the device studies conducted in HBR patients. However, since nearly all the new-generation DES platforms were extensively represented in P2Y12 inhibitor monotherapy trials without any safety concerns, the subsequent type of single antiplatelet therapy should not be considered an issue for stent selection [36, 37].

7.6 Conclusions

With significant improvement in stent design and clinical outcomes, DES is now considered the standard of care in all patients undergoing PCI. This is in response to a significant body of evidence demonstrating the safety and efficacy of newer-generation DES when compared to BMS. For HBR patients, individualized strategies should be developed to determine the duration of DAPT after PCI, taking into consideration patient-specific bleeding and thrombotic risks. In HBR patients requiring short-DAPT, the use of specific DES investigated in this clinical setting should be preferred.

References

1. Neumann F-J, Sousa-Uva M, Ahlsson A, Alfonso F, Banning AP, Benedetto U, Byrne RA, Collet J-P, Falk V, Head SJ, et al. 2018 ESC/EACTS guidelines on myocardial revascularization. Eur Heart J. 2019;40:87–165. https://doi.org/10.1093/eurheartj/ehy394.
2. Stefanini GG, Holmes DR. Drug-eluting coronary-artery stents. N Engl J Med. 2013;368:254–65. https://doi.org/10.1056/nejmra1210816.
3. Schömig A, Neumann F-J, Kastrati A, Schühlen H, Blasini R, Hadamitzky M, Walter H, Zitzmann-Roth E-M, Richardt G, Alt E, et al. A randomized comparison of antiplatelet and anticoagulant therapy after the placement of coronary-artery stents. 1996;334 https://doi.org/10.1056/NEJM199604253341702.
4. Camenzind E, Steg PG, Wijns W. A cause for concern. Circulation. 2007;115:1440–55. https://doi.org/10.1161/circulationaha.106.666800.
5. Urban P, Mehran R, Colleran R, Angiolillo DJ, Byrne RA, Capodanno D, Cuisset T, Cutlip D, Eerdmans P, Eikelboom J, et al. Defining high bleeding risk in patients undergoing percutaneous coronary intervention. Circulation. 2019;140:240–61. https://doi.org/10.1161/circulationaha.119.040167.
6. Cao D, Mehran R, Dangas G, Baber U, Sartori S, Chandiramani R, Stefanini GG, Angiolillo DJ, Capodanno D, Urban P, et al. Validation of the academic research consortium high bleeding risk definition in contemporary PCI patients. J Am Coll Cardiol. 2020;75:2711–22. https://doi.org/10.1016/j.jacc.2020.03.070.
7. Piccolo R, Oliva A, Avvedimento M, Franzone A, Windecker S, Valgimigli M, Esposito G, Jüni P. Mortality after bleeding versus myocardial infarction in coronary artery disease: a systematic review and meta-analysis. EuroIntervention. 2021;17 https://doi.org/10.4244/EIJ-D-20-01197.
8. Costa F, Van Klaveren D, Feres F, James S, Räber L, Pilgrim T, Hong M-K, Kim H-S, Colombo A, Steg PG, et al. Dual antiplatelet therapy duration based on ischemic and bleeding risks after coronary stenting. J Am Coll Cardiol. 2019;73:741–54. https://doi.org/10.1016/j.jacc.2018.11.048.
9. Bleeding Risk, Dual Antiplatelet Therapy Cessation, and Adverse Events After Percutaneous Coronary Intervention. The PARIS Registry – PubMed. Circ Cardiovasc Interv. 2020;13 https://doi.org/10.1161/CIRCINTERVENTIONS.119.008226.
10. Valgimigli M, Patialiakas A, Thury A, McFadden E, Colangelo S, Campo G, Tebaldi M, Ungi I, Tondi S, Roffi M, et al. Zotarolimus-eluting versus bare-metal stents in uncertain drug-eluting stent candidates. J Am Coll Cardiol. 2015;65:805–15. https://doi.org/10.1016/j.jacc.2014.11.053.
11. Urban P, Meredith IT, Abizaid A, Pocock SJ, Carrié D, Naber C, Lipiecki J, Richardt G, Iñiguez A, Brunel P, et al. Polymer-free drug-coated coronary stents in patients at high bleeding risk. N Engl J Med. 2015;373:2038–47. https://doi.org/10.1056/nejmoa1503943.
12. Varenne O, Cook S, Sideris G, Kedev S, Cuisset T, Carrié D, Hovasse T, Garot P, El Mahmoud R, Spaulding C, et al. Drug-eluting stents in elderly patients with coronary artery disease (SENIOR): a randomised single-blind trial. Lancet. 2018;391:41–50. https://doi.org/10.1016/s0140-6736(17)32713-7.
13. Ariotti S, Adamo M, Costa F, Patialiakas A, Briguori C, Thury A, Colangelo S, Campo G, Tebaldi M, Ungi I, et al. Is bare-metal stent implantation still justifiable in high bleeding risk patients undergoing percutaneous coronary intervention?: a pre-specified analysis from the ZEUS trial. J Am Coll Cardiol Intv. 2016;9:426–36. https://doi.org/10.1016/j.jcin.2015.11.015.
14. Naber CK, Urban P, Ong PJ, Valdes-Chavarri M, Abizaid AA, Pocock SJ, Fabbiocchi F, Dubois C, Copt S, Greene S, Morice M-C. Biolimus-A9 polymer-free coated stent in high bleeding risk patients with acute coronary syndrome: a *Leaders Free ACS* substudy. Eur Heart J. 2016;38:ehw203. https://doi.org/10.1093/eurheartj/ehw203.
15. Garot P, Morice M-C, Tresukosol D, Pocock SJ, Meredith IT, Abizaid A, Carrié D, Naber C, Iñiguez A, Talwar S, et al. 2-year outcomes of high bleeding risk patients after polymer-free drug-coated stents. J Am Coll Cardiol. 2017;69:162–71. https://doi.org/10.1016/j.jacc.2016.10.009.
16. Krucoff MW, Urban P, Tanguay J-F, McAndrew T, Zhang Y, Rao SV, Morice M-C, Price MJ, Cohen DJ, Abdel-Wahab M, et al. Global approach to high bleeding risk patients with polymer-free drug-coated coronary stents. Circ Cardiovasc Interv. 2020;13:e008603. https://doi.org/10.1161/CIRCINTERVENTIONS.119.008603.

17. Eberli FR, Stoll H-P, Urban P, Morice M-C, Brunel P, Maillard L, Lipiecki J, Cook S, Berland J, Hovasse T, et al. Polymer-free Biolimus-A9 coated thin strut stents for patients at high bleeding risk 1-year results from the LEADERS FREE III study. Catheter Cardiovasc Interv. 2022;99:593. https://doi.org/10.1002/ccd.29869.
18. Kirtane AJ, Stoler R, Feldman R, Neumann F-J, Boutis L, Tahirkheli N, Toelg R, Othman I, Stein B, Choi JW, et al. Primary results of the EVOLVE short DAPT study. Circ Cardiovasc Interv. 2021;14:14. https://doi.org/10.1161/circinterventions.120.010144.
19. Pivato CA, Reimers B, Testa L, Pacchioni A, Briguori C, Musto C, Esposito G, Piccolo R, Lucisano L, De Luca L, et al. One-month dual antiplatelet therapy after bioresorbable polymer everolimus-eluting stents in high bleeding risk patients. J Am Heart Assoc. 2022;11:11. https://doi.org/10.1161/jaha.121.023454.
20. Windecker S, Latib A, Kedhi E, Kirtane AJ, Kandzari DE, Mehran R, Price MJ, Abizaid A, Simon DI, Worthley SG, et al. Polymer-based or polymer-free stents in patients at high bleeding risk. N Engl J Med. 2020;382:1208–18. https://doi.org/10.1056/nejmoa1910021.
21. Kandzari DE, Kirtane AJ, Windecker S, Latib A, Kedhi E, Mehran R, Price MJ, Abizaid A, Simon DI, Worthley SG, et al. One-month dual antiplatelet therapy following percutaneous coronary intervention with zotarolimus-eluting stents in high-bleeding-risk patients. Circ Cardiovasc Interv. 2020;13:13. https://doi.org/10.1161/circinterventions.120.009565.
22. Valgimigli M, Wlodarczak A, Tölg R, Merkely B, Kelbæk H, Legutko J, Galli S, Godin M, Toth GG, Lhermusier T, et al. Biodegradable-polymer or durable-polymer stents in patients at high bleeding risk: a randomized. Open-Label Clin Trial Circ. 2023;148:989–99. https://doi.org/10.1161/circulationaha.123.065448.
23. Sakamoto A, Jinnouchi H, Torii S, Virmani R, Finn A. Understanding the impact of stent and scaffold material and strut design on coronary artery thrombosis from the basic and clinical points of view. Bioengineering. 2018;5:71. https://doi.org/10.3390/bioengineering5030071.
24. Koskinas KC, Chatzizisis YS, Antoniadis AP, Giannoglou GD. Role of endothelial shear stress in stent restenosis and thrombosis: pathophysiologic mechanisms and implications for clinical translation. J Am Coll Cardiol. 2012;59:1337–49. https://doi.org/10.1016/j.jacc.2011.10.903.
25. Madhavan MV, Howard JP, Naqvi A, Ben-Yehuda O, Redfors B, Prasad M, Shahim B, Leon MB, Bangalore S, Stone GW, Ahmad Y. Long-term follow-up after ultrathin vs. conventional 2nd-generation drug-eluting stents: a systematic review and meta-analysis of randomized controlled trials. Eur Heart J. 2021;42:2643–54. https://doi.org/10.1093/eurheartj/ehab280.
26. Paradies V, Maurina M, Tonino P, Hofma SH, Vos J, van Kuijk J-P, Oemrawsingh RM, Mafragi AA, Spano F, Pisters R, et al. Comparison of Supraflex Cruz 60 μm versus Ultimaster Tansei 80 μm stent struts in high bleeding risk PCI patients: study design and rational of compare 60/80 HBR trial. Am J Cardiol. 2023;206:230–7. https://doi.org/10.1016/j.amjcard.2023.08.046.
27. Smits PC. The primary endpoint results from the COMPARE 60/80 HBR trial. San Francisco: TCT 2023; 2023.
28. Naidu SS, Krucoff MW, Rutledge DR, Mao VW, Zhao W, Zheng Q, Wilburn O, Sudhir K, Simonton C, Hermiller JB. Contemporary incidence and predictors of stent thrombosis and other major adverse cardiac events in the year after XIENCE V implantation: results from the 8,061-patient XIENCE V United States study. J Am Coll Cardiol Intv. 2012;5:626–35. https://doi.org/10.1016/j.jcin.2012.02.014.
29. Mehran R, Cao D, Angiolillo DJ, Bangalore S, Bhatt DL, Ge J, Hermiller J, Makkar RR, Neumann FJ, Saito S, et al. 3- or 1-month DAPT in patients at high bleeding risk undergoing everolimus-eluting stent implantation. JACC Cardiovasc Interv. 2021;14:1870–83. https://doi.org/10.1016/j.jcin.2021.07.016.
30. Valgimigli M, Frigoli E, Heg D, Tijssen J, Jüni P, Vranckx P, Ozaki Y, Morice M-C, Chevalier B, Onuma Y, et al. Dual antiplatelet therapy after PCI in patients at high bleeding risk. N Engl J Med. 2021;385:1643–55. https://doi.org/10.1056/nejmoa2108749.
31. Smits PC, Frigoli E, Tijssen J, Jüni P, Vranckx P, Ozaki Y, Morice M-C, Chevalier B, Onuma Y, Windecker S, et al. Abbreviated antiplatelet therapy in patients at high bleeding risk with or without oral anticoagulant therapy after coronary stenting: an open-label, randomized. Control Trial Circ. 2021;144:1196–211. https://doi.org/10.1161/circulationaha.121.056680.
32. Valgimigli M, Smits PC, Frigoli E, Bongiovanni D, Tijssen J, Hovasse T, Mafragi A, Ruifrok WT, Karageorgiev D, Aminian A, et al. Duration of antiplatelet therapy after complex percutaneous coronary intervention in patients at high bleeding risk: a MASTER DAPT trial sub-analysis. Eur Heart J. 2022;43:3100–14. https://doi.org/10.1093/eurheartj/ehac284.
33. Lawton JS, Tamis-Holland JE, Bangalore S, Bates ER, Beckie TM, Bischoff JM, Bittl JA, Cohen MG, DiMaio JM, Don CW, et al. ACC/AHA/SCAI guideline for coronary artery revascularization: a report of the American College of Cardiology/American Heart Association Joint Committee on Clinical Practice Guidelines. Circulation. 2021;2022, 145 https://doi.org/10.1161/CIR.0000000000001038.
34. Byrne RA, Rossello X, Coughlan JJ, Barbato E, Berry C, Chieffo A, Claeys MJ, Dan G-A, Dweck MR, Galbraith M, et al. ESC guidelines for the management of acute coronary syndromes: developed by the task force on the management of acute coronary syndromes of the European Society of Cardiology (ESC). Eur Heart J. 2023;2023:44. https://doi.org/10.1093/eurheartj/ehad191.

35. Valgimigli M, Gragnano F, Branca M, Franzone A, Baber U, Jang Y, Kimura T, Hahn J-Y, Zhao Q, Windecker S, et al. P2Y12 inhibitor monotherapy or dual antiplatelet therapy after coronary revascularisation: individual patient level meta-analysis of randomised controlled trials. BMJ 2021-06-16;373. doi: https://doi.org/10.1136/bmj.n1332.
36. Dangas G, Baber U, Sharma S, Giustino G, Sartori S, Nicolas J, Goel R, Mehta SR, Cohen D, Angiolillo D, et al. Safety and efficacy of ticagrelor monotherapy according to drug-eluting stent type: the TWILIGHT-STENT study. EuroIntervention. 2022;17 https://doi.org/10.4244/EIJ-D-21-00721.
37. Capranzano P. The stent in the high-bleeding risk patient: antiplatelet monotherapy? Eur Heart J Suppl. 2022;24:I54. https://doi.org/10.1093/eurheartjsupp/suac074.

HBR in Interventional Cardiology: "The DCB Philosophy"

8

Matteo Sturla, Daniel Feldman, Andrea Scotti, Azeem Latib, and Juan F. Granada

8.1 Introduction and Historical Perspectives

The management of acute or chronic coronary artery disease (CAD) is complex and combines the use of medical therapy and revascularization, via percutaneous coronary intervention (PCI) or coronary artery bypass graft (CABG), based on a patient's clinical and anatomic scenario. Although drug-eluting stents (DES) are the tool of choice in PCI, these devices have several disadvantages. Among the disadvantages of DES include a platform and polymer that can lead to negative endothelial remodeling and a requirement of antiplatelet therapy to limit subsequent thrombotic events [1–7]. As a potential alternative or adjunct to DES, drug-coated balloons (DCB) provide potential advantages of delivering antiproliferative medications without implantation of a permanent metallic platform. This has the prospective of allowing for positive remodeling within the coronary artery [8, 9]. Additionally, the absence of a metallic platform reduces the use of subsequent antiplatelet agents and associated bleeding events, making this strategy particularly valuable in high-bleeding-risk (HBR) cohorts (Fig. 8.1) [10].

HBR patients, as defined in the ARC HBR article, are identified by a combination of clinical criteria and risk factors. This group includes individuals with a BARC 3 or 5 bleeding risk of >4% at 1 year or an ICH risk of >1% at 1 year [11]. Key factors contributing to this risk include advanced age, a history of bleeding, chronic kidney disease, and the use of anticoagulants or antiplatelet therapy. The comprehensive definition incorporates both major and minor criteria, emphasizing a tailored approach to assessing bleeding risk in these patients. Historically, patients with HBR have been notably underrepresented in PCI trials, despite constituting approximately one-third of the PCI demographic [11]. On the one hand, early post-PCI bleeding events pose a significant dilemma. On the other hand, the interruption of DAPT in this group dramatically elevates the risk of stent thrombosis, as much as 15-fold, which can have devastating consequences [12]. Stent thrombosis, particularly when it occurs early, is linked to a mortality rate approaching 50%, due to its association with large-territory myocardial infarction [13, 14]. These challenges underscore the need for alterna-

M. Sturla · D. Feldman · A. Scotti · A. Latib
Montefiore-Einstein Center for Heart and Vascular Care, Montefiore Medical Center, Albert Einstein College of Medicine, Bronx, NY, USA

J. F. Granada (✉)
Montefiore-Einstein Center for Heart and Vascular Care, Montefiore Medical Center, Albert Einstein College of Medicine, Bronx, NY, USA

Cardiovascular Research Foundation, New York, NY, USA
e-mail: jgranada@crf.org

B. Cortese, S. Rigattieri (eds.), *High Bleeding Risk Patients in Interventional Cardiology*,
https://doi.org/10.1007/978-3-031-87302-7_8

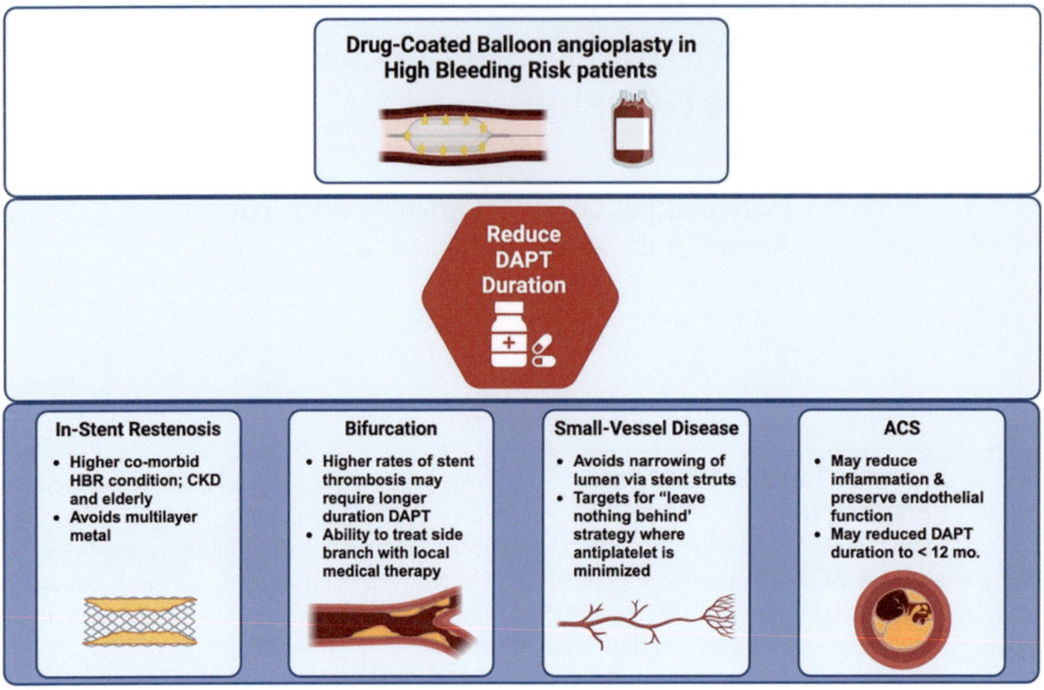

Fig. 8.1 Potential clinical advantages of drug-coated balloons in high-bleeding-risk patient population. *DAPT* dual antiplatelet, *HBR* high bleeding risk, *ACS* acute coronary syndrome

tive strategies in HBR patients, where the balance between preventing thrombosis and minimizing bleeding risk is delicate and critical. DCBs emerge as a promising option in this context, potentially mitigating the risks associated with permanent stents and extended DAPT use.

The evolution of PCI to the advent of DCB highlights a series of technological advancements addressing the limitations of previous methods. Balloon angioplasty, introduced in 1977 by Andreas Grüntzig, was a significant breakthrough in cardiology. This was followed by the development of bare-metal stents in 1986, which, while effective in reducing early vessel closure in POBA, suffered from high restenosis rates of 20–40% [15]. The early 2000s saw the introduction of DES aimed at reducing in-stent restenosis, which they did, but ISR issues persisted, affecting about 5% of PCIs [15, 16].

In response to these challenges, DCBs were developed. The innovation behind DCBs involved the use of paclitaxel, a highly lipophilic antiproliferative drug, known to inhibit microtubules assembly, effectively blocking cell cycle progression during mitosis. This drug was effectively delivered to the vessel wall using contrast media like iopromide as a carrier [17]. Early studies by Scheller et al. demonstrated the efficacy of this approach, showing that intracoronary application of paclitaxel dissolved in a contrast medium was safe and efficient in inhibiting in-stent restenosis [17].

These findings were substantiated by clinical trials, including the pivotal randomized study, PACCOCATH ISR for BMS restenosis [18]. The results showed a significant reduction in in-segment late luminal loss and lower restenosis rates in the paclitaxel-coated balloon group compared to uncoated balloons. This success led to the exploration of DCBs for single-lesion treatment, further proving their efficacy in reducing neointimal proliferation. Over time, several studies supported the safety and efficacy of DCBs, underscoring their potential in reducing the duration of dual antiplatelet therapy and avoiding issues like chronic inflammation and thrombosis associated with durable polymers in stents. The adoption of DCBs marked a significant shift in treating CAD, offering a solution that directly addresses the limitations of prior PCI techniques, and thus opened a new chapter in interventional cardiology. This chapter delves into the intricate relationship between DCBs and high-bleeding-risk patients, exploring the nuanced benefits, practical applications, and the evolving landscape of evidence supporting their use in contemporary practice.

8.2 Drug-Coated Balloon Angioplasty

8.2.1 Drug-Coated Balloon Technical Perspective

As mentioned, the rationale for DCB is the ability to deliver antiproliferative medications without the need for permanent device. DCBs are semi-compliant balloon catheters coated with an antiproliferative drug. When deployed, these lipophilic agents can be delivered to the vessel wall even with a short balloon inflation time. This local distribution of the antiproliferative agents allow for higher levels of drug delivery than systemic administration would allow [18–20].

Several principles are paramount for the efficacy of DCBs. The agents must be formed homogenously along the carrier balloon, the medication must remain stable through production and storage, premature loss of therapeutic agents during deployment prior to reaching the target vessel should be minimized and efficient release from the carrier balloon, and transfer to the vessel wall is crucial.

In the present era, paclitaxel and sirolimus are commercially available antiproliferative agents used with DCB [21]. Paclitaxel affects cell division via irreversible binding to and stabilization of microtubules thus halting mitosis [21, 22]. Sirolimus is an mTOR inhibitor that prevents several subsequent downstream pathways that upregulate cell cycle progression [21, 23, 24]. Ultimately both agents influence the inflammatory milieu that leads to de novo atherosclerotic disease as well as neointimal hyperplasia and neo-atherosclerosis for the treatment of in-stent restenosis (ISR) for bare-metal stents (BMS) and DES, respectively [21–25].

Due to the low level of systemic absorption, the difference in bleeding between these two agents is negligible; additionally, there is limited head-to-head data comparing these two technologies [26–28]. However, some commercially available DCB vary by guiding catheter sheath size. For example, the paclitaxel DCB, the SeQuent Please Neo (B. Braun), is compatible with a 5-Fr guiding catheter, whereas the sirolimus DCB, Magic Touch SCB (Concept Medical), is only compatible with a 6-Fr guiding catheter which leads to the potential for higher bleeding risk associated with catheter size [29, 30]. This theoretical difference is limited to the technical specifications of these two products and does not extend to other products on the market as well as future products in development (Table 8.1). The ongoing TRANSFORM I Trial directly compares these two technologies and should shed light on any differences, including bleeding risk [31].

8.2.2 Drug-Coated Balloon Lesion Preparation and Delivery

Lesion preparation is an important factor in any PCI; however, it carries a higher weight in treatment with DCB to ensure efficient balloon delivery and drug administration. In uncomplicated lesions, expert consensus suggests 1:1 balloon-to-artery predilation with a semi- or noncompliant balloon [10]. For more complex lesions, adjunctive devices may be required, such as specialty balloons (high-pressure noncompliant, cutting, and scoring balloons), atherectomy devices (rotational, orbital, and laser), lithotripsy, or prolonged dilation.

Table 8.1 Commercially available drug-coated balloons

Company	Device	Drug	Dosage	Additive/excipient
B. Braun (Germany)	SeQuent Please	Paclitaxel	3	Iopromide
Medtronic (United States)	Prevail (previously In. Pact)	Paclitaxel	3.5	Urea
Biosensors International (Singapore)	BioStream	Paclitaxel	3	Shellac
Biotronik (Switzerland)	Pantera Lux	Paclitaxel	3	BTHC
Boston Scientific (Massachusetts)	Agent	Paclitaxel	2	ATBC
Aachen Resonance (Germany)	Elutax SV	Paclitaxel	2.2	No additive
Blue Medical (Netherlands)	Protégé	Paclitaxel	3	Unknown
Minvasys (France)	Danubio	Paclitaxel	2.5	BTHC
iVascular (Spain)	Essential Pro	Paclitaxel	3	Unknown
Cardionovum (Germany)	Restore	Paclitaxel	3	Shellac
Nano Therapeutics (India)	Curex PTCA	Paclitaxel	2.3	BTHC
Bard (New Jersey)	Lutonix	Paclitaxel	2	Polysorbate/sorbitol
B.Braun (Germany)	SeQuent SCB	Sirolimus (crystalline)	4	–
Concept Medical (Florida)	Magic Touch	Sirolimus	1.3	Phospholipid
Cordis (United States)	Selution	Sirolimus	1	Micro-reservoirs

BTCH n-butyryl-tri-n-hexyl citrate, *NDGA* nordihydroguaiaretic acid, *ATBC* acetyl tributyl citrate

To ensure effective delivery of DCB, the following factors should be confirmed prior to deployment as angiographic outcomes are typically not of same caliber as DES [32, 33]:

1. A fully inflated balloon of the correct size for the vessel.
2. ≤30% residual stenosis
3. TIMI (thrombolysis in myocardial infarction) flow grade 3.
4. Absence of flow-limiting dissection (type A and B dissections are acceptable).

If needed physiologic testing can be used to confirm adequate functional result and absence of flow-limiting dissection [34]. The FFR cutoff may be able to be lowered in DCB due to the potential for positive remodeling [35]. Present expert guidelines suggest an FFR threshold of 0.80 [10].

Kleber et al. were the first to describe the delayed positive effects of paclitaxel DCB in a study of 58 lesions that found additional lumen gain at follow-up from intervention within the treated length as well as the adjacent 5-mm area (Fig. 8.2) [9]. It is presumed that inhibition of smooth muscle proliferation and upregulation of pro-apoptotic factors leading to thinning of the tunica media is the reason for late lumen enlargement. This has been reproduced by several other investigators [36, 37]. In addition, there may be positive vessel remodeling with an increase in vessel diameter, as plaque evolve, to preserve lumen area [38].

When delivering DCB, care should be taken as to not disrupt the drug-balloon interface. It is recommended to extend the DCB coverage 2 mm proximally and distally from the prepared lesion [10].

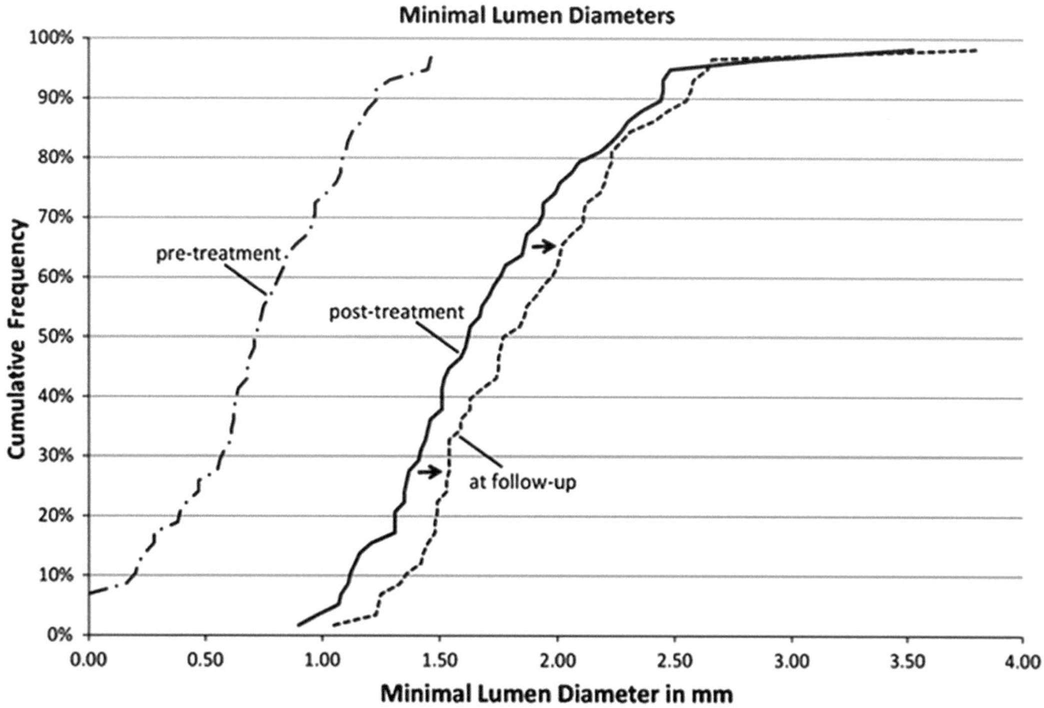

Fig. 8.2 Late lumen enlargement after DCB. Minimal lumen diameter of the lesion site during pre-, post-, and follow-up angiography (Kleber et al.). (From Ref. [9] with permission)

8.3 Clinical Scenarios for Drug-Coated Balloon Angioplasty

The appropriate indication for DCB is dependent on the patient profile, the anatomic distribution of the disease, and the clinical scenario. While most of the investigation for DCB efficacy has surrounded the anatomic intervention, it is important to recognize a patient-specific approach that includes individual bleeding risk. Bleeding after PCI is one of the most relevant adverse outcomes as it has been associated with an increase in mortality as high as sevenfold [39]. This is particularly important in the present era as octogenarians and those who are taking oral anticoagulation (OAC) are more frequently undergoing PCI [40–42]. Here we review the most common angiographic factors where DCB have proven efficacious that may apply to those with HBR.

8.3.1 In-Stent Restenosis

Intracoronary stent restenosis (ISR) is the progressive luminal re-narrowing of stented segments, or immediately adjacent area, by 50% of stent diameter [43]. The pathophysiology of these lesions is related to both (1) biologic processes, which include intimal injury and neointimal formation in BMS and chronic inflammation and neoatherosclerosis in DES, as well as (2) mechanical processes, including stent fracture, stent under-expansion, stent malappostion, suboptimal stent size, and uncovered stent struts [44, 45].

In the present era, the preferred treatment of ISR is with a "stent-in-stent" approach [46, 47]. However, this strategy leads to multiple layers of metal and may necessitate more aggressive antiplatelet use. Indeed, many clinical factors predictive of ISR, such as chronic kidney disease and older age, are also associated with high bleeding risk [11, 48, 49]. This has made DCB an attractive alternative. Furthermore, DCB may be better suited at treating neointimal hyperplasia, a typical cause of ISR. The effect of DCB may be dampened in patients with ISR of DES (as compared to BMS) due to the additional effects of neoatherosclerosis and perhaps drug resistance, although DCB is still efficacious in this population [50–52].

DCB have been shown to be effective and safe at treating ISR in multiple RCTs [53–56]. A patient-level meta-analysis comparing DES and DCB in ISR showed a nonsignificant but numerically lower event rate at 3 years in DCBs. A significant 30% increase in TLR was apparent in the DES arm [56]. This may have to do with the fact that the stent also imposes a significant mechanical impact on the vessel wall where the DCB only delivers the drug. This was elegantly taken into perspective by Tanaka et al. which showed the importance of lesion preparation on outcomes with DCB [57].

DCBs have been shown to be particularly effective at treating ISR with focal patterns of ISR, ISR of BMS, and may also be favorable with multilayer ISR and when a major side branch is involved to avoid jailing [48, 50, 58]. However, as DCB often does not achieve adequate final minimal luminal diameter, intravascular imaging should be used to ensure efficacy or consideration to DES crossover [10, 48, 50, 51].

Presently European and Japanese guidelines offer Class I, level of evidence A recommendations for the use of DCB in ISR [59, 60]. Additionally, an expert consensus from the European Association of Percutaneous Cardiovascular Interventions (EAPCI) recommends preference for DCB over DES in the treatment of ISR in lesions of BMS, multiple metal layers, or large side branches. Alternatively, DES may be preferred in lesions with stent fractures, diffuse ISR extending beyond the stent edges, or in cases of significant residual dissection or impaired flow after a balloon-only approach [61].

8.3.2 Small-Vessel Disease

DCB have also been trialed in the treatment of de novo CAD. The profile with the greatest theoretical benefit for de novo "leave nothing behind strategy" is small-vessel disease (SVD). These lesions typically have the highest rates of restenosis, and stenting may further reduce the lumen via metallic struts [62, 63]. Additionally, it has been shown that neointimal hyperplasia is independent of vessel size, and subsequent ISR after stent placement may be particularly deleterious in these vessels [64, 65]. DCB may have additional benefits in these lesions, which tend to be diffuse, as they are able to deliver drugs in a homogenous and uniform fashion.

Thus far outcomes for the use of DCB in SVD have been mixed, and interpretation of the data is difficult due to the nonstandardized definition of SVD as well as the different treatment protocols and intervention technologies used across the trials [66–72]. Within the HBR population, there is little data on outcomes. In a subgroup analysis of vessels <3 mm from the DEBUT trial, which compared DCB to BMS in de novo CAD, there was less risk of cardiovascular mortality, MI, and target lesion revascularization with a DCB intervention [73]. The largest trial to evaluate outcomes of DCB in SVD that included a HBR population was the BASKET-SMALL 2 trial. This study showed that HBR status attenuated the benefit of DCB in bleeding outcomes. However overall, there was no difference in adverse outcomes between DCB and DES in the HBR subgroup [68]. The recent patient-level ANDROMEDA meta-analysis showed for the first time a significant reduction in MACE compared with those treated with DES, the result being mainly driven by lower occurrence of target vessel myocardial infarction and target vessel and lesion revascularization. Interesting, the landmark analysis suggested consistent effects between DCB and DES over time, and sensitivity analyses did not reveal significant differences between DCB and second-generation DES [74].

8.3.3 Bifurcation Lesions

Bifurcation lesions are commonly encountered and associated with lower procedural success and higher rates of complications, including ISR and in-stent thrombosis [75, 76]. Specific challenges in these lesions include the bifurcation angles, carinal shift during procedures, differences in vessel diameters, and technical challenges when attempting to deploy two stents if necessary [77]. Specifically, bifurcation lesions that are treated with a two stent technique (in the main branch and side branch) have overlapping metal and thus have increased thrombogenic potential. In these instances dual antiplatelet (DAPT) strategies are understudied; however they may require prolonged DAPT, even extending beyond 1 year [78, 79]. Alternatively, lesions treated with provisional stenting, with a single stent placed in the main branch (MB), and the side branch (SB) treated with angioplasty alone may be undertreated. For this reason, DCB have potential benefit in the treatment of SB alongside MB DES or alternatively DCB-only intervention in both the MB and SB. The hybrid approach with DES in MB and DCB in SB has been studied and shown to be an effective strategy, while the DCB-only has been relatively understudied [80–82]. However, this latter approach may have the potential to safely reduce DAPT duration to one month, which is an advantage for HBR patients. In a subgroup analysis of bifurcation lesions from the DEBUT trial, which compared DCB to BMS in de-novo CAD, there was less risk of cardiovascular mortality, MI, and target lesion revascularization with a DCB intervention [73].

8.4 Antiplatelet Therapy Considerations

Current guidelines for antiplatelet therapy post-DCB intervention align with those established for DES. In patients with high bleeding risk who have stable CAD and are treated with DCBs, there is a Class IIa recommendation for a 3-month regimen of DAPT with clopidogrel and a Class IIb recommendation for a shorter, 1-month course of clopidogrel-based DAPT [83]. The body of high-quality evidence advocating for shorter durations of DAPT post-PCI has notably expanded in recent years [84–88]. This accumulation of positive trial outcomes is anticipated to substantially influence subsequent updates of clinical guidelines. Nevertheless, a critical gap persists in the specific context of DAPT duration following DCB PCI. This aspect remains inadequately addressed in the existing literature, with a conspicuous absence of robust, well-powered randomized controlled trials. Concurrently, current American clinical guidelines have yet to articulate definitive positions on the use of DCBs or the intricacies of antiplatelet therapy in this context, reflecting the relatively nascent integration of DCB technology in coronary interventions.

The initial rationale for DAPT was to avert stent thrombosis, a concept evolving since seminal work in the late 1990s [15]. Originally, the combination of aspirin with clopidogrel, or ticlopidine in earlier studies, was deemed essential for a period of 14 to 28 days post-BMS placement to mitigate this risk [89]. The rapid endothelialization of BMS, attributed to the absence of antiproliferative agents or polymer layers, significantly reduces the likelihood of late stent thrombosis. However, the introduction of DES marked a paradigm shift, primarily aimed at addressing the high restenosis rates associated with BMS. Intriguingly, first-generation DES demonstrated non-negligible rates of very late stent thrombosis, occurring more than a year post-procedure, a phenomenon potentially linked to the inhibition of endothelialization by the potent antiproliferative drugs they deliver [90]. Despite these risks, the incidence of late morbidity or mortality has not markedly escalated, likely offset by the reduced necessity for repeated revascularization and the diminished incidence of in-stent restenosis. The remarkably low rates of stent thrombosis in DES PCI are also partially attributable to consistent adherence to DAPT. Contemporary stent thrombosis rates with durable polymer-DES in unselected populations, following standard DAPT regimens, are impressively low, ranging from 0.4% to 0.5% at 1 year and under 1% at 5 years [91]. However, the balance between bleeding and thrombotic risk in patients predisposed to bleeding events stills begs attention.

Growing evidence supporting shorter DAPT durations in HBR patients using contemporary DES is growing with evidence pointing towards reduction in bleeding events without compromising ischemic events. Trials such as ONYX-ONE, SENIOR, LEADERS FREE, and ZEUS have demonstrated low definitive DES stent thrombosis rates of 1–2% at 1 year in this context [87, 92–94]. Advances in stent technology and procedural techniques, including high-pressure stent post-dilation and improved DAPT regimens, have contributed to these low rates, particularly within the first year post-PCI. However, it's noted that higher rates may occur in STEMI patients or after complex PCI procedures. Notably, an international expert consensus group advocates for a 4-week DAPT duration following DCB PCI in de novo lesions, a recommendation supported by trials like DEBUTE and BASKET SMALL 2, which reported no acute vessel closure in DCB arms [10, 68, 73]. This underscores the procedure's safety and eases the anxiety that metal scaffolding is superior in keeping the vessel open acutely.

The avoidance of foreign material implantation in the vessel during DCB PCI offers several notable advantages, particularly in the context of antiplatelet therapy. This approach presents a viable option for DAPT cessation in scenarios of bleeding events or the need for urgent surgery within the first month post-PCI, an option that remains considerably risky in patients with newly implanted DES. This flexibility is particularly beneficial for patients with HBR, affording a safer and more adaptable therapeutic strategy.

Furthermore, emerging data have begun to elucidate the feasibility and safety of a single antiplatelet therapy (SAPT) regimen after DCB PCI, particularly in HBR patients, challenging the conventional reliance on DAPT [95]. Interestingly, in the periprocedural setting, a significant portion of these patients received cangrelor due to its rapid onset and termination of therapeutic effects on the ADP receptor, thereby attenuating the risk of periprocedural bleeding in this susceptible group. Of the 172 patients enrolled, there were no occurrences of acute or subacute vessel closures, with rates of stent thrombosis, myocardial infarction, and mortality aligning with findings from previous studies [95]. This emerging evidence suggests that SAPT post-DCB might offer a safe, efficacious alternative, particularly advantageous for HBR patients. However, the limitations inherent in this study are significant, necessitating further exploration through larger and robust randomized trials before the widespread adoption of this therapeutic strategy can be confidently advocated.

8.5 Conclusions

In this chapter, we focused on the expanding role of DCBs in managing HBR patients. The DCB approach, by abstaining from permanent implants, presents a compelling alternative in minimizing extended antiplatelet therapy, thereby mitigating bleeding risks. This is especially crucial for HBR patients, who are often precariously balanced between thrombotic and bleeding complications. Evidence from trials such as DEBUTE and BASKET SMALL 2, which advocate for abbreviated durations of DAPT, signals a paradigm shift towards safer and more adaptable therapeutic strategies in this patient cohort.

The DEBATE trial, a pivotal ongoing study, is set to further illuminate this evolving landscape. This trial is exploring the efficacy and safety of DCBs coupled with shorter DAPT regimens, in contrast to longer DAPT durations with DES. Targeting a patient demographic with inherent bleeding risks, including those on anticoagulation therapy or elderly patients, the DEBATE trial aims to provide a more nuanced understanding of the optimal duration and strategy of antiplatelet therapy in this context. This study is significant not just for its potential to affirm the non-inferiority of the DCB strategy compared to the traditional DES approach but also for its exploration into the realms of stable

CAD and acute coronary syndromes in patients at HBR.

As we eagerly await the outcomes of the DEBATE trial, the field of interventional cardiology is on the cusp of a transformative era. The potential for DCBs to offer a safer, more effective treatment option for HBR patients is substantial, and the results of this trial could catalyze a shift in clinical practice guidelines and patient management strategies. The intersection of technological innovation, clinical research, and patient-centric care in the realm of DCB usage exemplifies the dynamic nature of this field and underscores the potential for significant advancements in the treatment of CAD.

References

1. Gutierrez E, Flammer AJ, Lerman LO, Elizaga J, Lerman A, Fernandez-Aviles F. Endothelial dysfunction over the course of coronary artery disease. Eur Heart J. 2013;34:3175–81.
2. Kim JW, Suh SY, Choi CU, et al. Six-month comparison of coronary endothelial dysfunction associated with sirolimus-eluting stent versus paclitaxel-eluting stent. JACC Cardiovasc Interv. 2008;1:65–71.
3. Luscher TF, Steffel J, Eberli FR, et al. Drug-eluting stent and coronary thrombosis: biological mechanisms and clinical implications. Circulation. 2007;115:1051–8.
4. Nakazawa G, Ladich E, Finn AV, Virmani R. Pathophysiology of vascular healing and stent mediated arterial injury. EuroIntervention. 2008;(4 Suppl C):C7-10.
5. Pendyala LK, Yin X, Li J, Chen JP, Chronos N, Hou D. The first-generation drug-eluting stents and coronary endothelial dysfunction. JACC Cardiovasc Interv. 2009;2:1169–77.
6. Angiolillo DJ, Galli M, Collet JP, Kastrati A, O'Donoghue ML. Antiplatelet therapy after percutaneous coronary intervention. EuroIntervention. 2022;17:e1371–96.
7. Cao D, Chandiramani R, Chiarito M, Claessen BE, Mehran R. Evolution of antithrombotic therapy in patients undergoing percutaneous coronary intervention: a 40-year journey. Eur Heart J. 2021;42:339–51.
8. Cortese B, Silva Orrego P, Agostoni P, et al. Effect of drug-coated balloons in native coronary artery disease left with a dissection. JACC Cardiovasc Interv. 2015;8:2003–9.
9. Kleber FX, Schulz A, Waliszewski M, et al. Local paclitaxel induces late lumen enlargement in coronary arteries after balloon angioplasty. Clin Res Cardiol. 2015;104:217–25.
10. Jeger RV, Eccleshall S, Wan Ahmad WA, et al. Drug-coated balloons for coronary artery disease: third report of the International DCB Consensus Group. JACC Cardiovasc Interv. 2020;13:1391–402.
11. Urban P, Mehran R, Colleran R, et al. Defining high bleeding risk in patients undergoing percutaneous coronary intervention. Circulation. 2019;140:240–61.
12. Mehran R, Baber U, Steg PG, et al. Cessation of dual antiplatelet treatment and cardiac events after percutaneous coronary intervention (PARIS): 2 year results from a prospective observational study. Lancet (London, England). 2013;382:1714–22.
13. Jeger RV, Pfisterer ME, Sørensen R, et al. Tradeoff between bleeding and stent thrombosis in different dual antiplatelet therapy regimes: importance of case fatality rates and effective treatment durations. Am Heart J. 2014;168:698–705.
14. Almalla M, Schröder J, Hennings V, Marx N, Hoffmann R. Long-term outcome after angiographically proven coronary stent thrombosis. Am J Cardiol. 2013;111:1289–94.
15. Byrne RA, Joner M, Kastrati A. Stent thrombosis and restenosis: what have we learned and where are we going? The Andreas Grüntzig Lecture ESC 2014. Eur Heart J. 2015;36:3320–31.
16. Buccheri D, Piraino D, Andolina G, Cortese B. Understanding and managing in-stent restenosis: a review of clinical data, from pathogenesis to treatment. J Thorac Dis. 2016;8:E1150–62.
17. Scheller B, Speck U, Schmitt A, Böhm M, Nickenig G. Addition of paclitaxel to contrast media prevents restenosis after coronary stent implantation. J Am Coll Cardiol. 2003;42:1415–20.
18. Scheller B, Hehrlein C, Bocksch W, et al. Treatment of coronary in-stent restenosis with a paclitaxel-coated balloon catheter. N Engl J Med. 2006;355:2113–24.
19. Scheller B, Speck U, Abramjuk C, Bernhardt U, Bohm M, Nickenig G. Paclitaxel balloon coating, a novel method for prevention and therapy of restenosis. Circulation. 2004;110:810–4.
20. Alfonso F, Scheller B. State of the art: balloon catheter technologies – drug-coated balloon. EuroIntervention. 2017;13:680–95.
21. Palma G, Sanchez-Jimenez EF, Lazar L, Cortese B. Should paclitaxel be considered an old generation DCB? The limus era. RCM. 2021;22:1323–30.
22. Herdeg C, Oberhoff M, Baumbach A, et al. Local paclitaxel delivery for the prevention of restenosis: biological effects and efficacy in vivo. J Am Coll Cardiol. 2000;35:1969–76.
23. Marx SO, Marks AR. Bench to bedside: the development of rapamycin and its application to stent restenosis. Circulation. 2001;104:852–5.
24. Martinet W, De Loof H, De Meyer GRY. mTOR inhibition: a promising strategy for stabilization of atherosclerotic plaques. Atherosclerosis. 2014;233:601–7.

25. Elgendy IY, Gad MM, Elgendy AY, et al. Clinical and angiographic outcomes with drug-coated balloons for de novo coronary lesions: a meta-analysis of randomized clinical trials. J Am Heart Assoc. 2020;9:e016224.
26. Cao Z, Li J, Fang Z, Feierkaiti Y, Zheng X, Jiang X. The factors influencing the efficiency of drug-coated balloons. Front Cardiovasc Med. 2022;9:947776.
27. Axel DI, Kunert W, Goggelmann C, et al. Paclitaxel inhibits arterial smooth muscle cell proliferation and migration in vitro and in vivo using local drug delivery. Circulation. 1997;96:636–45.
28. Clever YP, Peters D, Calisse J, et al. Novel sirolimus-coated balloon catheter: in vivo evaluation in a porcine coronary model. Circ Cardiovasc Interv. 2016;9:e003543.
29. Mehta SK, Frutkin AD, Lindsey JB, et al. Bleeding in patients undergoing percutaneous coronary intervention: the development of a clinical risk algorithm from the National Cardiovascular Data Registry. Circ Cardiovasc Interv. 2009;2:222–9.
30. Dauerman HL, Rao SV, Resnic FS, Applegate RJ. Bleeding avoidance strategies. Consensus and controversy. J Am Coll Cardiol. 2011;58:1–10.
31. Ono M, Kawashima H, Hara H, et al. A prospective multicenter randomized trial to assess the effectiveness of the MagicTouch sirolimus-coated balloon in small vessels: rationale and design of the TRANSFORM I trial. Cardiovasc Revasc Med. 2021;25:29–35.
32. Kleber FX, Mathey DG, Rittger H, Scheller B. German drug-eluting Balloon Consensus G. How to use the drug-eluting balloon: recommendations by the German Consensus Group. EuroIntervention. 2011;(7 Suppl K):K125-8.
33. Kleber FX, Rittger H, Bonaventura K, et al. Drug-coated balloons for treatment of coronary artery disease: updated recommendations from a consensus group. Clin Res Cardiol. 2013;102:785–97.
34. Koo B-K, Hwang D, Park S, et al. Practical application of coronary physiological assessment. JACC: Asia. 0
35. Shin ES, Bang LH, Jun EJ, et al. Provisional drug-coated balloon treatment guided by physiology on de novo coronary lesion. Cardiol J. 2021;28:615–22.
36. Ann SH, Balbir Singh G, Lim KH, Koo BK, Shin ES. Anatomical and physiological changes after paclitaxel-coated balloon for atherosclerotic de novo coronary lesions: serial IVUS-VH and FFR study. PLoS One. 2016;11:e0147057.
37. Her AY, Ann SH, Singh GB, et al. Serial morphological changes of side-branch ostium after paclitaxel-coated balloon treatment of de novo coronary lesions of main vessels. Yonsei Med J. 2016;57:606–13.
38. Glagov S, Weisenberg E, Zarins CK, Stankunavicius R, Kolettis GJ. Compensatory enlargement of human atherosclerotic coronary arteries. N Engl J Med. 1987;316:1371–5.
39. Palmerini T, Bacchi Reggiani L, Della Riva D, et al. Bleeding-related deaths in relation to the duration of dual-antiplatelet therapy after coronary stenting. J Am Coll Cardiol. 2017;69:2011–22.
40. Rajani R, Lindblom M, Dixon G, et al. Evolving trends in percutaneous coronary intervention. Br J Cardiol. 2011;18:73–6.
41. Abadie BQ, Cannon CP, Cavender MA. Novel oral anticoagulants following percutaneous coronary intervention. Circ Cardiovasc Interv. 2020;13:e008465.
42. January CT, Wann LS, Calkins H, et al. 2019 AHA/ACC/HRS focused update of the 2014 AHA/ACC/HRS guideline for the management of patients with atrial fibrillation: a report of the American College of Cardiology/American Heart Association Task Force on Clinical Practice Guidelines and the Heart Rhythm Society. J Am Coll Cardiol. 2019;74:104–32.
43. Cutlip DE, Windecker S, Mehran R, et al. Clinical end points in coronary stent trials: a case for standardized definitions. Circulation. 2007;115:2344–51.
44. Shlofmitz E, Iantorno M, Waksman R. Restenosis of drug-eluting stents: a new classification system based on disease mechanism to guide treatment and state-of-the-art review. Circ Cardiovasc Interv. 2019;12:e007023.
45. Dangas GD, Claessen BE, Caixeta A, Sanidas EA, Mintz GS, Mehran R. In-stent restenosis in the drug-eluting stent era. J Am Coll Cardiol. 2010;56:1897–907.
46. Alfonso F, Byrne RA, Rivero F, Kastrati A. Current treatment of in-stent restenosis. J Am Coll Cardiol. 2014;63:2659–73.
47. Writing Committee M, Lawton JS, Tamis-Holland JE, et al. 2021 ACC/AHA/SCAI guideline for coronary artery revascularization: a report of the American College of Cardiology/American Heart Association Joint Committee on Clinical Practice Guidelines. J Am Coll Cardiol. 2022;79:e21–e129.
48. Giustino G, Colombo A, Camaj A, et al. Coronary in-stent restenosis: JACC state-of-the-art review. J Am Coll Cardiol. 2022;80:348–72.
49. Graham MM, Ghali WA, Faris PD, et al. Survival after coronary revascularization in the elderly. Circulation. 2002;105:2378–84.
50. Giacoppo D, Alfonso F, Xu B, et al. Drug-coated balloon angioplasty versus drug-eluting stent implantation in patients with coronary stent restenosis. J Am Coll Cardiol. 2020;75:2664–78.
51. Alfonso F, Perez-Vizcayno MJ, Cardenas A, et al. A prospective randomized trial of drug-eluting balloons versus everolimus-eluting stents in patients with in-stent restenosis of drug-eluting stents: the RIBS IV Randomized Clinical Trial. J Am Coll Cardiol. 2015;66:23–33.
52. Byrne RA, Cassese S, Windisch T, et al. Differential relative efficacy between drug-eluting stents in patients with bare metal and drug-eluting stent restenosis; evidence in support of drug resistance: insights from the ISAR-DESIRE and ISAR-DESIRE 2 trials. EuroIntervention. 2013;9:797–802.
53. Byrne RA, Neumann FJ, Mehilli J, et al. Paclitaxel-eluting balloons, paclitaxel-eluting stents, and balloon

angioplasty in patients with restenosis after implantation of a drug-eluting stent (ISAR-DESIRE 3): a randomised, open-label trial. Lancet. 2013;381:461–7.
54. Indermuehle A, Bahl R, Lansky AJ, et al. Drug-eluting balloon angioplasty for in-stent restenosis: a systematic review and meta-analysis of randomised controlled trials. Heart. 2013;99:327–33.
55. Unverdorben M, Vallbracht C, Cremers B, et al. Paclitaxel-coated balloon catheter versus paclitaxel-coated stent for the treatment of coronary in-stent restenosis: the three-year results of the PEPCAD II ISR study. EuroIntervention. 2015;11:926–34.
56. Giacoppo D, Alfonso F, Xu B, et al. Paclitaxel-coated balloon angioplasty vs. drug-eluting stenting for the treatment of coronary in-stent restenosis: a comprehensive, collaborative, individual patient data meta-analysis of 10 randomized clinical trials (DAEDALUS study). Eur Heart J. 2020;41:3715–28.
57. Tanaka A, Latib A, Jabbour RJ, et al. Impact of angiographic result after predilatation on outcome after drug-coated balloon treatment of in-stent coronary restenosis. Am J Cardiol. 2016;118:1460–5.
58. Wang X, Lu W, Wang X, et al. Drug-coated balloon angioplasty: predicting outcomes based on different patterns of drug-eluting stent restenosis. Int J Cardiovasc Imaging. 2020;36:171–8.
59. Nakamura M, Yaku H, Ako J, et al. JCS/JSCVS 2018 guideline on revascularization of stable coronary artery disease. Circ J. 2022;86:477–588.
60. Neumann FJ, Sousa-Uva M, Ahlsson A, et al. 2018 ESC/EACTS guidelines on myocardial revascularization. Eur Heart J. 2019;40:87–165.
61. Stefanini GG, Alfonso F, Barbato E, et al. Management of myocardial revascularisation failure: an expert consensus document of the EAPCI. EuroIntervention. 2020;16:e875–90.
62. Siontis GC, Piccolo R, Praz F, et al. Percutaneous coronary interventions for the treatment of stenoses in small coronary arteries: a network meta-analysis. JACC Cardiovasc Interv. 2016;9:1324–34.
63. Elezi S, Kastrati A, Neumann FJ, Hadamitzky M, Dirschinger J, Schomig A. Vessel size and long-term outcome after coronary stent placement. Circulation. 1998;98:1875–80.
64. Ellis SG, Popma JJ, Lasala JM, et al. Relationship between angiographic late loss and target lesion revascularization after coronary stent implantation: analysis from the TAXUS-IV trial. J Am Coll Cardiol. 2005;45:1193–200.
65. Mauri L, Orav EJ, Kuntz RE. Late loss in lumen diameter and binary restenosis for drug-eluting stent comparison. Circulation. 2005;111:3435–42.
66. Cortese B, Di Palma G, Guimaraes MG, et al. Drug-coated balloon versus drug-eluting stent for small coronary vessel disease: PICCOLETO II Randomized Clinical Trial. JACC Cardiovasc Interv. 2020;13:2840–9.
67. Cortese B, Micheli A, Picchi A, et al. Paclitaxel-coated balloon versus drug-eluting stent during PCI of small coronary vessels, a prospective randomised clinical trial. PICCOLETO Study Heart. 2010;96:1291–6.
68. Jeger RV, Farah A, Ohlow MA, et al. Drug-coated balloons for small coronary artery disease (BASKET-SMALL 2): an open-label randomised non-inferiority trial. Lancet. 2018;392:849–56.
69. Latib A, Colombo A, Castriota F, et al. A randomized multicenter study comparing a paclitaxel drug-eluting balloon with a paclitaxel-eluting stent in small coronary vessels: the BELLO (balloon elution and late loss optimization) study. J Am Coll Cardiol. 2012;60:2473–80.
70. Sanz Sanchez J, Chiarito M, Cortese B, et al. Drug-coated balloons vs drug-eluting stents for the treatment of small coronary artery disease: a meta-analysis of randomized trials. Catheter Cardiovasc Interv. 2021;98:66–75.
71. Silverio A, Buccheri S, Venetsanos D, et al. Percutaneous treatment and outcomes of small coronary vessels: a SCAAR report. JACC Cardiovasc Interv. 2020;13:793–804.
72. Tian J, Tang YD, Qiao S, et al. Two-year follow-up of a randomized multicenter study comparing a drug-coated balloon with a drug-eluting stent in native small coronary vessels: the RESTORE Small Vessel Disease China Trial. Catheter Cardiovasc Interv. 2020;95(Suppl 1):587–97.
73. Rissanen TT, Uskela S, Eränen J, et al. Drug-coated balloon for treatment of de-novo coronary artery lesions in patients with high bleeding risk (DEBUT): a single-blind, randomised, non-inferiority trial. Lancet (London, England). 2019;394:230–9.
74. Fezzi S, Giacoppo D, Fahrni G, Latib A, Alfonso F, Colombo A, Mahfoud F, Scheller B, Jeger R, Cortese B. Individual patient data meta-analysis of paclitaxel-coated balloons vs. drug-eluting stents for small-vessel coronary artery disease: the ANDROMEDA study. Eur Heart J. 2025;46(17):1586–1599. https://doi.org/10.1093/eurheartj/ehaf002. PMID: 39981922.
75. Al Suwaidi J, Berger PB, Rihal CS, et al. Immediate and long-term outcome of intracoronary stent implantation for true bifurcation lesions. J Am Coll Cardiol. 2000;35:929–36.
76. Latib A, Colombo A. Bifurcation disease: what do we know, what should we do? JACC Cardiovasc Interv. 2008;1:218–26.
77. Feldman D, Beerkens F, Nicolas J, et al. Defining key features of complex coronary lesions: an evidence based review of clinical practice. Part I: Bifurcations, left main disease, and calcifications. RCM. 2022;23
78. Jang WJ, Ahn SG, Song YB, et al. Benefit of prolonged dual antiplatelet therapy after implantation of drug-eluting stent for coronary bifurcation lesions: results from the Coronary Bifurcation Stenting Registry II. Circ Cardiovasc Interv. 2018;11:e005849.
79. De Filippo O, Kang J, Bruno F, et al. Benefit of extended dual antiplatelet therapy duration in acute coronary syndrome patients treated with drug eluting stents for coronary bifurcation lesions

(from the BIFURCAT Registry). Am J Cardiol. 2021;156:16–23.
80. Megaly M, Rofael M, Saad M, Shishehbor M, Brilakis ES. Outcomes with drug-coated balloons for treating the side branch of coronary bifurcation lesions. J Invasive Cardiol. 2018;30:393–9.
81. Worthley S, Hendriks R, Worthley M, et al. Paclitaxel-eluting balloon and everolimus-eluting stent for provisional stenting of coronary bifurcations: 12-month results of the multicenter BIOLUX-I study. Cardiovasc Revasc Med. 2015;16:413–7.
82. Berland J, Lefevre T, Brenot P, et al. DANUBIO – a new drug-eluting balloon for the treatment of side branches in bifurcation lesions: six-month angiographic follow-up results of the DEBSIDE trial. EuroIntervention. 2015;11:868–76.
83. Valgimigli M, Bueno H, Byrne RA, et al. 2017 ESC focused update on dual antiplatelet therapy in coronary artery disease developed in collaboration with EACTS. Eur Heart J. 2018;39:213–60.
84. Vranckx P, Valgimigli M, Jüni P, et al. Ticagrelor plus aspirin for 1 month, followed by ticagrelor monotherapy for 23 months vs aspirin plus clopidogrel or ticagrelor for 12 months, followed by aspirin monotherapy for 12 months after implantation of a drug-eluting stent: a multicentre, open-label, randomised superiority trial. Lancet. 2018;392:940–9.
85. Valgimigli M, Frigoli E, Heg D, et al. Dual antiplatelet therapy after PCI in patients at high bleeding risk. N Engl J Med. 2021;385:1643–55.
86. Mehran R, Baber U, Sharma SK, et al. Ticagrelor with or without aspirin in high-risk patients after PCI. N Engl J Med. 2019;381:2032–42.
87. Windecker S, Latib A, Kedhi E, et al. Polymer-based or polymer-free stents in patients at high bleeding risk. N Engl J Med. 2020;382:1208–18.
88. Hahn J-Y, Song YB, Oh J-H, et al. Effect of P2Y12 inhibitor monotherapy vs dual antiplatelet therapy on cardiovascular events in patients undergoing percutaneous coronary intervention: the SMART-CHOICE Randomized Clinical Trial. JAMA. 2019;321:2428–37.
89. Leon MB, Baim DS, Popma JJ, et al. A clinical trial comparing three antithrombotic-drug regimens after coronary-artery stenting. N Engl J Med. 1998;339:1665–71.
90. Biondi-Zoccai GGL, Lotrionte M, Agostoni P, et al. A systematic review and meta-analysis on the hazards of discontinuing or not adhering to aspirin among 50,279 patients at risk for coronary artery disease. Eur Heart J. 2006;27:2667–74.
91. Lee S-J, Choi D-W, Suh Y, et al. Long-term clinical outcomes between biodegradable and durable polymer drug-eluting stents: a Nationwide Cohort Study. Front Cardiovasc Med. 2022;9:873114.
92. Varenne O, Cook S, Sideris G, et al. Drug-eluting stents in elderly patients with coronary artery disease (SENIOR): a randomised single-blind trial. Lancet (London, England). 2018;391:41–50.
93. Urban P, Meredith IT, Abizaid A, et al. Polymer-free drug-coated coronary stents in patients at high bleeding risk. N Engl J Med. 2015;373:2038–47.
94. Valgimigli M, Patialiakas A, Thury A, et al. Zotarolimus-eluting versus bare-metal stents in uncertain drug-eluting stent candidates. J Am Coll Cardiol. 2015;65:805–15.
95. Räsänen A, Kärkkäinen JM, Eranti A, Eränen J, Rissanen TT. Percutaneous coronary intervention with drug-coated balloon-only strategy combined with single antiplatelet treatment in patients at high bleeding risk: single center experience of a novel concept. Catheter Cardiovasc Interv. 2023;101:569–78.

Drug-Coated Balloons (DCB): Clinical Data from Registries to Randomized Trials

9

Alexandre Abizaid, Brunna Pileggi, and Pedro C. Melo

Abbreviations

PCI	percutaneous coronary intervention
POBA	plain old balloon angioplasty
BMS	bare-metal stents
DES	drug-eluting stents
ISR	in-stent restenosis
CABG	coronary artery bypass grafting
DCB	drug-coated balloons
DAPT	dual antiplatelet therapy
SMC	smooth muscle cell
SCB	sirolimus-coated balloons
PCB	paclitaxel-coated balloons
LLL	late lumen loss
SVD	small vessel disease
HBR	high bleeding risk
MI	myocardial infarction
SAPT	single-antiplatelet therapy
MACE	major adverse cardiac events
TLR	target lesion revascularization
ACS	acute coronary syndrome

A. Abizaid (✉)
University of São Paulo Medical School – FMUSP, Ribeirão Preto, Brazil

Interventional Cardiology at the Heart Institute of Sao Paulo (InCor), São Paulo, Brazil

B. Pileggi · P. C. Melo
Interventional Cardiology at the Heart Institute of Sao Paulo (InCor), São Paulo, Brazil
e-mail: brunna.pileggi@hc.fm.usp.br

9.1 Introduction

The history of percutaneous coronary intervention (PCI) began in 1977 when Andreas Gruentzig pioneered the plain old balloon angioplasty (POBA). Following, bare-metal stents (BMS) emerged to overcome the main challenges and limitations of POBA, such as acute elastic recoil and flow-limiting dissections. However, the long-term efficacy of PCI was limited by high rates of in-stent restenosis [1, 2]. Drug-eluting stents (DES) revolutionized the field of interventional cardiology, significantly reducing neointimal hyperplasia and the consequent in-stent restenosis (ISR). More recently, second-generation DES, with thinner struts; lower doses of antiproliferative drugs; and more biocompatible polymers resulted in better vascular healing and endothelization, with reduced rates of stent thrombosis (Fig. 9.1) [3, 4].

Despite significant technological advancements in DES platforms, and the more frequent use of intravascular imaging and calcium modification techniques, stent failure remains common in scenarios such as extensive calcification and long coronary lesions. This results in PCI having a more modest long-term efficacy than coronary artery bypass grafting (CABG). Additionally, the annual rate of stent-related events (i.e., target lesion revascularization or stent thrombosis) remains steady over 1% between the fifth and tenth years following PCI [5, 6].

B. Cortese, S. Rigattieri (eds.), *High Bleeding Risk Patients in Interventional Cardiology*, https://doi.org/10.1007/978-3-031-87302-7_9

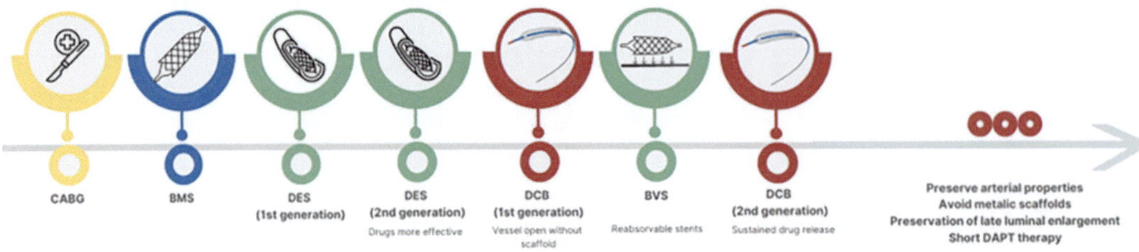

Fig. 9.1 Advancements in technologies for coronary revascularization. *CABG* coronary artery bypass grafting. *BMS* bare-metal stent, *DES* drug-eluting stent, *DCB*, drug-coated ballon, *BVS* bioresorbable vascular scaffold

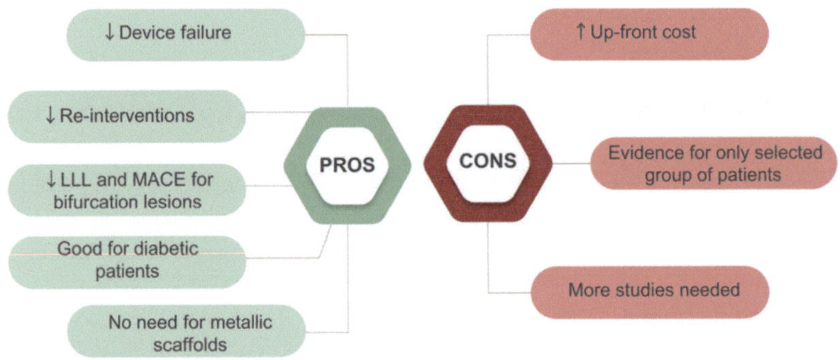

Fig. 9.2 Pros and cons of DCB angioplasty. *LLL* late lumen loss, *MACE* major adverse cardiovascular events

Drug-coated balloons (DCB) have been increasingly used for coronary revascularization in multiple clinical contexts. This approach integrates balloon angioplasty with the controlled delivery of antiproliferative drugs (e.g., sirolimus and paclitaxel) preserving vasomotion and enabling adaptive remodeling. Unlike permanent metal scaffold implants, DCBs mitigate the risk of vascular constriction and distortion, thereby maintaining vascular architecture integrity, and most importantly, without leaving any scaffold behind [7, 8]. Since stents have no functional role once an artery has healed and there is a non-neglectable residual risk of stent-related adverse events in the late follow-up, DCBs would be preferred over permanent implants if they achieve similar acute results in a broader angiographic spectrum.

DCB angioplasty also facilitates a shorter duration of dual antiplatelet therapy (DAPT), potentially lowering the risk of bleeding [9]. Consequently, the shift toward "intervention without metal scaffolds implantation" holds a special promise for patients at high bleeding risk, potentially enhancing outcomes by providing an effective acute result while reducing post-PCI bleeding and tardy ischemic events (Fig. 9.2).

9.2 Drug-Coated Balloons: Technical Aspects

DCB-only angioplasty is a relatively simple procedure in which a balloon catheter coated with an antiproliferative drug is inflated (0.8–1.0/1.0) at nominal pressures for 30–120 seconds. Adequate lesion preparation with balloon pre-dilation, scoring balloon, rotational atherectomy, or intravascular lithotripsy is strongly recommended before DCB dilation of complex lesions.

While inflated, the larger surface of the balloon in contact with the vessel wall allows a more even drug-tissue transfer compared to DES, yielding an effective inhibition of smooth muscle cell (SMC) proliferation and migration [10, 11]. Paclitaxel and sirolimus are the two antiproliferative drugs coating DCBs currently available on the market. Despite that, the technologies might significantly differ in terms of balloon design and polymeric matrix, making it difficult to assert that there is a class effect of DCBs.

Paclitaxel, the first antiproliferative medication used on DCB's coating, acts through the inhibition of cellular mitosis by binding to microtubes, and its highly lipophilic nature facilitates drug transfer to the cell membrane. On the other hand, sirolimus has a more desirable cytostatic nature, a wider therapeutic window, and has been associated with a long-lasting sustained effect [12, 13]. Sirolimus' mechanism of action relies on the mammalian target of rapamycin (mTOR) inhibition, ultimately restricting SMC proliferation and migration. Different comparisons between sirolimus-coated balloons (SCB) and paclitaxel-coated balloons (PCB) have revealed similar late lumen loss (LLL) and clinical events at 12 months [14, 15].

DCB is widely regarded as the preferred treatment for ISR, with substantial evidence supporting its benefits in managing small vessel disease (SVD) [16]. However, the clinical efficacy of DCB in coronary de novo stenosis and challenging clinical subsets of patients require further investigation. This chapter examines the latest evidence on the use of DCB for treating HBR patients.

9.3 DCB-PCI in High-Bleeding-Risk Patients

More than 40% of patients undergoing PCI with current-generation DES are at high bleeding risk (HBR), with increased mortality and myocardial infarction (MI) rates compared to non-HBR patients [17]. Post-PCI management of HBR patients is the subject of extensive debate among interventional cardiologists, as they challenge paradigms regarding the duration and choice of DAPT, as well as drug combination options, and the selection of the ideal medication when transitioning to single-antiplatelet therapy (SAPT) [18, 19, 20]. In 2019, Urban et al. published the Academic Research Consortium for High Bleeding Risk (ARC-HBR) establishing the most widely adopted high bleeding risk definition [21]. The ACR-HBR criteria were validated in large-scale "real-world" registries with thousands of patients who underwent PCI, showing a significant stepwise increase in bleeding risk corresponding to the number of criteria met [22, 23].

Retrospective registries have indicated a low rate of target-lesion revascularization following DCB-PCI, coupled with the advantage of requiring a shorter duration of DAPT [24]. A 4-week DAPT duration following DCB-PCI was previously proven safe and has been recommended by specialist consensus [25, 26]. More recent evidence supports that the second antiplatelet agent can even be dropped in the presence of unexpected bleeding or urgent surgery with relevant safety and efficacy [27]. Furthermore, in a comprehensive single-center registry encompassing 487 PCI procedures performed with DCBs, the median DAPT duration was 1 month. Notably, 4% of these procedures were conducted with single-antiplatelet therapy due to extremely high bleeding risk with a minimal incidence of thrombotic complications (0.2% of acute vessel closure) [28].

Räsänen et al. published a single-center registry with 172 elderly patients (87% of HBR) assessing the safety and efficacy of using single-antiplatelet therapy (SAPT) following DCB PCI to treat mainly de novo lesions in large vessels. The 12-month MACE rate was 1.4% in stable CAD and 7.1% in ACS. The rate of ischemia-driven TLR was 0% in stable CAD and 3.0% in ACS at 12 months, and the 12-month rate of

BARC type 2–5 bleeding was 10.5% [29]. These findings on DCB PCI followed by SAPT will be tested in the DEBATE trial which is currently recruiting (NTC04814212).

The DEBUT trial was a randomized, single-blind, non-inferiority trial involving patients at high bleeding risk undergoing PCI. Two hundred eight patients with de novo lesions (2.5–4.0 mm) in native coronaries or bypass grafts were randomized to receive either a paclitaxel-coated balloon or a bare-metal stent (BMS). Both groups received DAPT for 1 month regardless of acute or stable presentation. At 9-month follow-up, major adverse cardiac events (MACE) occurred less often with DCB treatment (1 vs. 14%). Similarly, target lesion revascularization (TLR) was less frequent with DCB (0 vs. 6%). The DEBUT trial's results supported the safety and efficacy of DCB-PCI in large de novo lesions in HBR patients receiving 1 month of DAPT. The main limitations of the study were the imbalance of randomization regarding diabetes and the use of BMS as a competitor [30].

A recent post hoc analysis of the BASKET-SMALL 2 trial, with 155 high-bleeding-risk patients among the 758 originally randomized, revealed that HBR was significantly associated with higher mortality rates at 3 years (HR 3.09; $p < 0.001$). For major adverse cardiac events (MACE), there were no significant differences between DCB and DES in the overall population, regardless of the bleeding risk (HR 1.16; $p = 0.719$ for HBR vs. non-HBR, HR 0.96; $p = 0.863$). Major bleeding events overall tended to be nonsignificantly lower after DCB versus DES (1.6% versus 3.7%; $P = 0.064$) [31].

Cortese et al. also investigated the safety and efficacy of a SAPT in solo-DCB angioplasty, comparing it to a standard DAPT in a HBR population, and found similar rates of MACE at 1 year (9 vs. 10%, HR 1.03, CI 0.53–1.98), with no cases of acute vessel closure in both groups. The SAPT group shower reduced rates of BARC 2–5 bleedings (9 vs. 9%, HR 0.80, CI 0.38–0.98) [32].

The ongoing PICCOLETO IV-EPIC trial is randomizing HBR or elderly patients who undergone DCB angioplasty to SAPT and DAPT and along with the DEBATE trial will shed light on this therapeutic strategy in HBR patients.

Ongoing DCB trials specifically involving HBR patients are presented in Table 9.1, whereas in Table 9.2 we present promising trials related to the use of DCBs in the general population.

Table 9.1 Ongoing trials regarding DCB and HBR patients

Trial	NCT	Status	Study population	Number of participants	Randomization	Key outcomes	Follow-up
DCB-HBR	NCT05221931	Recruiting	Denovo coronary lesion	1350	DCB vs. DES	TVF at 24 mo. CV death at 24 mo. TV-MI at 24 mo. TLR at 24 mo. ST at 24 mo.	24 months
DEBATE	NCT04814212	Recruiting	Stable CAD or ACS	546	DCB vs. DES	Composite of MACE and BARC 2–5 bleeding at 12 mo. BARC 35 bleedings at 12, 24, and 36 mo. CV death at 12, 24, and 36 mo. TVF at 12, 24, and 36 mo. TLR at 12, 24, and 36 mo.	36 months
DEBORA	NCT04885816	Completed	Elective PCI	Unknown	DCB vs. DES	TLF at 12 mo. CV death at 12 mo. TV-MI at 12 mo.	12 months
PARIS	NCT06321757	Recruiting	Small native vessel coronary artery disease	501	DCB Standard DAPT. Short DAPT.	Effectiveness of DCB (MACE) at 12 mo. CV death at 12 mo. TLR at 12 mo. TVF at 12 mo. TV-MI at 12 mo. Major bleeding at 12 mo.	12 months
Ticagrelor as SAPT after DCB	NCT06088433	Recruiting	Primary coronary small vessel disease	234	DCB SAPT (ticagrelor). DAPT (ASA plus clopidogrel)	MACE at 12 mo. MACE at 1 mo. Thromboelastogram at 12 mo.	12 months
PICCOLETO IV-EPIC	NCT06761422	Recruiting	Stable or unstable CAD	412	Solo-DCB PCI randomized to the following: SAPT. DAPT.	MACE at 12 mo. NACE at 12 mo.	12 months

ASA aspirin, *ACS* acute coronary syndrome, *BARC* bleeding academic research consortium, *CAD* coronary artery disease, *CV* cardiovascular, *DAPT* dual antiplatelet therapy, *DCB* drug-coated ballon, *DES* drug-eluting stent, *HBR* high bleeding risk, *MACE* major adverse cardiovascular events, *PCI* percutaneous coronary intervention, *SAPT* single-antiplatelet therapy, *TLR* target lesion revascularization, *TVF* target vessel failure, *TV-MI* target vessel myocardial infarction

Table 9.2 Ongoing trials regarding DCB in general population

Trial	NCT	Status	Study population	Number of participants	Randomization	Key outcomes	Follow-up
ISAR-DESIRE5	NCT05544864	Recruiting	In-stent restenosis seen by OCT	376	DES (Xience, Abbott vascular) vs. PCB (Boston Scientific)	MACE at 24 mo. TLR at 24 mo. TLF at 24 mo. ST at 24 mo.	24 months
DCB with IVUS	NCT04475978	Recruiting	STEMI	208	DCB with IVUS vs. angiography	LLL at 9 mo. TLF at 12 mo.	12 months
TRANSFORM I	NCT03913832	Active, not recruiting	De novo coronary artery lesions in small vessels	121	SCB (magic touch, concept medical) vs. PCB (SeQuent please TM, B.Braun)	Net gain (mm) in 6mo. LLL at 6 mo. Restenosis rate at 6 mo. Cardiac death 1, 6, and 12 mo. TV-MI at 1, 6, and 12 mo. TLR at 1, 6, and 12 mo.	12 months
TRANSFORM II	NCT04893291	Recruiting	De novo coronary artery lesions in small to medium vessels	1820	SCB (magic touch, concept medical) vs. EES	TLF at 12 mo. NACE at 12 mo. Cardiac death at 60 mo. TVR at 60 mo.	60 months
DCB for CTO	NCT04744571	Completed	CTO located in epicardial coronary artery	200	DCB vs. DES	LLL at 12 mo. MACE at 12 mo.	12 months
DCB vs. DES guided by OCT	NCT04664283	Unknown*	De novo coronary artery lesions in large vessels (non-inferiority)	254	DCB vs. DES	LLL at 12 mo. Device-related ischemic events at 12 mo. Patient-related ischemic events at 12 mo.	12 months
PRO-DAVID	NCT04403048	Unknown†	De novo bifurcation lesion with affected side branch	800	Standard procedure vs. DCB	MACE at 12 mo. ST at 12 mo. Angiographic success immediately after procedure	12 months
D-LESION LONG	NCT03155971	Unknown§	De novo lesions of main coronary arteries	60	Single arm (PCB)	Minimal lumen diameter by QCA at 9 mo.	9 months

CTO chronic total occlusion, *DCB* drug-coated ballon, *DES* drug-eluting stent, *EES* everolimus-eluting stent, *IVUS* intravascular ultrasound, *LLL* late lumen loss, *MACE*, major adverse cardiovascular events, *NACE* net adverse clinical events, *OCT* optical coherence tomography, *PCB* paclitaxel-coated ballon, *QCA* quantitative coronary angiography, *SCB* sirolimus-coated ballon, *ST* stent thrombosis, *STEMI* ST-segment elevated myocardial infarction, *TLF* target lesion failure, *TLR* target vessel revascularization, *TV-MI* target vessel myocardial infarction

*Last updated in December, 2020

§ Last updated in May 20

† Last updated in May, 2020

9.4 Conclusion and Future Perspectives

DCB technology has emerged as an appealing alternative for patients deemed unsuitable for conventional DAPT due to HBR. The current evidence underscores the safety of shorter DAPT durations with low rates of acute vessel closure and MACE. In addition, there is a signal of potential reduction of bleeding events. The DEBUT trial, a clinical study particularly devoted to HBR patients with large-vessel de novo lesions, showed minimal adverse cardiac events with the DCB-only strategy and reduced MACE rated in comparison to BMS. Despite these promising results, several aspects of DCB application in HBR patients still require further exploration, and the optimal duration of DAPT following DCB-PCI remains a subject of ongoing research.

In conclusion, while retrospective registries and smaller studies have provided encouraging data, large-scale randomized controlled trials are necessary to confirm the long-term benefits and safety of DCBs against DES, before establishing DCBs as the frontline therapy for HBR patients with coronary artery disease.

References

1. Grüntzig AR, Senning Å, Siegenthaler WE. Nonoperative dilatation of coronary-artery stenosis: percutaneous transluminal coronary angioplasty. N Engl J Med. 1979 Jul 12;301(2):61–8.
2. Fischman DL, Leon MB, Baim DS, Schatz RA, Savage MP, Penn I, Detre K, Veltri L, Ricci D, Nobuyoshi M, Cleman M. A randomized comparison of coronary-stent placement and balloon angioplasty in the treatment of coronary artery disease. N Engl J Med. 1994 Aug 25;331(8):496–501.
3. Kirtane AJ, Gupta A, Iyengar S, Moses JW, Leon MB, Applegate R, Brodie B, Hannan E, Harjai K, Jensen LO, Park SJ. Safety and efficacy of drug-eluting and bare metal stents: comprehensive meta-analysis of randomized trials and observational studies. Circulation. 2009 Jun 30;119(25):3198–206.
4. Planer D, Smits PC, Kereiakes DJ, Kedhi E, Fahy M, Xu K, Serruys PW, Stone GW. Comparison of everolimus-and paclitaxel-eluting stents in patients with acute and stable coronary syndromes: pooled results from the SPIRIT (a clinical evaluation of the XIENCE V Everolimus eluting coronary stent system) and COMPARE (a trial of Everolimus-eluting stents and paclitaxel-eluting stents for coronary revascularization in daily practice) trials. J Am Coll Cardiol Intv. 2011 Oct;4(10):1104–15.
5. Fearon WF, Zimmermann FM, De Bruyne B, Piroth Z, van Straten AH, Szekely L, Davidavičius G, Kalinauskas G, Mansour S, Kharbanda R, Östlund-Papadogeorgos N. Fractional flow reserve–guided PCI as compared with coronary bypass surgery. N Engl J Med. 2022 Jan 13;386(2):128–37.
6. Brugaletta S, Gomez-Lara J, Ortega-Paz L, Jimenez-Diaz V, Jimenez M, Jiménez-Quevedo P, Diletti R, Mainar V, Campo G, Silvestro A, Maristany J. 10-year follow-up of patients with everolimus-eluting versus bare-metal stents after ST-segment elevation myocardial infarction. J Am Coll Cardiol. 2021 Mar 9;77(9):1165–78.
7. Richelsen RK, Overvad TF, Jensen SE. Drug-eluting balloons in the treatment of coronary de novo lesions: a comprehensive review. Cardiol Ther. 2016 Dec;5:133–60.
8. Patel S, Svermova T, Burke-Gaffney A, Bogle RG. Drug-eluting balloons with provisional bail-out or adjunctive stenting in de novo coronary artery lesions—a systematic review and meta-analysis. Cardiovasc Diagn Ther. 2018 Apr;8(2):121.
9. Sorrentino S, Claessen BE, Chandiramani R, Guedeney P, Vogel B, Baber U, Rau V, Wang J, Krucoff M, Kozuma K, Ge J. Long-term safety and efficacy of durable polymer cobalt-chromium everolimus-eluting stents in patients at high bleeding risk: a patient-level stratified analysis from four postapproval studies. Circulation. 2020 Mar 17;141(11):891–901.
10. Speck U, Stolzenburg N, Peters D, Scheller B. How does a drug-coated balloon work? Overview of coating techniques and their impact. J Cardiovasc Surg. 2016 Feb 1;57(1):3–11.
11. Granada JF, Stenoien M, Buszman PP, Tellez A, Langanki D, Kaluza GL, Leon MB, Gray W, Jaff MR, Schwartz RS. Mechanisms of tissue uptake and retention of paclitaxel-coated balloons: impact on neointimal proliferation and healing. Open Heart. 2014 Aug 1;1(1):e000117.
12. Scheller B, Hehrlein C, Bocksch W, Rutsch W, Haghi D, Dietz U, Böhm M, Speck U. Treatment of coronary in-stent restenosis with a paclitaxel-coated balloon catheter. N Engl J Med. 2006 Nov 16;355(20):2113–24.
13. Clever YP, Peters D, Calisse J, Bettink S, Berg MC, Sperling C, Stoever M, Cremers B, Kelsch B, Böhm M, Speck U. Novel sirolimus–coated balloon catheter: in vivo evaluation in a porcine coronary model. Circ Cardiovasc Interv. 2016 Apr;9(4):e003543.
14. Ali RM, Abdul Kader MA, Wan Ahmad WA, Ong TK, Liew HB, Omar AF, Mahmood Zuhdi AS, Nuruddin AA, Schnorr B, Scheller B. Treatment of coronary drug-eluting stent restenosis by a sirolimus- or paclitaxel-coated balloon. Cardiovasc Interv. 2019 Mar 25;12(6):558–66.

15. Briguori C, Visconti G, Golino M, Focaccio A, Scarpelli M, Nuzzo S, Biondi-Zoccai G. Paclitexel versus sirolimus-coated balloon in the treatment of coronary instent restenosis. Panminerva Med. 2021 Nov 11;65(3):327–34.
16. Bondesson P, Lagerqvist B, James SK, Olivecrona GK, Venetsanos D, Harnek J. Comparison of two drug-eluting balloons: a report from the SCAAR registry. EuroIntervention. 2012 Aug 1;8(4):444–9.
17. Généreux P, Giustino G, Witzenbichler B, Weisz G, Stuckey TD, Rinaldi MJ, Neumann FJ, Metzger DC, Henry TD, Cox DA, Duffy PL. Incidence, predictors, and impact of post-discharge bleeding after percutaneous coronary intervention. J Am Coll Cardiol. 2015 Sep 1;66(9):1036–45.
18. Zhang WJ, Qiao X, Liang XY, Li Y, Yang RR, Wang ZL. Efficacy and safety of short-term 1–3 months versus standard 12 months dual antiplatelet therapy in patients undergoing percutaneous coronary intervention: a meta-analysis of randomized clinical trials. Platelets. 2021 Jul 4;32(5):582–90.
19. Mehran R, Baber U, Sharma SK, Cohen DJ, Angiolillo DJ, Briguori C, Cha JY, Collier T, Dangas G, Dudek D, Džavík V. Ticagrelor with or without aspirin in high-risk patients after PCI. N Engl J Med. 2019 Nov 21;381(21):2032–42.
20. Cui K, Lyu S, Song X, Yuan F, Xu F, Zhang M, Wang W, Zhang D, Dai J. Drug-eluting balloon versus bare-mental stent and drug-eluting stent for de novo coronary artery disease: a systematic review and meta-analysis of 14 randomized controlled trials. PLoS One. 2017 Apr 26;12(4):e0176365.
21. Urban P, Mehran R, Colleran R, Angiolillo DJ, Byrne RA, Capodanno D, Cuisset T, Cutlip D, Eerdmans P, Eikelboom J, Farb A. Defining high bleeding risk in patients undergoing percutaneous coronary intervention: a consensus document from the academic research consortium for high bleeding risk. Circulation. 2019 July 16;140(3):240–61.
22. Cao D, Mehran R, Dangas G, Baber U, Sartori S, Chandiramani R, Stefanini GG, Angiolillo DJ, Capodanno D, Urban P, Morice MC. Validation of the academic research consortium high bleeding risk definition in contemporary PCI patients. J Am Coll Cardiol. 2020 Jun 2;75(21):2711–22.
23. Corpataux N, Spirito A, Gragnano F, Vaisnora L, Galea R, Svab S, Gargiulo G, Zanchin T, Zanchin C, Siontis GC, Praz F. Validation of high bleeding risk criteria and definition as proposed by the academic research consortium for high bleeding risk. Eur Heart J. 2020 Oct 7;41(38):3743–9.
24. Cortese B, Testa L, Heang TM, Ielasi A, Bossi I, Latini RA, Lee CY, Perez IS, Milazzo D, Caiazzo G, Tomai F, Benincasa S, Nuruddin AA, Stefanini G, Buccheri D, Seresini G, Singh R, Karavolias G, Cacucci M, Sciahbasi A, Ocaranza R, Menown IBA, Torres A, Sengottvelu G, Zanetti A, Pesenti N, Colombo A; EASTBOURNE Investigators. Sirolimus-Coated Balloon in an All-Comer Population of Coronary Artery Disease Patients: The EASTBOURNE Prospective Registry. JACC Cardiovasc Interv. 2023 Jul 24;16(14):1794-1803. https://doi.org/10.1016/j.jcin.2023.05.005. PMID: 37495352.
25. Jeger RV, Eccleshall S, Wan Ahmad WA, Ge J, Poerner TC, Shin ES, Alfonso F, Latib A, Ong PJ, Rissanen TT, Saucedo J. Drug-coated balloons for coronary artery disease: third report of the international DCB consensus group. Cardiovasc Interv. 2020 Jun 22;13(12):1391–402.
26. Cortese B, Berti S, Biondi-Zoccai G, Colombo A, Limbruno U, Bedogni F, Cremonesi A, Silva PL, Sgueglia GA. Drug-coated balloon treatment of coronary artery disease: a position paper of the Italian Society of Interventional Cardiology. Catheter Cardiovasc Interv. 2014 Feb 15;83(3):427–35.
27. Cortese B, D'Ascenzo F, Fetiveau R, Balian V, Blengino S, Fineschi M, Rogacka R, Lettieri C, Pavei A, D'Amico M, Poli A, Di Palma G, Latini RA, Orrego PS, Seregni R. Treatment of coronary artery disease with a new-generation drug-coated balloon: final results of the Italian Elutax SV rEgistry-DCB-RISE. J Cardiovasc Med (Hagerstown). 2018;19:247–52.
28. Uskela S, Kärkkäinen JM, Eränen J, Siljander A, Mäntylä P, Mustonen J, Rissanen TT. Percutaneous coronary intervention with drug-coated balloon-only strategy in stable coronary artery disease and in acute coronary syndromes: an all-comers registry study. Catheter Cardiovasc Interv. 2019 Apr 1;93(5):893–900.
29. Räsänen A, Kärkkäinen JM, Eranti A, Eränen J, Rissanen TT. Percutaneous coronary intervention with drug-coated balloon-only strategy combined with single antiplatelet treatment in patients at high bleeding risk: single center experience of a novel concept. Catheter Cardiovasc Interv. 2023 Feb;101(3):569–78.
30. Rissanen TT, Uskela S, Eränen J, Mäntylä P, Olli A, Romppanen H, Siljander A, Pietilä M, Minkkinen MJ, Tervo J, Kärkkäinen JM. Drug-coated balloon for treatment of de-novo coronary artery lesions in patients with high bleeding risk (DEBUT): a single-blind, randomised, non-inferiority trial. Lancet. 2019 Jul 20;394(10194):230–9.
31. Scheller B, Rissanen TT, Farah A, Ohlow MA, Mangner N, Wöhrle J, Möbius-Winkler S, Weilenmann D, Leibundgut G, Cuculi F, Gilgen N. Drug-coated balloon for small coronary artery disease in patients with and without high-bleeding risk in the BASKET-SMALL 2 trial. Circ Cardiovasc Interv. 2022 Apr;15(4):e011569.
32. Cortese B, Serruys PW. Single-antiplatelet treatment after coronary angioplasty with drug-coated balloon. J Am Heart Assoc. 2023;12:e028413.

10 Is There a Potential Advantage of DCB Over DES, on the Long Term?

Takamasa Tanaka, Kenji Kawai, Renu Virmani, Bernardo Cortese, and Aloke V. Finn

10.1 Introduction

Percutaneous coronary intervention (PCI) has evolved over the past 40 years, with PCI becoming the most common treatment for patients with symptomatic coronary artery disease. While coronary stents are a mainstay in the treatment of PCI, they require appropriate antiplatelet therapy to prevent thrombosis formation in part because of the permanent implant of "foreign" metal material. Dual antiplatelet therapy (DAPT) is currently a well-known standard regimen after PCI involving aspirin and a P2Y212 inhibitor such as clopidogrel, ticagrelor, or prasugrel. While the DAPT trial has shown that continuing DAPT for an extended period (i.e., > 1 year) after PCI reduces the risk of stent thrombosis [1], long-term (i.e., 12 months or greater) DAPT has a well-documented increased risk of bleeding complications compared with short-term (1–3 months) DAPT [2]. Therefore, it is always necessary to consider the trade-off between the prevention of thrombotic events, including stent thrombosis and the risk of bleeding complications after the PCI, especially in patients at high bleeding risk (HBR). Although it is reasonable to predict and assess bleeding and thrombotic risks for individual patients and choose the appropriate duration of DAPT based on risk stratification, the appropriate antiplatelet regimen is still controversial in HBR patients because thrombogenicity in the lesion is affected not only by types of antiplatelet therapy but also by device factors such as strut thickness, the presence of polymer coating, and types of antiproliferative drugs, as well as lesion, factors i.e., thrombotic lesion or calcified lesion, etc. [3, 4].

Drug-coated balloons (DCB) are becoming more widely used not only for in-stent restenosis but also for de novo coronary artery lesions [5]. The most advantageous aspect of DCBs compared to DES is that they contain no metal scaffold which may lead to quicker healing with much lower risk of target lesion thrombosis. Therefore, DCB technologies have the potential to contribute to shortening the duration of DAPT in HBR patients who undergo PCI. In recent decades, evidence supporting short-term DAPT

T. Tanaka · K. Kawai · R. Virmani
CVPath Institute, Gaithersburg, MD, USA
e-mail: ttanaka@cvpath.org; kkawai@cvpath.org; rvirmani@cvpath.org

B. Cortese
University Hospitals Harrington Heart & Vascular Institute, Cleveland, OH, USA

Fondazione Ricerca e Innovazione Cardiovascolare, Milan, Italy

DCB Academy, Milan, Italy

A. V. Finn (✉)
CVPath Institute, Gaithersburg, MD, USA

University of Maryland, School of Medicine, Baltimore, MD, USA
e-mail: afinn@cvpath.org

B. Cortese, S. Rigattieri (eds.), *High Bleeding Risk Patients in Interventional Cardiology*,
https://doi.org/10.1007/978-3-031-87302-7_10

following PCI using new generation DES has been emerging through randomized and non-randomized trials. More recently, similar types of data are beginning to emerge for DCBs. This chapter provides a comprehensive review of the current understanding of HBR patients, antiplatelet therapy in these patients, and how device and lesion factors may determine which approach is best from the clinical, histological, and biological perspectives.

10.2 Clinical Evidence For Short-Term DAPT After DES

DAPT is administrated before or immediately after PCI and continues for a certain period and then shifts to single antiplatelet therapy with cessation of one of the two types of antiplatelet agents (i.e., either ASA or P2Y12 inhibitor) with P2Y12 most commonly being discontinued. In the current guidelines, the recommendation for the duration of antiplatelet therapy depends upon the clinical presentation with a division between those with stable or unstable symptoms/lesions. In 2017, the European Society of Cardiology (ESC) and the American College of Cardiology/American Heart Association (ACC/AHA) recommended a new standard guideline for the duration of DAPT following PCI: 6 months for patients with stable CAD and 12 months for patients with ACS. Nonetheless, the decision about DAPT duration also requires consideration of patient characteristics because prolonging DAPT leads to severe bleeding, especially in HBR patients. To avoid this risk, many trials have explored the safety of short-term DAPT in these patients. Table 10.1 shows the summary of recent trials supporting short DAPT after PCI in both HBR and non-HBR patients [6–26].

10.2.1 DAPT After DES Implantation in Stable Coronary Artery Disease

Attempts to shorten the duration of DAPT have undergone dramatic changes over the past decade, beginning with comparisons of 6- and 12-month DAPT and then transitioning to attempts to validate the feasibility of even shorter DAPT durations in the range of 1 or 3 months. Many trials have examined the safety of 1-month DAPT. In the STOPDAPT-2 (Short and Optimal Duration of Dual Antiplatelet Therapy After Everolimus-Eluting Cobalt-Chromium Stent) trial [20], the investigators examined whether 1 month of DAPT followed by clopidogrel monotherapy significantly lowered the rate of a composite of cardiovascular and bleeding events compared with 12 months of DAPT with aspirin and clopidogrel. The trial was conducted in patients with mainly stable angina and was not limited to HBR patients but showed that an approach of 1-month DAPT followed by SAPT was noninferior to 12 months DAPT, resulting in lower bleeding; yet, there were no differences in ischemic endpoints. Among HBR patients undergoing CoCr-EES implantation, a very short DAPT regimen of 1 month resulted in a significant reduction in major bleeding and non-inferior ischemic outcomes compared with DAPT up to 3 months [27, 28]. In the LEADERS FREE trial, a polymer-free biolimus-coated stent was superior in safety and efficacy endpoints to a bare-metal stent in patients at high bleeding risk who received 1 month of the DAPT [29]. In a later trial termed Onyx-ONE, HBR patients were randomized to either a polymer-based zotarolimus-eluting stent followed by 1 month of DAPT or a polymer-free drug-coated stent. The result of 12 months showed non-inferiority between the two groups as a result of composite outcomes including cardiac death, myocardial infarction, and stent thrombosis [30]. The development of the recent new-generation DES has led to greater data supporting the efficacy and safety of a strategy that discontinues DAPT within 1–3 months. One must keep in mind that most of the patients in these trials presented stable angina although some trials enrolled up to 1/3 of patients with acute coronary syndromes (ACS).

10.2.2 DAPT After DES Implantation in Acute Coronary Syndrome

Compared to patients with stable CAD, several trials have shown that short duration DAPT is still challenging in patients with ACS. In the SMART-

Table 10.1 Trials of short DAPT after PCI

Trial	Year	Patents, n	ACS	Discontinuation	DAPT duration	Outcomes
EXCELLENT	2011	1443		P2Y12 inhibitor	6 month vs 12 month	Non-inferior
RESET	2012	2117		P2Y12 inhibitor	3 month vs 12 month	Non-inferior
OPTIMIZE	2013	3119		P2Y12 inhibitor	3 month vs 12 month	Non-inferior
SECURITY	2014	1399		P2Y12 inhibitor	6 month vs 12 month	Non-inferior
ISAR-SAFE	2015	4000		P2Y12 inhibitor	6 month vs 12 month	Non-inferior
I-LOVE-IT 2	2016	1829		P2Y12 inhibitor	6 month vs 12 month	Non-inferior
IVUS-XPL	2016	1400		P2Y12 inhibitor	6 month vs 12 month	Non-inferior
NIPPON	2017	2772		P2Y12 inhibitor	6 month vs 18 month	Non-inferior
ITALIC	2017	1822		P2Y12 inhibitor	6 month vs 24 month	Non-inferior
OPTIMA-C	2018	1368		P2Y12 inhibitor	6 month vs 12 month	Non-inferior
DAPT-STEMI	2018	870	ACS	P2Y12 inhibitor	6 month vs 12 month	Non-inferior
SMART-DATE	2018	2712	ACS	P2Y12 inhibitor	6 month vs 12 month	Non-inferior
GLOBAL LEADERS	2018	15,968		Aspirin	1 month vs 12 month	Non-inferior
REDUCE-ACS	2019	1496	ACS	P2Y12 inhibitor	3 month vs 12 month	Non-inferior
STOPDAPT2	2019	3045		Aspirin	1 month vs 12 month	Non-inferior
SMART-CHOICE	2019	3000		Aspirin	3 month vs 12 month	Non-inferior
TWILIGHT	2019	9006		Aspirin	3 month vs 15 month	Non-inferior
IDEAL-LM	2019	818		P2Y12 inhibitor	4 month vs 12 month	Non-inferior
TICO	2020	3056	ACS	Aspirin	3 month vs 12 month	Non-inferior
ONE-MONTH DAPT	2020	3020		P2Y12 inhibitor	1 month vs 6–12 month	Non-inferior
STOPDAPT-ACS	2022	4169	ACS	Aspirin	1–2 month vs 12 month	Non-superior
STOPDAPT3	2023	5966		Aspirin	0 month vs 1 month	Non-superior
TARGET DAPT		2446		P2Y12 inhibitor	3 month vs 12 month	

Abbreviation: *ACS* acute coronary syndrome, *DAPT* dual antiplatelet therapy, *PCI* percutaneous coronary intervention

DATE trial, the 6-month DAPT group showed non-inferiority to the 12-month continuation group for major cardiovascular events in patients with ACS after DES implantation. However, the 6-month DAPT duration group had a significantly higher incidence of one of the secondary endpoints, myocardial infarction, than the 12-month duration DAPT group [17]. The STOPDAPT-2ACS trial enrolled high-risk patients with ACS (56% STEMI) who underwent successful PCI using CoCr-EES and randomized them to either 1-month DAPT followed by clopidogrel SAPT or 12-month DAPT with ASA and clopidogrel. The trial failed to show that clopidogrel monotherapy for 1–2 months of DAPT was non-inferior to 12 months of DAPT with aspirin and clopidogrel for cardiovascular events despite a reduction in bleeding events [26]. This was mainly because of an increase in cardiovascular events in the short-term DAPT group.

Meanwhile, in the Master DAPT trial, 1-month DAPT after biodegradable-polymer sirolimus-eluting stent (Ultimaster) implantation was non-inferior to ≥3 months DAPT for preventing the occurrence of net adverse clinical events and major adverse cardiac or cerebral events. Despite the fact that in this trial, more than half of the patients enrolled had ACS, including NSTEMI, STEMI, or UAP with myocardial infarction (Killip class II, III, or IV), 1-month DAPT was superior to standard therapy for limiting major or clinically relevant nonmajor bleeding events [31]. The STOPDAPT3 trial showed that 1 month of prasugrel monotherapy without aspirin after CoCr-EES implantation in patients with HBR or ACS was not superior to DAPT with aspirin and prasugrel for bleeding 4.47 and 4.41% but was non-inferior to DAPT for the cardiovascular endpoint (4.12% versus 3.69%, HR 1.12, 95% CI 0.87–1.45; p for noninferiority = 0.01). In addition, the prevalence of subacute definite or probable stent thrombosis was higher in the prasugrel monotherapy arm at 30 days compared with DAPT. Although the optimal duration of DAPT in ACS patients implanted with newer-generation DES remains controversial, it is understandable that until more definitive evidence is available, the guideline recommendation of 3–6 months of DAPT for ACS patients at high bleeding risk implanted with DES is reasonable.

10.3 Delayed Healing in the Lesion of Unstable Plaque After Stenting

In addition to the stent itself, underlying plaque morphology can affect not only the stent healing process but also in non-stented regions predisposed toward plaque progression and ACS from these non-stented plaques. Understanding the histologic healing process after stenting and the mechanisms of plaque progression in unstable lesions helps to interpret the results of clinical trials showing challenges in shortening the duration of DAPT in patients with ACS. A histological study in the first-generation DES era demonstrated that the culprit lesion of plaque rupture in ACS is one of the factors leading to delayed healing. When stents are placed over culprit lesions and non-culprit lesions in patients with stable coronary artery disease, healing is less delayed (Fig. 10.1) [4, 32]. Culprit lesions from AMI patients who underwent stent implantation and were > 30 days out had less neointimal growth and greater inflammation, fibrin deposition, and uncovered struts compared with areas of the same stent not covering the site of plaque rupture and to stented lesions from matched patients with stable angina having underlying fibro-atheromatous plaque as the culprit. The previous studies showed that delayed healing response and incomplete neointimal strut coverage are associated with the risk of late stent thrombosis following first-generation DES implantation [33, 34]. In human autopsy data, the cobalt-chromium everolimus-eluting stent (CoCr-EES), which is a second generation DES, demonstrated greater strut coverage with less inflammation, less fibrin deposition, and less late and very late stent thrombosis compared with first-generation SES and PES [32]. The development of the new-generation DES has undoubtedly revealed

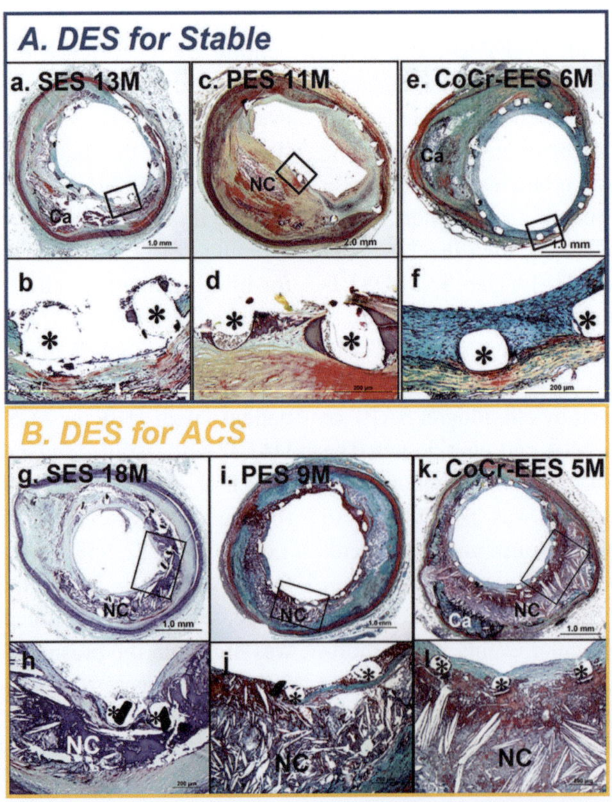

superior safety and improved efficacy compared with BMS and first-generation DES, but even with these advances, second-generation DES still requires a minimum 1 month of DAPT in stable angina patients and 6 months or greater DAPT in patients with ACS. This protects against most thrombotic events at the culprit stented site as well as at other sites of unstable plaque formation.

10.4 General Understanding of Thrombogenicity on Medical Devices After PCI

Thrombus formation is a common cause of failure for blood-contacting medical devices such as DES. Since a stent is a foreign material which is permanently implanted into the lesion, it is important to obtain deeper knowledge of how blood-contacting medical devices initiate clotting and how best to manage it. The combination of intravascular vessel wall damage due to PCI procedures, stasis of flow, and the presence of a hypercoagulable state all can induce thrombosis. These three factors are interrelated, leading to the progression of thrombus formation.

The pathogenesis of thrombus formation on medical devices contacting blood is associated with the complex pathway of coagulation on the interface between devices and blood (Fig. 10.2). Artificial surfaces promote clotting through various processes such as protein adsorption, platelet adhesion, leukocytes, red blood cells, thrombin generation, and complement activation [35]. Protein adsorption on the surface of medical devices modulates the reactions, subsequently initiating thrombus formation events such as platelet adhesion, activation, and aggregation. Fibrinogen is one of the plasma proteins which adhere to artificial surfaces, followed by fibronectin and von Willebrand factor, facilitating platelet adhesion. This sets off a cascade, including factor XII activation; the resulting factor XIIa converts pre-kallikrein to kallikrein and initiates coagulation and thrombin generation. This interplay between complement and coagulation pathways amplifies thrombosis, making the protein monolayer a dynamic modulator on artificial surfaces [36]. In addition to inducing fibrin deposition on the surface, thrombin mediates the adhesion of platelets, leukocytes,

Fig. 10.1 Culprit lesion in AMI is one of the factors for delayed healing. Representative images of sirolimus-eluting stent (SES), paclitaxel-eluting stent (PES), and cobalt-chromium everolimus-eluting stent (CoCr-EES) implanted for stable coronary artery disease (CAD; A: **a** to **f**) and for acute coronary syndromes (ACS; B: **g** to **l**). Seen in (**a**) and (**b**) are histological sections from a 53-year-old man with SES implanted in the proximal left anterior descending coronary artery for 13 months. A low-power image (**a**) shows mild neointimal growth and underlying fibrocalcific plaque. Focal uncovered struts are highlighted in high-power (**b**). *Stent strut. Shown in (**c**) and (**d**) are histological sections from a 71-year-old man with PES implanted in the right coronary artery 11 months antemortem. A low-power image (**c**) shows mild to moderate neointimal proliferation and underlying fibroatheroma. Note uncovered struts with persistent peri-strut fibrin deposition shown at the high-power image (**d**). Seen in (**e**) and (**f**) are histological sections from a 60-year-old man who received CoCr-EES in the mid left circumflex artery 6 months antemortem. A low-power image (**e**) shows mild neointimal proliferation and underlying fibrocalcific plaque. All struts are covered with proteoglycan-rich neointima with the absence of fibrin, which is highlighted in a high-power image (**f**). Shown in (**g**) and (**h**) are histological sections from a 74-year-old woman who received SES in the proximal left anterior descending coronary artery for acute myocardial infarction 18 months antemortem, who died of diffuse severe coronary artery disease. A low-power image (**g**) shows mild neointimal proliferation. Note focal uncovered struts and strut penetration into the necrotic core (NC; **h**). In (**i**) and (**j**) histological sections from a 64-year-old woman can be observed with PES implanted in the right coronary artery for acute myocardial infarction 9 months antemortem, who died of congestive heart failure. A low-power image (**i**) shows patent lumen with stent struts surrounded by fibrin and an underlying NC. Note uncovered struts with fibrin deposition that overlie the NC (**j**). Seen in (**k**) and (**l**) are histological sections from a 67-year-old man who received CoCr-EES in the proximal left anterior descending coronary artery for non-ST-segment elevation acute myocardial infarction 5 months antemortem, who died of noncardiac causes. A low-power image (**k**) shows mild neointimal proliferation and an underlying large NC. All struts are covered with a thin neointima overlying the NC, which is highlighted in the high-power image in (**l**). All histological sections are stained with Movat pentachrome. DES indicates drug-eluting stents. (Modified with permission from Otsuka F, et al., 2014 [32])

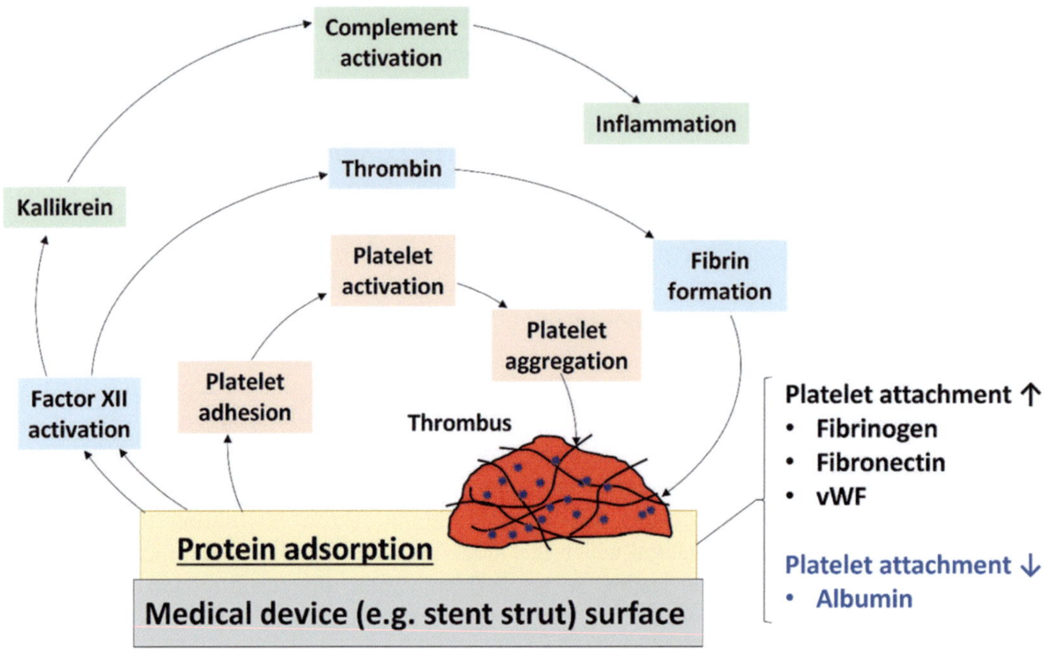

Fig. 10.2 Relationship between medical devices and thrombogenicity. Blood-contacting medical device-associated thrombosis. Protein absorbed to the surface of medical devices induces platelets to adhere, activate, and aggregate. Factor XII adsorbed to the surface undergoes autoactivation, and the resulting factor XIIa converts prekallikrein to kallikrein initiating coagulation and thrombin generation. In addition to inducing fibrin deposition on the surface, thrombin promotes platelet activation. Platelet aggregates deposited on the surface are stabilized by fibrin strands to form a platelet-fibrin thrombus. Kallikrein, thrombin, and other coagulation enzymes activate complement and induce a local inflammatory response. (Modified with permission from Jaffer H, et al., 2015 [35])

and red blood cells to the surfaces of medical devices. Platelet clusters adhered to the surface are reinforced by fibrin fibers, creating a platelet-fibrin clot. Adherent platelets promote leukocyte adhesion to adsorbed fibrinogen via CD11b/CD18 [37] and activated complement components [38]. Kallikrein, thrombin, and other coagulation enzymes trigger complement activation, leading to a localized inflammatory response. Strategies to minimize protein and cell adhesion are rooted in the understanding that protein binding to surfaces is influenced by electrostatic and hydrophobic interactions between the adsorbed protein and the artificial surface. Scientists have explored various synthetic and natural materials to manipulate these processes. In contrast to plasma proteins like fibrinogen and γ-globulin, albumin leads to less platelet adhesion [39, 40].

10.5 Developments and Challenges of Current DESs in HBR Patients

10.5.1 Thromboresistance of Polymer Loaded on DES

The type and duration of antiplatelet therapy and the antithrombotic properties of the implanted stent itself are also important aspects of preventing stent thrombosis in patients with high bleeding risk [41, 42]. Early endothelial coverage after stent implantation is an important process for healing and preventing stent thrombosis [33]. The rate of endothelial coverage is dependent on several factors, including strut thickness, type of polymer, type of drug, and amount of drug. In patients at HBR, promotion of adequate endothelial coverage is particularly important to prevent thrombus formation [41, 42]. With the evolution of DES over the past 30 years, clinical trials suggest that the newer generation of DES has improved biologic synthesis compared to the first generation, allowing for better neointima and reduced ST risk with uncoated struts [20, 21].

On the other hand, it has also been shown that the polymer coating of the DES itself may contribute to a protective process against thrombus formation [43]. Preclinical studies have revealed the impact of the components of the newer generation of stents on their antithrombotic properties, demonstrating the lower thrombogenicity of the newer generation of DES due to the polymer coating and thin struts [44–46]. This provides rationale for considering the antithrombotic properties of stents in PCI in patients at high bleeding risk. Kolandaivelu et al. showed that BMS has greater thrombogenicity compared to polymer-coated DES in an in vitro flow loop model [44]. Furthermore, the experimental series of studies using flow loops has shown that the type of polymer loaded on DES has potential to show individual differences with respect to thrombogenicity, as well as substantial differences between durable and biodegradable polymers (Fig. 10.3) [46]. In DES loaded with durable poly-

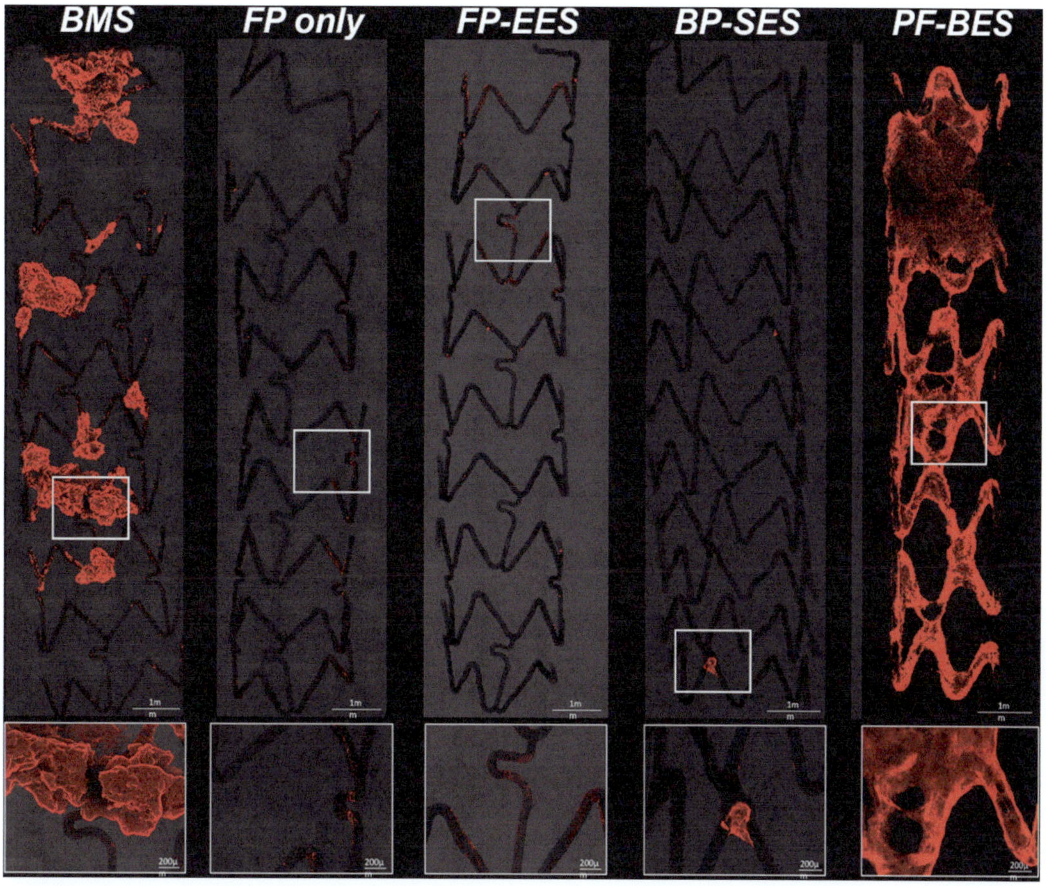

Fig. 10.3 Confocal microscopic images with immunofluorescent staining. Representative confocal microscopic images of bare-metal stent (BMS), fluoropolymer (FP)-only, FP-coated everolimus-eluting stents (FP-EES), biodegradable polymer sirolimus-eluting stents (BP-SES), and polymer-free Biolimus A9-coated stents (PF-BCS) with immunofluorescent staining against dual platelet markers (CD61/CD42b) in a swine shunt model. Low- and high-power confocal microscopic images showing the least thrombus-occupied area in stents with fluoropolymer (FP-only and FP-EES) as compared with the other stents. Note minimal thrombus is only observed in the link portion of FP-only and FP-EES, whereas large thrombus covers almost all the struts in PF-BCS. (Modified with permission from Torii S, et al., 2019 [46])

mers, the fluoropolymer (FP) EES is the strongest thromboresistant polymer in the DES. The integrity of the FP coating and the fluoropassivation phenomenon could contribute to the higher thromboresistance compared to the biodegradable polymer (BP) DES. The favorable antithrombotic effect of fluoropolymer coatings has been confirmed under both antithrombotic therapies simulating DAPT and SAPT [46–48].

10.5.2 Quality of Endothelial Coverage

While abluminal-coated polymers were developed to improve the rate of endothelial coverage, the bare-metal surface in direct contact with blood can cause acute thrombus formation from clot aggregation [46]. However, clinical data provide no evidence of a significant difference in thrombus formation between durable and biodegradable polymers, either in the acute or chronic phase. This suggests that in patients at high risk of bleeding, improvement in the "quality" of the endothelial coating of the stent may also be an important factor in reducing the risk of thrombus formation. In a previous preclinical study, a biodegradable polymer sirolimus-eluting stent coated with Albumin (Ultimaster®; Terumo Corporation, Tokyo, Japan) showed better VE-cadherin, an expression compared to DP-EES (Fig. 10.4) [49]. Evans blue staining showed that endothelial barrier function was impaired in all DES compared to C-PzF at 28 days. There are reports that exposure to mammalian rapamycin target inhibitors such as sirolimus and everolimus impairs endothelial barrier function via Ca2 + -mediated activation of protein kinase Cα and disruption of VE-cadherin junction formation in the downstream endothelium [50].

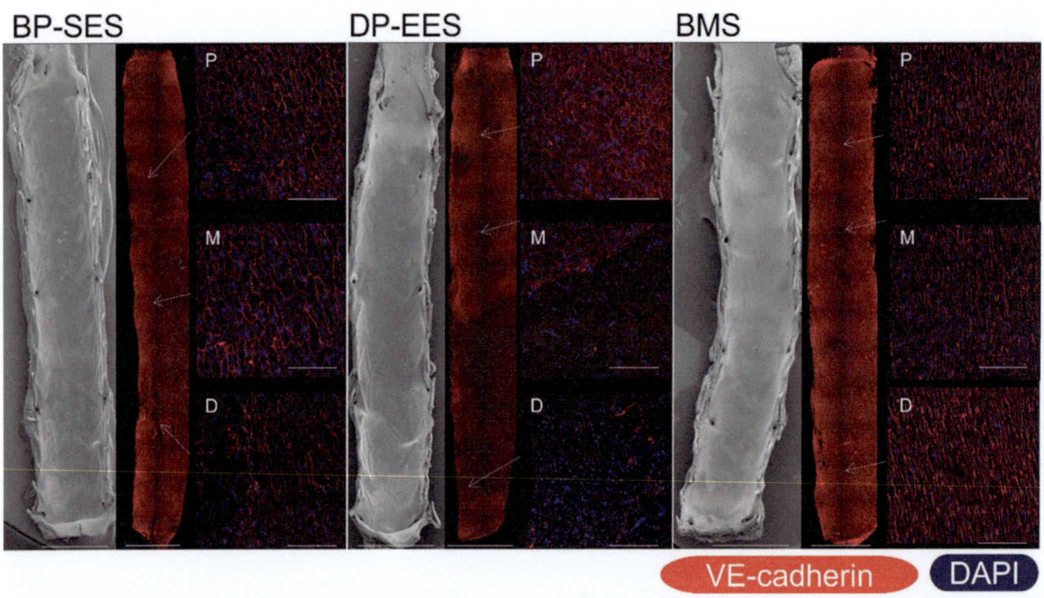

Fig. 10.4 Low- and high-power images of confocal images. Representative low- and high-power images of confocal images in each stent type with corresponding low-power scanning electron microscopy (SEM) images at 120 days. The red channel is vascular endothelial (VE)-cadherin, and the blue channel is DAPI (nuclear counterstain). Boxed areas in each low-power image are shown in correspondingly labeled high-power images on the right. Struts are fully covered for all types of stents by SEM. However, in both drug-eluting stents, some areas (P and D in biodegradable polymer sirolimus-eluting stents (BP-SES)) and more obvious in M and D in durable polymer-coated everolimus-eluting stents (DP-EES) showed lower VE-cadherin expression, whereas it was fully expressed in bare-metal stent (BMS). The dotted yellow line in the low-power image of DP-EES outlines a relatively large VE-cadherin-negative area. Scale bars in low-power confocal microscopic images and SEM images ¼ 2 mm. Scale bars in high-power confocal microscopic images ¼ 200 mm. (Modified with permission from Mori H, et al., 2017 [49])

Endothelial barrier function after DES implantation also contributes to antithrombotic potential, which is an important aspect related to the regimen of antiplatelet therapy in HBR patients.

Therefore, stent selection to minimize the risk of thrombus formation in patients at high bleeding risk is critical. Factors such as types of polymers loaded on DES, rate of endothelial coverage, and quality of the endothelial coverage on DES are key to improving antithrombotic performance in patients with HBR, and further study of DES performance based on clinical and preclinical trials is essential to improve treatment strategies for patients with HBR by facilitating the improvement of antithrombotic performance.

10.6 Advantages of DCB Technology Compared to DES in HBR Patients

DCB may have advantages over stents in terms of vascular healing and need for DAPT. The concept of the DCBs is to suppress neointimal proliferation by antiproliferative drugs, a similar concept to DES. However, the greatest advantage of DCB is that there is no permanent metallic stent scaffold after the treatment, the so-called leave nothing behind strategy. This strategy can potentially lower both acute and late complications associated with stent placement, such as stent thrombosis and in-stent restenosis. These advantages of DCB can be useful for lesions which are unsuitable for stent implantation such as small vessels, bifurcations, etc. but also for a patient who has a history of a metallic allergy or HBR indicators.

In general, the main causes of restenosis after balloon angioplasty are acute vessel recoil and late neointimal growth due to proliferation of smooth muscle cells. This neointimal growth occurs within the first 7 days to 3 months following the procedure in humans [51, 52]. DES consists of metallic scaffold and coated polymer which provide a slow drug release and transportation to vessel wall, resulting in preventing acute vessel recoil and suppressing the neointimal proliferation. The effect of the antiproliferative drugs must be maintained during smooth muscle cell migration and proliferation. While DCB has no permanent polymeric scaffold to control drug release, the innovation of transporter excipient technologies and carriers in DCBs has also allowed for effective drug release and delivery to the vessel wall.

DCB can either be loaded with one of two types of drugs in the clinical setting: paclitaxel or sirolimus. Paclitaxel (PTX) is the most widely used antiproliferative drug for DCBs. PTX is highly lipophilic properties, which allow passive absorption through cell membranes and sustained action within the target vessel wall [53]. Clinical trials have confirmed the efficacy of PTX DCBs both for coronary and above-the-knee indications [54–56]. Sirolimus (SRL) has the advantages of less drug toxicity and effective suppression of inflammation compared to PTX. The use of sirolimus in DCBs has only succeeded with improved excipients, formulation, and encapsulation of sirolimus with biodegradable or phospholipid based particles. Recent small clinical trials have also demonstrated the efficacy and safety of sirolimus DCBs, but more data are needed [57, 58].

10.7 Evidence of DCB in HBR Patients

10.7.1 The Efficacy of DCB

In the current guideline, DCBs are recommended as class IA especially for ISR (European Society of Cardiology [ESC] guidelines: 2018 ESC/EACTS guidelines) [59]. DCBs have been shown to be superior to POBA for restenosis after BMS or DES implantation [60–63]. A recent RCT meta-analysis showed that DCB and DES have similar efficacy and safety in the treatment of BMS-ISR. Since stent implantation is challenging, especially for small vessels, DCBs have an advantage in the treatment in small size vessels with de novo lesions. Large registry-based studies showed low target lesion revascularization rates and low risk of acute vessel occlusion [56, 64], supporting the use of DCBs in de novo lesions. The BASKET-SMALL2 trial with a 3-year follow-up also showed the safety and efficacy of DCBs as compared to current DESs in the treatment of coronary arteries <3 mm regardless of the presence of bleeding risk, while there was a trend toward a reduction in major bleeding events at 3 years in patients treated with DCBs [65] This result is a supporting case for the advantage of using DCBs for CAD patients with HBR compared to DES in terms of reducing bleeding events. On the other hand, the effect of DCB is limited in comparison to DES in de novo lesions with large reference vessel diameters (≥3.0 mm) [66].

The DEBUT trial demonstrated that DCB is superior to BMS in patients at high bleeding risk (HBR) [67]. In the PEPCAD NSTEMI trial, DCBs demonstrated non-inferiority to metallic stents (i.e., BMS or DES) with respect to TLF at 9 months. However, a considerable number of patients who received DCB-only treatment required additional stent implantation as "bailout" stenting was unavoidable [68]. The "leave nothing behind" strategy was also the strongest disadvantage in treatment of DCB only. The presence of a dissection after POBA was associated with increased events of thrombosis, reocclusion, and restenosis [69]. Optimal lesion preparation was one of the most important factors to maintain the effect of DCB. Type A to C dissections without flow limitation after DCB treatment was associated with sealing the dissections at follow-up as well as inhibition of the neointimal hyperplasia on angiographic follow-up at 6 months [70]. Therefore, during the DCB treatment, the intimal dissection without a flow limitation was a key finding to determine whether additional stenting was necessary. However, medial dissection, intramural hematoma, or extramedial injury should be treated with "bailout" stenting to prevent the revascularization at the late phase after the treatment.

Although several studies have reported on the efficacy of DCB in ACS, the evidence on the application of DCBs in patients with ACS is still controversial. The BASKET-SMALL2 trial showed that the sustained efficacy and safety of the DCB in both ACS and CCS was demonstrated at a 3-year follow-up [71]. In a retrospective study in which 52% of subjects had HBR, a DCB-only strategy with the option of provisional stenting was shown to be safe and effective for de novo coronary lesions in both stable CAD and ACS [72]. At present, DCB treatment for ACS lesions is preferred for use on selected lesions in HBR patients. Further studies on the effects of DCB in large vessels (≥3.0 mm) as well as ACS patients are warranted. Table 10.2 summarizes studies examining the duration of DAPT after the DCB treatment in patients with stable CAD and ACS [56, 64–68, 73–78]. The recently published patient level meta-analysis ANDROMEDA showed how in patients undergoing PCI for de novo small vessels, PCB angioplasty was associated with a reduction in MACE as compared to DES at 3 year follow-up [79].

10.7.2 Histopathologic Findings After DCB Treatment

We have recently evaluated the pathological findings after DCB treatment in preclinical studies. Saami K et al. demonstrated pathologic findings of the vascular response to a low-dose 2-mg/mm^2 paclitaxel-coated balloon (Lutonix®; BD, USA) in a swine femoral artery model (Fig. 10.5) [80]. The endothelial layer was almost completely healed, and mild medial SMC loss was observed at 28 days posttreatment with DCB. There was a peak in medial SMC loss at 90 days reflecting the drug effect, which was still evident at 180 days. Furthermore, the area of medial SMC loss, proteoglycan, and collagen deposition was significantly greater than that of uncoated balloon angioplasty as a control group at 90 days, reaching a maximum. These results indicate the efficacy of DCB with sustained healing through 180 days. Meanwhile, inflammation was low at 28 days and absent at 180 days. The changes in the intima consisted of only rare fibrin deposition and loss of endothelium at 28 days in both the DCB and control group. There was no significant thinning of the vessel wall or thrombosis observed at any time point following DCB treatment.

We have also shown that the neointimal fibrin deposition is lower in DCB treatment than in

Table 10.2 Randomized trials of DCB for de novo coronary artery lesions

Trial	Patients, n	Design	RVD (mm)	HBR (%)	ACS (%)	DAPT duration	F/U duration	TLR (%)	Bleeding (%)
PICOLETO (2010)	57	DCB vs PES	$\le$ 2.75	N/A	55 (UA)	1 month in DCB 3 month in DES 12 month in UA	9 month	32.1 vs 10.3	N/A
Bello (2012)	182	DCB vs PES	<2.8	N/A	23 (UA)	1 month in DCB 3 month in BMS 12 month in DES	6 month 3 year	4.4 vs 7.6 7 vs 13	N/A N/A
Funatsu et al. (2017)	135	DCB vs POBA	2.0–2.75	N/A	Including UA	$\ge$ 12 weeks	24 week	2.3 vs 10.3	N/A
RESTORE SVD China (2018)	230	DCB vs nDES	2–2.75		80 (UA)	$\ge$ 6 months	12 month 24 month	4.4 vs 2.6 5.2 vs 2.8	N/A N/A
BASKET-SMALL2 (2018)	758	DCB vs nDES	2.0–3.0	20	28	1 month in DCB 3 month in DES 12 month in ACS	12 month 3 year	3.4 vs 4.5 9 vs 9	1.1 vs 2.4 2 vs 4
DEBUT (2019)	208	DCB vs BMS	2.5–4.0	100	46	1 month	9 month	0 vs 6	13 vs 10
PEPCAD NSTEMI (2020)	210	DCB vs BMS/nDES	2.5–3.5	N/A	100	12 month	9 month	1.0 vs 0.9	N/A
PICCOLETO II (2020)	232	DCB vs EES	2.0–2.75		45	1 month in DCB 6 month in DES 12 month in ACS	12 month	5.6 vs 5.6	0 vs 0

Abbreviation: *ACS* acute coronary syndrome, *BMS* bare-metal stent, *DAPT* dual antiplatelet therapy, *DCB* drug-coated balloon, *nDES* new-generation drug-eluting stent, *EES* everolimus-eluting stent, *HBR* high bleeding risk, *POBA* plain balloon angioplasty, *PES* paclitaxel-eluting stent, *RVD* reference vessel diameter, *TLR* target lesion revascularization, *UA* unstable angina

DES implantation at 1 month after each procedure [81]. Previous investigation demonstrated the mechanism of late thrombosis such as delayed endothelial coverage and excessive fibrin deposition which is associated with abnormal vascular response [82].

These pathologic findings are evaluated using healthy swine and do not take into consideration all the complexities of the human artery. However, these preclinical studies suggest that the DCB treatment has the potential of a shorter duration of the DAPT compared with stent implantation not only due to the drug's effect suppressing neointimal proliferation but also by its ability to shorten the duration needed for complete reendothelialization.

10.7.3 DAPT Duration After DCB

The duration of DAPT in patients who undergo DCB treatment is still a work in progress. The European Society of Cardiology Guidelines on DAPT recommend to continue DAPT for

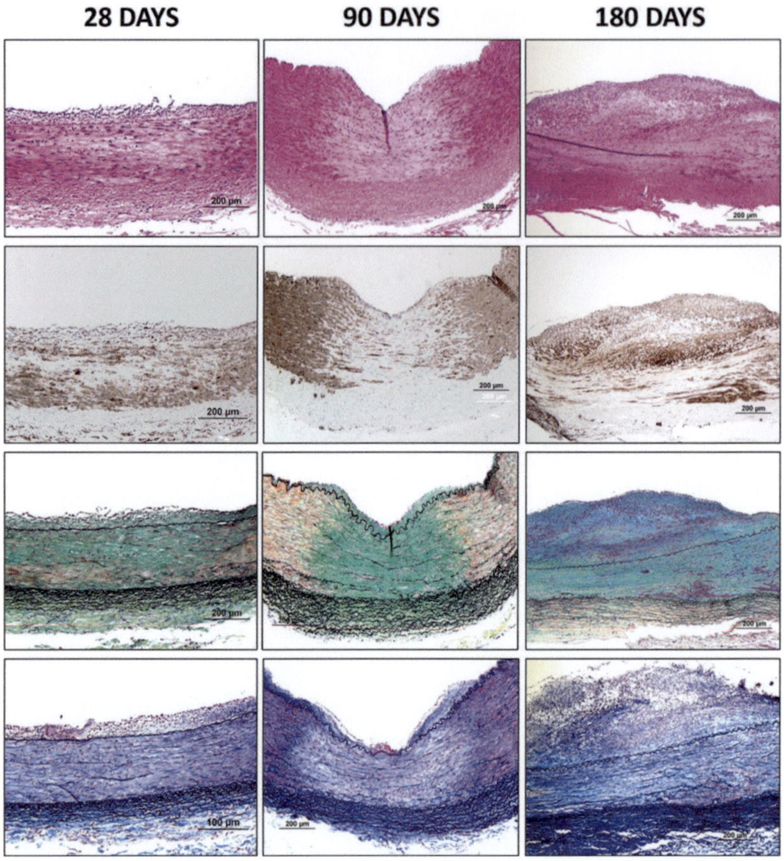

Fig. 10.5 Representative images of the medial response following DCB treatment. Representative images of the medial response following DCB treatment H&E (top row) and smooth muscle cell actin (second row) stains show the peak of smooth muscle cell loss at 90 days. In the parallel rows, proteoglycan and collagen replacement can be observed at 90 and 180 days by the Movat (third row) and Masson's Trichrome (bottom row) stains. (Modified with permission from Yazdani, S.K., et al., 2014 [80])

6 months in patients with stable CAD and with de novo lesion or ISR lesions. In HBR patients with stable CAD, duration of DAPT is recommended to be 1–3 months. However, in patients with ACS who received stent implantation, DAPT with a P2Y12 inhibitor and aspirin is recommended for 12 months unless contraindicated. In cases of HBR patients with ACS, P2Y12 inhibitor therapy should be discontinued 6 months after the DAPT administration [83]. However, the initial consensus from Germany reported that DAPT is recommended to continue for 4 weeks after DCB treatment to the ISR lesion. For smaller de novo coronary artery lesions, it is recommended to continue DAPT for at least 4 weeks after PCI with DCB alone, and aspirin 100 mg per day should be continued as long as possible. In patients with ACS, the duration of DAPT is recommended for 12 months with DCB as well as stent implantation with either BMS or DES [84, 85]. Although there are still no studies investigating DCB treatment with SAPT in large cohorts, several retrospective studies demonstrate that the frequency of BARC 2–5 bleeding after DCB with SAPT is 6–10% [86, 87], which is lower compared to other studies performed in patients with high bleeding risk who underwent DES implantation [29]. The "leave nothing behind" strategy using DCB leads to a shorter period of inflammatory response without a metallic scaffold. This strategy has potential to prevent metallic stent induced delay in healing and creates potential for shorter durations of DAPT use. While there is no doubt that DCBs are the ideal device in terms of shortening DAPT compared to DES, as noted above, DCBs have not demonstrated long-term results comparable to DES in all lesions except ISR and small vessels. At the present moment, the use of DCB is limited to only specific types of lesions; it is

important to understand which lesions are eligible for the use of DCB to treat patients with HBR. Further studies are warranted to explore the effect of DCB on the types of target lesions as well as in patients with ACS.

10.8 Summary and Perspective

This chapter reviewed the evidence regarding short-term DAPT after DCB and DES, providing a comprehensive review of factors of which heighten risk for thrombosis. While DCBs may have an advantage for the treatment of small vessels and bifurcation lesions, it is still less certain for outcomes in patients with thrombotic lesions treated with DCBs. It is important to understand the substantial structural differences in DCBs and DESs that may have a significant impact on posttreatment predisposition toward thrombosis. In addition, it is important to understand that DCB technologies are still developing, and there is limited data about results in a variety of lesions as well as the use of DAPT or SAPT compared to DES. Technical advancement and further investigation of additional evidence are needed to ascertain the role of DCB in patients with HBR.

Disclosure
R.V. and A.V.F. have received institutional research support from 480 Biomedical; 4C Medical; 4Tech; Abbott; Accumedical; Amgen; Biosensors; Boston Scientific; Cagent Vascular; Cardiac Implants; CeloNova; Claret Medical; Concept Medical; Cook; CSI; DuNing, Inc.; Edwards LifeSciences; Emboline; Endotronix; Envision Scientific; Gateway; Leducq Foundation Grant; Lifetech; Limflo; Lutonix/Bard; MedAlliance; Medtronic; Mercator; Meril; Microport Medical; Microvention; Mitraalign; Mitra Assist; NAMSA; Nanova; Neovasc; NIH (HL141425); NIPRO; Novogate; Occlutech; OrbusNeich Medical; Phenox; Profusa; Protembis; Qool; Recor; Senseonics; Shockwave; Sinomed; Spectranetics; Surmodics; Symic; Vesper; and W. L. Gore; Xeltis. A.V.F. has received honoraria from Abbott Vascular; Biosensors; Boston Scientific; Celonova; Cook Medical; CSI; Lutonix Bard; Sinomed; and Terumo Corporation and is a consultant to Amgen; Abbott Vascular; Boston Scientific; Celonova; Cook Medical; Lutonix Bard; and Sinomed. R.V. has received honoraria from Abbott Vascular; Biosensors; Boston Scientific; CeloNova; Cook Medical; Cordis; CSI; Lutonix Bard; Medtronic; OrbusNeich Medical; ReCor; Sino Medical Technology; Spectranetics; Terumo Corporation; and W. L. Gore and is a consultant for Abbott Vascular; Boston Scientific; CeloNova; Cook Medical; Cordis; CSI; Edwards Lifesciences; Lutonix Bard; Medtronic; OrbusNeich Medical; ReCor; Sino Medical Sciences Technology; Spectranetics; Surmodics; Terumo Corporation; and W. L. Gore; Xeltis.

References

1. Mauri L, et al. Twelve or 30 months of dual antiplatelet therapy after drug-eluting stents. N Engl J Med. 2014;371(23):2155–66.
2. Palmerini T, et al. Mortality in patients treated with extended duration dual antiplatelet therapy after drug-eluting stent implantation: a pairwise and Bayesian network meta-analysis of randomised trials. Lancet. 2015;385(9985):2371–82.
3. Torii S, et al. Vascular responses to coronary calcification following implantation of newer-generation drug-eluting stents in humans: impact on healing. Eur Heart J. 2020;41(6):786–96.
4. Nakazawa G, et al. Delayed arterial healing and increased late stent thrombosis at culprit sites after drug-eluting stent placement for acute myocardial infarction patients: an autopsy study. Circulation. 2008;118(11):1138–45.
5. Cortese B, et al. Sirolimus-coated balloon in an all-comer population of coronary artery disease patients: the EASTBOURNE prospective registry. JACC Cardiovasc Interv. 2023;16(14):1794–803.
6. Gwon HC, et al. Six-month versus 12-month dual antiplatelet therapy after implantation of drug-eluting stents: the efficacy of Xience/Promus versus cypher to reduce late loss after stenting (EXCELLENT) randomized, multicenter study. Circulation. 2012;125(3):505–13.
7. Kim BK, et al. A new strategy for discontinuation of dual antiplatelet therapy: the RESET Trial (Real safety and efficacy of 3-month dual antiplatelet therapy following Endeavor zotarolimus-eluting stent implantation). J Am Coll Cardiol. 2012;60(15):1340–8.
8. Feres F, et al. Three vs twelve months of dual antiplatelet therapy after zotarolimus-eluting stents: the OPTIMIZE randomized trial. JAMA. 2013;310(23):2510–22.

9. Colombo A, et al. Second-generation drug-eluting stent implantation followed by 6- versus 12-month dual antiplatelet therapy: the SECURITY randomized clinical trial. J Am Coll Cardiol. 2014;64(20):2086–97.
10. Schulz-Schüpke S, et al. ISAR-SAFE: a randomized, double-blind, placebo-controlled trial of 6 vs. 12 months of clopidogrel therapy after drug-eluting stenting. Eur Heart J. 2015;36(20):1252–63.
11. Han Y, et al. Six versus 12 months of dual antiplatelet therapy after implantation of biodegradable polymer sirolimus-eluting stent: randomized substudy of the I-LOVE-IT 2 Trial. Circ Cardiovasc Interv. 2016;9(2):e003145.
12. Hong SJ, et al. 6-month versus 12-month dual-antiplatelet therapy following long everolimus-eluting stent implantation: the IVUS-XPL randomized clinical trial. JACC Cardiovasc Interv. 2016;9(14):1438–46.
13. Nakamura M, et al. Dual antiplatelet therapy for 6 versus 18 months after biodegradable polymer drug-eluting stent implantation. JACC Cardiovasc Interv. 2017;10(12):1189–98.
14. Didier R, et al. 6- versus 24-month dual antiplatelet therapy after implantation of drug-eluting stents in patients nonresistant to aspirin: final results of the ITALIC trial (Is there a life for DES after discontinuation of clopidogrel). JACC Cardiovasc Interv. 2017;10(12):1202–10.
15. Lee BK, et al. Safety of six-month dual antiplatelet therapy after second-generation drug-eluting stent implantation: OPTIMA-C randomised clinical trial and OCT substudy. EuroIntervention. 2018;13(16):1923–30.
16. Kedhi E, et al. Six months versus 12 months dual antiplatelet therapy after drug-eluting stent implantation in ST-elevation myocardial infarction (DAPT-STEMI): randomised, multicentre, non-inferiority trial. BMJ. 2018;363:k3793.
17. Hahn JY, et al. 6-month versus 12-month or longer dual antiplatelet therapy after percutaneous coronary intervention in patients with acute coronary syndrome (SMART-DATE): a randomised, open-label, non-inferiority trial. Lancet. 2018;391(10127):1274–84.
18. Vranckx P, et al. Ticagrelor plus aspirin for 1 month, followed by ticagrelor monotherapy for 23 months vs aspirin plus clopidogrel or ticagrelor for 12 months, followed by aspirin monotherapy for 12 months after implantation of a drug-eluting stent: a multicentre, open-label, randomised superiority trial. Lancet. 2018;392(10151):940–9.
19. De Luca G, et al. Final results of the randomised evaluation of short-term dual antiplatelet therapy in patients with acute coronary syndrome treated with a new-generation stent (REDUCE trial). EuroIntervention. 2019;15(11):e990–8.
20. Watanabe H, et al. Effect of 1-month dual antiplatelet therapy followed by clopidogrel vs 12-month dual antiplatelet therapy on cardiovascular and bleeding events in patients receiving PCI: The STOPDAPT-2 randomized clinical trial. JAMA. 2019;321(24):2414–27.
21. Hahn JY, et al. Effect of P2Y12 inhibitor monotherapy vs dual antiplatelet therapy on cardiovascular events in patients undergoing percutaneous coronary intervention: the SMART-CHOICE randomized clinical trial. JAMA. 2019;321(24):2428–37.
22. Mehran R, et al. Ticagrelor with or without aspirin in high-risk patients after PCI. N Engl J Med. 2019;381(21):2032–42.
23. Lemmert ME, et al. Reduced duration of dual antiplatelet therapy using an improved drug-eluting stent for percutaneous coronary intervention of the left main artery in a real-world, all-comer population: rationale and study design of the prospective randomized multicenter IDEAL-LM trial. Am Heart J. 2017;187:104–11.
24. Kim BK, et al. Effect of ticagrelor monotherapy vs ticagrelor with aspirin on major bleeding and cardiovascular events in patients with acute coronary syndrome: the TICO randomized clinical trial. JAMA. 2020;323(23):2407–16.
25. Hong SJ, et al. 1-month dual-antiplatelet therapy followed by aspirin monotherapy after polymer-free drug-coated stent implantation: one-month DAPT trial. JACC Cardiovasc Interv. 2021;14(16):1801–11.
26. Watanabe H, et al. Comparison of clopidogrel monotherapy after 1 to 2 months of dual antiplatelet therapy with 12 months of dual antiplatelet therapy in patients with acute coronary syndrome: the STOPDAPT-2 ACS randomized clinical trial. JAMA Cardiol. 2022;7(4):407–17.
27. Mehran R, et al. 3- or 1-month DAPT in patients at high bleeding risk undergoing everolimus-eluting stent implantation. JACC Cardiovasc Interv. 2021;14(17):1870–83.
28. Valgimigli M, et al. Duration of dual antiplatelet therapy for patients at high bleeding risk undergoing PCI. J Am Coll Cardiol. 2021;78(21):2060–72.
29. Urban P, et al. Polymer-free drug-coated coronary stents in patients at high bleeding risk. N Engl J Med. 2015;373(21):2038–47.
30. Windecker S, et al. Polymer-based or polymer-free stents in patients at high bleeding risk. N Engl J Med. 2020;382(13):1208–18.
31. Valgimigli M, et al. Dual antiplatelet therapy after PCI in patients at high bleeding risk. N Engl J Med. 2021;385(18):1643–55.
32. Otsuka F, et al. Pathology of second-generation everolimus-eluting stents versus first-generation sirolimus- and paclitaxel-eluting stents in humans. Circulation. 2014;129(2):211–23.
33. Joner M, et al. Pathology of drug-eluting stents in humans: delayed healing and late thrombotic risk. J Am Coll Cardiol. 2006;48(1):193–202.
34. Cook S, et al. Correlation of intravascular ultrasound findings with histopathological analysis of thrombus aspirates in patients with very late drug-eluting stent thrombosis. Circulation. 2009;120(5):391–9.
35. Jaffer IH, et al. Medical device-induced thrombosis: what causes it and how can we prevent it? J Thromb Haemost. 2015;13(Suppl 1):S72–81.

36. Gorbet MB, Sefton MV. Biomaterial-associated thrombosis: roles of coagulation factors, complement, platelets and leukocytes. Biomaterials. 2004;25(26):5681–703.
37. Wright SD, et al. Complement receptor type three (CD11b/CD18) of human polymorphonuclear leukocytes recognizes fibrinogen. Proc Natl Acad Sci USA. 1988;85(20):7734–8.
38. Kazatchkine MD, Carreno MP. Activation of the complement system at the interface between blood and artificial surfaces. Biomaterials. 1988;9(1):30–5.
39. Park K, Mosher DF, Cooper SL. Acute surface-induced thrombosis in the canine ex vivo model: importance of protein composition of the initial monolayer and platelet activation. J Biomed Mater Res. 1986;20(5):589–612.
40. Kim SW, et al. Platelet adhesion to polymer surfaces. Trans Am Soc Artif Intern Organs. 1974;20(b):449–55.
41. Richter Y, Edelman ER. Cardiology is flow. Circulation. 2006;113(23):2679–82.
42. LaDisa JF Jr, et al. Alterations in regional vascular geometry produced by theoretical stent implantation influence distributions of wall shear stress: analysis of a curved coronary artery using 3D computational fluid dynamics modeling. Biomed Eng Online. 2006;5:40.
43. Palmerini T, et al. Long-term safety of drug-eluting and bare-metal stents: evidence from a comprehensive network meta-analysis. J Am Coll Cardiol. 2015;65(23):2496–507.
44. Kolandaivelu K, et al. Stent thrombogenicity early in high-risk interventional settings is driven by stent design and deployment and protected by polymer-drug coatings. Circulation. 2011;123(13):1400–9.
45. Otsuka F, et al. Acute Thrombogenicity of a Durable Polymer Everolimus-Eluting Stent Relative to Contemporary Drug-Eluting Stents With Biodegradable Polymer Coatings Assessed Ex Vivo in a Swine Shunt Model. JACC Cardiovasc Interv. 2015;8(9):1248–60.
46. Torii S, et al. Acute thrombogenicity of fluoropolymer-coated versus biodegradable and polymer-free stents. EuroIntervention. 2019;14(16):1685–93.
47. Jinnouchi H, et al. Thromboresistance and functional healing in the COBRA PzF stent versus competitor DES: implications for dual antiplatelet therapy. EuroIntervention. 2019;15(4):e342–53.
48. Sato Y, et al. Acute thrombogenicity of fluoropolymer coated stents versus competitive drug-eluting stents under single antiplatelet therapy. Int J Cardiol. 2021;338:42–9.
49. Mori H, et al. Endothelial barrier protein expression in biodegradable polymer sirolimus-eluting versus durable polymer everolimus-eluting metallic stents. JACC Cardiovasc Interv. 2017;10(23):2375–87.
50. Habib, A., et al., Sirolimus-FKBP12.6 impairs endothelial barrier function through protein kinase C-α activation and disruption of the p120-vascular endothelial cadherin interaction. Arterioscler Thromb Vasc Biol, 2013. 33(10): p. 2425–2431.
51. Virmani R, et al. Drug eluting stents: are human and animal studies comparable? Heart. 2003;89(2):133–8.
52. Nikol S, Huehns TY, Höfling B. Molecular biology and post-angioplasty restenosis. Atherosclerosis. 1996;123(1–2):17–31.
53. Kolodgie FD, et al. Comparison of particulate embolization after femoral artery treatment with IN.PACT admiral versus lutonix 035 paclitaxel-coated balloons in healthy swine. J Vasc Interv Radiol. 2016;27(11):1676–1685.e2.
54. Laird JA, et al. Long-term clinical effectiveness of a drug-coated balloon for the treatment of femoropopliteal lesions. Circ Cardiovasc Interv. 2019;12(6):e007702.
55. Wöhrle J, et al. SeQuent please world wide registry: clinical results of SeQuent please paclitaxel-coated balloon angioplasty in a large-scale, prospective registry study. J Am Coll Cardiol. 2012;60(18):1733–8.
56. Jeger RV, et al. Drug-coated balloons for small coronary artery disease (BASKET-SMALL 2): an open-label randomised non-inferiority trial. Lancet. 2018;392(10150):849–56.
57. Ali RM, et al. Treatment of coronary drug-eluting stent restenosis by a sirolimus- or paclitaxel-coated balloon. JACC Cardiovasc Interv. 2019;12(6):558–66.
58. Cortese B, Di Palma G, Latini R. Magic touch®: preliminary clinical evidence with a novel sirolimus drug coated balloon. Minerva Cardioangiol. 2018;66(4):508–17.
59. Neumann FJ, et al. 2018 ESC/EACTS Guidelines on myocardial revascularization. Eur Heart J. 2019;40(2):87–165.
60. Scheller B, et al. Long-term follow-up after treatment of coronary in-stent restenosis with a paclitaxel-coated balloon catheter. JACC Cardiovasc Interv. 2012;5(3):323–30.
61. Habara S, et al. A multicenter randomized comparison of paclitaxel-coated balloon catheter with conventional balloon angioplasty in patients with bare-metal stent restenosis and drug-eluting stent restenosis. Am Heart J. 2013;166(3):527–33.
62. Habara S, et al. Effectiveness of paclitaxel-eluting balloon catheter in patients with sirolimus-eluting stent restenosis. JACC Cardiovasc Interv. 2011;4(2):149–54.
63. Rittger H, et al. A randomized, multicenter, single-blinded trial comparing paclitaxel-coated balloon angioplasty with plain balloon angioplasty in drug-eluting stent restenosis: the PEPCAD-DES study. J Am Coll Cardiol. 2012;59(15):1377–82.
64. Cortese B, et al. Drug-coated balloon versus drug-eluting stent for small coronary vessel disease: PICCOLETO II randomized clinical trial. JACC Cardiovasc Interv. 2020;13(24):2840–9.
65. Scheller B, et al. Drug-coated balloon for small coronary artery disease in patients with and without high-

bleeding risk in the BASKET-SMALL 2 trial. Circ Cardiovasc Interv. 2022;15(4):e011569.
66. Zhang Y, et al. Duration of dual antiplatelet therapy after implantation of drug-coated balloon. Front Cardiovasc Med. 2021;8:762391.
67. Rissanen TT, et al. Drug-coated balloon for treatment of de-novo coronary artery lesions in patients with high bleeding risk (DEBUT): a single-blind, randomised, non-inferiority trial. Lancet. 2019;394(10194):230–9.
68. Scheller B, et al. Bare metal or drug-eluting stent versus drug-coated balloon in non-ST-elevation myocardial infarction: the randomised PEPCAD NSTEMI trial. EuroIntervention. 2020;15(17):1527–33.
69. Cowley MJ, et al. Acute coronary events associated with percutaneous transluminal coronary angioplasty. Am J Cardiol. 1984;53(12):12c–6c.
70. Cortese B, et al. Effect of drug-coated balloons in native coronary artery disease left with a dissection. JACC Cardiovasc Interv. 2015;8(15):2003–9.
71. Mangner N, et al. Safety and efficacy of drug-coated balloons versus drug-eluting stents in acute coronary syndromes: a prespecified analysis of BASKET-SMALL 2. Circ Cardiovasc Interv. 2022;15(2):e011325.
72. Uskela S, et al. Percutaneous coronary intervention with drug-coated balloon-only strategy in stable coronary artery disease and in acute coronary syndromes: An all-comers registry study. Catheter Cardiovasc Interv. 2019;93(5):893–900.
73. Cortese B, et al. Paclitaxel-coated balloon versus drug-eluting stent during PCI of small coronary vessels, a prospective randomised clinical trial. The PICCOLETO Study. Heart. 2010;96(16):1291–6.
74. Latib A, et al. A randomized multicenter study comparing a paclitaxel drug-eluting balloon with a paclitaxel-eluting stent in small coronary vessels: the BELLO (Balloon Elution and Late Loss Optimization) study. J Am Coll Cardiol. 2012;60(24):2473–80.
75. Jeger RV, et al. Long-term efficacy and safety of drug-coated balloons versus drug-eluting stents for small coronary artery disease (BASKET-SMALL 2): 3-year follow-up of a randomised, non-inferiority trial. Lancet. 2020;396(10261):1504–10.
76. Latib A, et al. 3-year follow-up of the Balloon Elution and Late Loss Optimization Study (BELLO). JACC Cardiovasc Interv. 2015;8(8):1132–4.
77. Tang Y, et al. Drug-coated balloon versus drug-eluting stent for small-vessel disease: the RESTORE SVD China randomized trial. JACC Cardiovasc Interv. 2018;11(23):2381–92.
78. Funatsu A, et al. A multicenter randomized comparison of paclitaxel-coated balloon with plain balloon angioplasty in patients with small vessel disease. Clin Res Cardiol. 2017;106(10):824–32.
79. Fezzi S, Giacoppo D, Fahrni G, et al. Individual patient data meta-analysis of paclitaxel-coated balloons vs. drug-eluting stents for small-vessel coronary artery disease: the ANDROMEDA study. Eur Heart J. Published online February 21, 2025. https://doi.org/10.1093/eurheartj/ehaf002.
80. Yazdani SK, et al. Vascular, downstream, and pharmacokinetic responses to treatment with a low dose drug-coated balloon in a swine femoral artery model. Catheter Cardiovasc Interv. 2014;83(1):132–40.
81. Torii S, et al. Biologic drug effect and particulate embolization of drug-eluting stents versus drug-coated balloons in healthy swine femoropopliteal arteries. J Vasc Interv Radiol. 2018;29(7):1041–1049.e3.
82. Nakazawa G. Stent thrombosis of drug eluting stent: pathological perspective. J Cardiol. 2011;58(2):84–91.
83. Valgimigli M, et al. 2017 ESC focused update on dual antiplatelet therapy in coronary artery disease developed in collaboration with EACTS: the Task Force for dual antiplatelet therapy in coronary artery disease of the European Society of Cardiology (ESC) and of the European Association for Cardio-Thoracic Surgery (EACTS). Eur Heart J. 2018;39(3):213–60.
84. Kleber FX, et al. Drug-coated balloons for treatment of coronary artery disease: updated recommendations from a consensus group. Clin Res Cardiol. 2013;102(11):785–97.
85. Kleber FX, et al. How to use the drug-eluting balloon: recommendations by the German consensus group. EuroIntervention. 2011;7(Suppl K):K125–8.
86. Cortese B, Serruys PW. Single-antiplatelet treatment after coronary angioplasty with drug-coated balloon. J Am Heart Assoc. 2023;12(6):e028413.
87. Räsänen A, et al. Percutaneous coronary intervention with drug-coated balloon-only strategy combined with single antiplatelet treatment in patients at high bleeding risk: Single center experience of a novel concept. Catheter Cardiovasc Interv. 2023;101(3):569–78.

11 Protected PCI in High-Bleeding-Risk Patients

Pedro Rafael Vieira de Oliveira Salerno, Gabriel Tensol Rodrigues Pereira, Bernardo Cortese, and Luis Augusto Palma Dallan

11.1 Introduction

The advances in percutaneous coronary intervention (PCI) have revolutionized the management of coronary artery disease (CAD), offering improved therapeutic options for patients previously deemed ineligible for intervention [1]. These developments have not only broadened the range of interventional cardiology but have also challenged previous assumptions about patient selection and procedural complexity [2].

In this scenario, complex and high-risk intervention in indicated patients (CHIP) has become a central theme of discussion, marked by considerable uncertainty. Traditionally, CHIP is conceived as having three core components [3].

1. Patients factors (patient comorbidities and surgical ineligibility).
2. Complicated heart disease (adverse hemodynamics, depressed ventricular function, and concurrent valve disease).
3. Complex PCI (complexity of coronary anatomy including adequacy of distal targets).

Further classifications, such as the one proposed by Fujimoto et al., attempt to provide more granularity to the CHIP definition, and subdivide them into definite CHIP, possible CHIP, and non-CHIP. Due to the challenges involved in tackling CHIPs, the use of mechanical circulatory support (MCS) in patients undergoing high-risk PCI has been practiced for more than 40 years [3]. This strategy of undergoing high-risk PCI and attempting to ensure hemodynamic support by reducing left ventricular systolic work and myocardial oxygen demand, while ensuring sustained systemic and coronary perfusion, was named "protected PCI." [2] However, appropriate patient selection and planning is crucial for protected PCI. This is particularly important for challenging subgroups such as those patients with high bleeding risk (HBR). Therefore, in this chapter, we will focus on protected PCI in HBR patients.

P. R. V. de Oliveira Salerno · G. Tensol Rodrigues Pereira · L. A. P. Dallan (✉)
University Hospitals Cleveland Medical Center, Cleveland, OH, USA

Case Western Reserve University, Cleveland, OH, USA
e-mail: gabriel.tensolrodriguespereira@uhhospitals.org

B. Cortese
University Hospitals Harrington Heart & Vascular Institute, Cleveland, OH, USA

Fondazione Ricerca e Innovazione Cardiovascolare, Milan, Italy

DCB Academy, Milan, Italy

B. Cortese, S. Rigattieri (eds.), *High Bleeding Risk Patients in Interventional Cardiology*,
https://doi.org/10.1007/978-3-031-87302-7_11

11.2 High-Bleeding-Risk Definition

Patients with HBR pose a significant challenge to PCI due to the often pro-hemorrhagic nature of the procedure and post-procedural interventions [4]. In 2019, the Academic Research Consortium for High Bleeding Risk (ARC-HBR) published the "Defining High Bleeding Risk in Patients Undergoing Percutaneous Coronary Intervention" consensus [4]. THE ARC-HBR criteria for HBR take into consideration 20 clinical criteria stratified into major or minor and considers a patient as having an HBR if he has at least 1 major or 2 minor criteria (Table 11.1) [4]. While a binary classification of HBR reduces the complexity of the definition, the cumulative impact of multiple risk factors on bleeding risk must not be neglected. [4]

11.3 Protected PCI in HBR

Managing CAD in patients with HBR presents a significant challenge. Frequently, HBR patients are deemed ineligible for coronary artery bypass graft (CABG) and therefore need PCI with drug-eluting stents [5]. However, this therapeutic approach requires dual antiplatelet therapy (DAPT), inevitably increasing the risk of bleeding [5]. When the patient factor of HBR is compounded with complicated heart disease or lesions characterized by increased PCI complexity, the clinical scenario transitions to that of CHIP. In such cases, MCS may be required during PCI. Unfortunately, the integration of MCS into PCI introduces an additional layer of complexity for patients HBR.

Currently, there are four main options for MCS in protected PCI: intra-aortic balloon pump (IABP), percutaneous left ventricular assist

Table 11.1 The Academic Research Consortium for High Bleeding Risk (ARC-HBR) criteria. HBR is defined as having at least one major criteria or two minor criteria

ARC-HBR criteria for HBR	
Major criteria	Minor criteria
	Age > 75 years
Anticipated use of long-term oral anticoagulation[a]	
Severe or end-stage CKD (eGFR <30 mL/min)	Moderate CKD (eGFR 30–59 mL/min)
Hemoglobin <11 g/dl	Hemoglobin 11–12.9 g/dl for males and 11–11.9 g/dl for females
Spontaneous bleeding requiring hospitalization or transfusion in the past 6 months or at any time, if recurrent	Spontaneous bleeding requiring hospitalization or transfusion within the past 12 not the meeting major criteria
Moderate or severe baseline thrombocytopenia (platelet count <100 × 10^9/L)	
Chronic bleeding diathesis	
	Long-term use of oral NSAIDs or steroids
Liver cirrhosis with portal hypertension	
Active malignancy (excluding non-melanoma skin cancer) within the past 12 months	
Previous spontaneous ICH (at any time) OR previous traumatic ICH within the past OR presence of a bAVM OR moderate or severe ischemic stroke within the past 6 months	Any ischemic stroke at any time not meeting the major criteria
Nondeferrable major surgery on DAPT	
Recent major surgery or major trauma within 30 days before PCI	

Abbreviations: *CKD* Chronic kidney disease, *eGFR* Estimated glomerular filtration rate, *ICH* Intracranial hemorrhage, *NSAIDs* nonsteroidal anti-inflammatory drug, *DAPT* Dual antiplatelet therapy, *bAVM* brain arteriovenous malformation

[a] Does not include vascular protection doses

devices (pLVAD), left atrial to aorta assist devices (LAAD), and veno-arterial extracorporeal membrane oxygenation (VA-ECMO) [2]. IABP and LVAD devices are the most commonly used. While the American College of Cardiology/American Heart Association 2021 guidelines give a 2b recommendation for the use of MCS in select high-risk patients with complex PCI, there are limited recommendations to aid in patient selection and personalized device definition [6]. Therefore, recommendations concerning the use of protected PCI in HBR lack the support of robust evidence and must be assessed in a case-by-case scenario.

More importantly, most studies were not designed to assess the use of protected PCI in a HBR scenario. In fact, several of them excluded patients with significant renal or liver disease, recent stroke or transient ischemic attack, and uncorrectable abnormal coagulation parameters, factors, and conditions that could be associated with a HBR. This was, for example, the case of the PROTECT trials, a series of trials analyzing protected PCI with the Impella 2.5 (Abiomed, Danvers, MA) pLVAD device [7]. PROTECT I was a prospective pilot study to demonstrate the feasibility of protected PCI with Impella that enrolled 20 patients from 7 United States (US) centers, and 2 deaths and 2 periprocedural myocardial infarctions (MI) were reported. Notably 40% of the patients developed hematomas in the access site, but no patients required transfusion or vascular repair [7]. The PROTECT II trial was a larger prospective, multicenter, randomized trial conducted in 112 sites in the United States, Canada, and Europe that enrolled 452 patients (only 69% of the planned patient enrollment) and aimed to compare Impella vs. IABP but was ended early due to the low enrolment, compromising the power of the study [8]. The study did not show a statistically significant difference in the 30-day incidence of major adverse events between the two groups [8]. However, at 90 days, there was a trend toward lower rates of major adverse events among patients supported by Impella 2.5, although this difference did not reach statistical significance [8].

In 2022, Kim et al. recommended an algorithm to guide patient selection and device choice (Fig. 11.1), suggesting that IABPs be preferred in patients with HBR due to the indispensable need for adequate anticoagulation in protected PCI with pLVAD, LAAD, and VA-ECMO. [2]

However, there are strategies that can be employed in planning for protected PCI procedures with Impella for patients with HBR, and these have been summarized in Fig. 11.2 [9]. In brief, a thorough patient assessment is key. Adequately assessing bleeding risk and patient comorbidities such as peripheral artery disease (PAD) are needed to personalize the procedures [9]. For example, in patients with a HBR, a single-access approach is preferred to limit puncture sites, and in PAD patients, the use of axillary access can be a viable alternative. [9] Additionally, the removal of the Impella device within the catheterization room and the use of vascular closure devices (VCD), such as the MANTA device, may aid in reducing access site bleeding complications. Anticoagulation strategies may also play a major role [9]. O'Neil et al., in a study that analyzed data from the PROTECT III (a post approval FDA-audited observational study trial), found a substantial decrease in bleeding complications necessitating transfusion among participants in the PROTECT III cohort compared to those in the historic PROTECT II cohort (1.8% versus 9.3%; $p < 0.001$) [10]. Suggesting that a potential explanation would be the decrease in the usage of glycoprotein IIb/IIIa inhibitors, which have been found to be linked to increased bleeding rates, regardless of the use of other antiplatelet medications [10]. They additionally noted that in PROTECT III, VCDs were the dominating closure method, which could have also contributed to the reduced access site bleeding complicatons [10].

Moreover, extrapolating evidence from unprotected PCI in HBR patients, there could be a benefit in using abbreviated DAPT regimens. Based on a meta-analysis conducted by Costa et al. that demonstrated that an abbreviated DAPT regimen (1 or 3 months) was associated with lower bleeding and cardiovascular mortality without

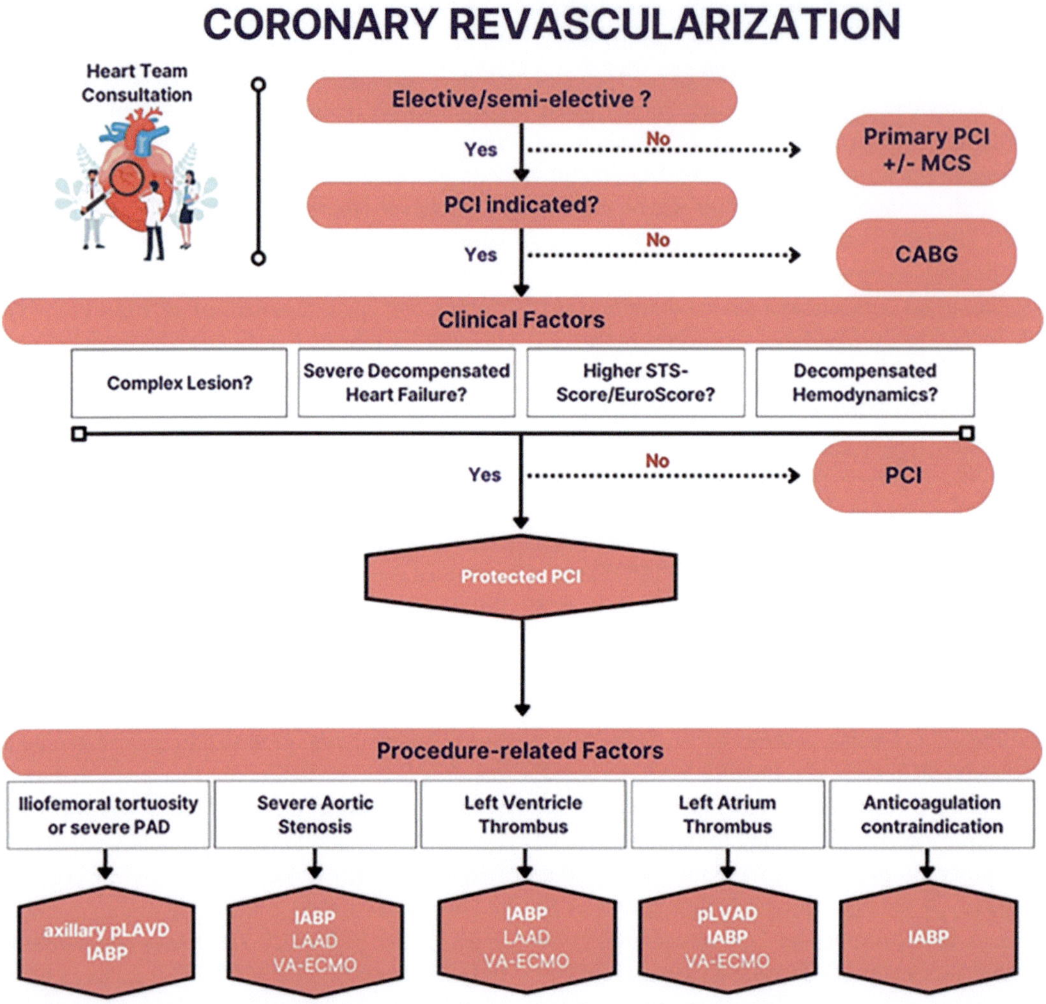

Fig. 11.1 Approach proposed by Kim et al. (2022) for patient selection for protected PCI depending on the clinical and procedure-related factors. Adapted from Kim SH, Baumann S, Behnes M, Borggrefe M, and Akin I. Patient Selection for Protected Percutaneous Coronary Intervention. *Interv Cardiol Clin*. 2022;11 (4):455–464. https://doi.org/10.1016/j.iccl.2022.07.001. Abbreviations: *IABP* Intra-aortic balloon pump, *pLVAD* Percutaneous left ventricular assist devices, *LAAD* Left atrial to aorta assist devices, *VA-ECMO* Veno-arterial extracorporeal membrane oxygenation, *PAD* Peripheral artery disease, *PCI* Percutaneous coronary intervention, *CABG* Coronary artery bypass graft

increasing ischemic events, when compared to a ≥ 6-month DAPT regimen. [11]

Nonetheless, HBR patients remained severely understudied, and therefore, trials and studies focusing on HBR patients undergoing protected PCI are greatly needed. The Safe Surveillance of PCI Under Mechanical Circulatory Support With the Saranas Early Bird Bleed Monitoring System (SAFE-MCS) is an ongoing multicenter, single-arm, open-label study designed to evaluate the safety of complex high-risk PCI using Impella and surveillance with the Saranas Early Bird Bleed Monitoring System (EBBMS) [12]. Its primary end point will be the incidence of access-site-related Bleeding Academic Research Consortium (BARC) type III or V bleeding and may contribute to a better understanding of the bleeding risk in patients undergoing Impella. However, its relatively small sample size and lack of randomization are important limitations.

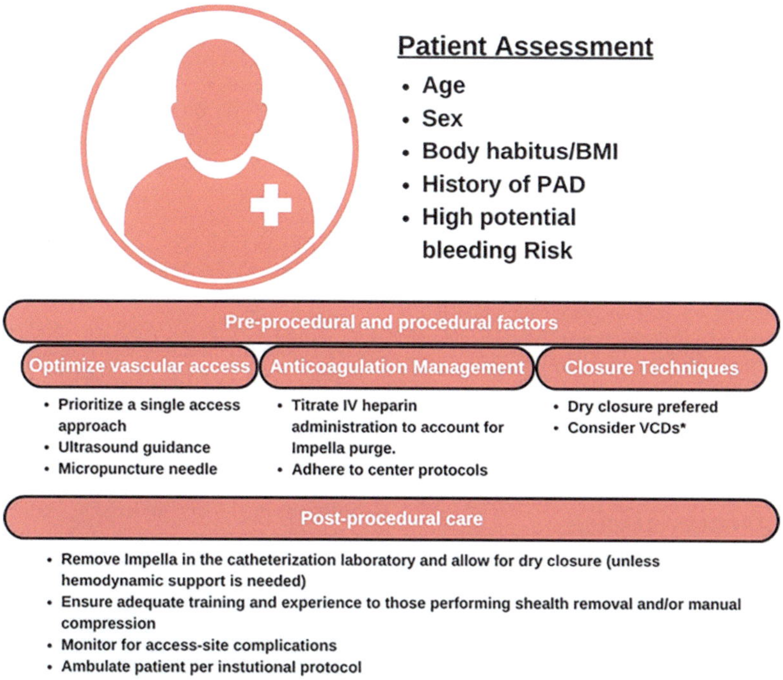

Fig. 11.2 Approach proposed by Vetrovec et al. (2022) of strategies for reducing vascular and bleeding risk for percutaneous left ventricular assist device-supported high-risk percutaneous coronary intervention. Adapted from Vetrovec GW, Kaki A, Wollmuth J, and Dahle TG. Strategies for Reducing Vascular and Bleeding Risk for Percutaneous Left Ventricular Assist Device-supported High-risk Percutaneous Coronary Intervention. Heart Int. 2022;16 (2):105–111. https://doi.org/10.17925/HI.2022.16.2.105. Abbreviations: *BMI* Body mass index, *CTA* computerized tomography angiography, *IV* Intravenous, *PAD* Peripheral arterial disease, *VCD* vascular closure device. * Examples of VCDs include the Manta Device and the Perclose Proglide.

Additionally, the study does not focus on patients with prior HBR.

The ongoing PROTECT 4 trial (Impella®-Supported PCI in High-Risk Patients With Complex Coronary Artery Disease and Reduced Left Ventricular Function, NCT04763200) is assessing the use of Impella® CP or 2.5 device during high-risk PCI in patients with reduced left ventricular function to understand symptoms improvement, heart function recovery, and complications as compared to standard care. Primary endpoint is the composite of all-cause death, stroke, MI, unplanned clinically driven revascularization, durable LVAD implant or heart transplant, or other hospitalization for cardiovascular causes though 3-year follow-up. Study completion with 1252 patients is expected by March 2026.

In conclusion, most of the evidence regarding the use of protected PCI in HBR patients must be extrapolated either from studies that reported bleeding complications in patients undergoing protected PCI or from studies conducted in HBR patients undergoing unprotected PCI. While the American College of Cardiology/American Heart Association 2021 guidelines tend to favor the use of LVAD as the preferred MCS device in protected PCI, in the context of HBR patients, several authors recommend the use of IABP. However, there are several strategies that can be implemented to reduce bleeding risk in patients undergoing protected PCI with a LVAD.

References

1. Hoole SP, Bambrough P. Recent advances in percutaneous coronary intervention. Heart. 2020;106(18):1380–6. https://doi.org/10.1136/heartjnl-2019-315707.
2. Kim SH, Baumann S, Behnes M, Borggrefe M, Akin I. Patient selection for protected percutaneous coronary intervention. Interv Cardiol Clin. 2022;11(4):455–64. https://doi.org/10.1016/j.iccl.2022.07.001.
3. Fujimoto Y, Sakakura K, Fujita H. Complex and high-risk intervention in indicated patients (CHIP) in contemporary clinical practice. Cardiovasc Interv Ther. 2023;38(3):269–74. https://doi.org/10.1007/s12928-023-00930-1.
4. Urban P, Mehran R, Colleran R, et al. Defining high bleeding risk in patients undergoing percutaneous coronary intervention. Circulation. 2019;140(3):240–61. https://doi.org/10.1161/CIRCULATIONAHA.119.040167.
5. Chiarito M, Kini A, Roumeliotis A, et al. Prevalence and impact of high bleeding risk in patients undergoing left Main artery disease PCI. JACC Cardiovasc Interv. 2021;14(22):2447–57. https://doi.org/10.1016/j.jcin.2021.08.056.
6. Lawton JS, Tamis-Holland JE, Bangalore S, et al. 2021 ACC/AHA/SCAI guideline for coronary artery revascularization: a report of the American College of Cardiology/American Heart Association joint committee on clinical practice guidelines. Circulation. 2022;145(3):e18–e114. https://doi.org/10.1161/CIR.0000000000001038.
7. Dixon SR, Henriques JPS, Mauri L, et al. A prospective feasibility trial investigating the use of the Impella 2.5 system in patients undergoing high-risk percutaneous coronary intervention (the PROTECT I trial). JACC Cardiovasc Interv. 2009;2(2):91–6. https://doi.org/10.1016/j.jcin.2008.11.005.
8. O'Neill WW, Kleiman NS, Moses J, et al. A prospective, randomized clinical trial of hemodynamic support with Impella 2.5 versus intra-aortic balloon pump in patients undergoing high-risk percutaneous coronary intervention. Circulation. 2012;126(14):1717–27. https://doi.org/10.1161/CIRCULATIONAHA.112.098194.
9. Vetrovec GW, Kaki A, Wollmuth J, Dahle TG. Strategies for reducing vascular and bleeding risk for percutaneous left ventricular assist device-supported high-risk percutaneous coronary intervention. Heart Int. 2022;16(2):105–11. https://doi.org/10.17925/HI.2022.16.2.105.
10. O'Neill WW, Anderson M, Burkhoff D, et al. Improved outcomes in patients with severely depressed LVEF undergoing percutaneous coronary intervention with contemporary practices. Am Heart J. 2022;248:139–49. https://doi.org/10.1016/j.ahj.2022.02.006.
11. Costa F, Montalto C, Branca M, et al. Dual antiplatelet therapy duration after percutaneous coronary intervention in high bleeding risk: a meta-analysis of randomized trials. Eur Heart J. 2023;44(11):954–68. https://doi.org/10.1093/eurheartj/ehac706.
12. Généreux P, Kaki A, Naguib M, et al. Design and rationale of the Safe surveillance of PCI under mechanical circulatory support with the Saranas early bird bleed monitoring system (SAFE-MCS) study. J Soc Cardiovasc Angiogr Interv. 2023;2(5):101049. https://doi.org/10.1016/j.jscai.2023.101049.

12 Contemporary Bypass Techniques in Hybrid Revascularization

Olatoye Olutola, Pablo Ruda Vega, and Marc Pelletier

12.1 Background

The principle of hybrid coronary revascularization (HCR) was first described in 1996 by Angelini [1]. Although HCR was performed infrequently for several years afterward, the number of patients treated with HCR has increased steadily. These procedures are performed by a team of cardiac surgeons and interventional cardiologists who function collaboratively, ideally with proficiency in advanced techniques in minimally invasive surgery and percutaneous coronary intervention (PCI).

Based on the guidelines of joint American societies on coronary artery bypass graft (CABG) and PCI, HCR is a procedure involving a coronary bypass of the left internal mammary artery (LIMA) to the left anterior descending (LAD) and PCI of at least one non-LAD coronary artery [2]. The 2011 American College of Cardiology Foundation (ACC)/American Heart Association (AHA) guidelines for CABG states that the primary purpose of performing HCR is to decrease the morbidity rate of traditional CABG in high-risk patients [3]. It is a class IIb recommendation for certain patient subsets at experienced centers [4]. In patients with multivessel coronary artery disease, hybrid revascularization combines minimally invasive CABG and PCI with the goal of obtaining complete revascularization with a combination of surgery and coronary stents, while minimizing surgical trauma. This requires collaboration between interventional cardiologists and cardiothoracic surgeons and capitalizes on the major advantage of both treatments, including the utilization of durable left internal mammary artery (LIMA) to left anterior descending artery (LAD) bypass graft, with the less invasive aspect of PCI in treating other stenoses [5]. Previous meta-analyses involving hybrid revascularization have demonstrated favorable outcomes, while suggesting shorter length of stay, improved recovery, and decreased need for blood transfusion [6]. However, patient selection is important, given the results of the SYNTAX trial which outlined the superiority of complete surgical revascularization in certain patients [7].

Despite the potential benefits of HCR, there are certain risks inherent to each type of procedure. The drawbacks of PCI can include inferior long-term outcomes with higher re-intervention rates, the need for dual antiplatelet therapy, and limited options for repeat stenting, including the

O. Olutola
Department of Surgery, University Hospitals, Cleveland Medical Center, Case Western Reserve University, Cleveland, OH, USA
e-mail: Olatoye.olutola@uhhospitals.org

P. R. Vega · M. Pelletier (✉)
Division of Cardiac Surgery, University Hospitals, Cleveland Medical Center, Case Western Reserve University, Cleveland, OH, USA
e-mail: pablo.rudavega@uhhospitals.org; marc.pelletier@uhhospitals.org

B. Cortese, S. Rigattieri (eds.), *High Bleeding Risk Patients in Interventional Cardiology*,
https://doi.org/10.1007/978-3-031-87302-7_12

possibility of requiring bypass grafting. In CABG patients, there are risks of general anesthesia, invasiveness, surgical trauma, and the need for mechanical ventilation. To optimize outcomes, coronary revascularization should offer minimal invasiveness to reduce risk and maximal durability to improve survival. The benefits and risks of hybrid revascularization should be discussed in a multidisciplinary setting with the patient, cardiologist, and the cardiac surgeon.

12.2 Definition and Key Concept in HCR

HCR is defined as a planned revascularization using a combination of PCI and CABG, in different coronary territories. The key concept of this approach is to perform a LIMA to LAD preferably through a minimally invasive approach combined with PCI, typically with a drug-eluting stent (DES) to non-LAD territories. The major reasoning with this approach is the combination of the well-established benefit of a LIMA to the LAD coupled with the less invasive approach of PCI. This gives patients the best of both worlds: durability and less invasiveness.

The two key principles for any potential HCR patient are the following:

1. Suitable LAD for grafting (especially for minimally invasive off-pump LIMA to LAD)
2. Suitable non-LAD vessels for DES

The major indications, contraindications, inclusion, and exclusion criteria are related to these two principles.

12.3 Indications

When considering patients for hybrid revascularization, we have found that they fall in four main categories:

1. Single-vessel disease involving the LAD (+/– diagonals). This is especially important in the case of heavily calcified LAD vessels, ostial LAD disease, complete total occlusion (CTO), and bifurcation lesions.
2. High-risk patients. Individuals with multivessel disease and good surgical anatomy, but with comorbidities that render standard CABG risky. Examples include patients that are elderly, frail, previous CVA, calcified ascending aorta, lack of surgical conduits, and high STS surgical risk.
3. Prognosis value: Patients with viable options for both PCI and CABG, but who after a heart team discussion, are felt to benefit prognostically from a LIMA to the LAD.
4. Patient preference: In the current era of transparency and patient discussion, some patients will refuse to have a sternotomy for valid and personal reasons but agree to a MIDCAB procedure to obtain a LIMA to the LAD with PCI of the other vessels. The reasoning is diverse and individualized to each patient; examples include aesthetic reasons, faster return to work, and personal or family needs.

12.4 Inclusion Criteria

Candidates for HCR have multivessel coronary artery disease (CAD) involving the LAD or the left main coronary artery with at least one other coronary artery stenosis amenable to PCI [8]. In patients with distal left main bifurcation disease, HCR will provide LIMA graft to LAD and DES from the left main into the proximal left circumflex artery. These patients are required to tolerate dual antiplatelet therapy (DAPT) for at least 3 months and up to ~12 months or longer.

Patients with high-risk conditions can be considered for HCR. This includes those with reduced left ventricular ejection fraction, recent myocardial infarction, and lack of non-LAD surgical targets. Others who may also benefit from HCR are those with carotid disease, lack of vein conduits, chronic kidney disease, and elderly patients with calcific aortas with a reduction in the risk of stroke [9]. Obese and diabetic patients also have a survival benefit of a LIMA graft without the risk of median sternotomy or sternal wound infection.

Table 12.1 Inclusion criteria and considerations in patients considered for hybrid coronary revascularization (HCR)

Inclusion criteria	Considerations
Suitable anatomy	Proximal LAD disease, left main disease
	Coronary arteries amenable to PCI
High mortality and morbidity risk with standard CABG	Advanced age
	Frailty
	Multiple comorbidities
	Important cerebrovascular impairment with history of cerebral stroke or paraplegia
	Serious carotid artery disease
	Pulmonary illness
Patients with increased risk of morbidity with a sternotomy	Previous sternotomy
	History of sternal infection
	Previous mediastinitis
	Sternal tumors
	Previous thoracic radiation exposure
	Severe obesity with diabetes
	Mobility impairment restricting rehabilitation
Specific cardiac risk factors	Impaired left ventricular function Recent myocardial infarction Unfavorable non-LAD targets or distal lesions in circumflex or right coronary artery
Other factors	Profound aortic or mitral annular calcification Unwillingness to undergo median sternotomy Non-suitable venous or arterial conduits other than LIMA

Finally, some patients prefer to avoid a sternotomy and opt for a hybrid approach. The general indications for HCR are listed in Table 12.1.

12.5 Exclusion Criteria

For some patients, hybrid revascularization is either not advisable or contraindicated. The reasons can be classified into clinical factors, technical factors for LIMA to LAD and clinical factors for PCI.

Clinical conditions can further be classified as either cardiac or noncardiac reasons. Specific examples related to cardiovascular issues include hemodynamically unstable patients who might benefit from being placed on cardiopulmonary bypass, those with a recent myocardial infarction, cardiogenic shock, and severe decompensated ischemic cardiomyopathy. Noncardiac medical conditions that can pose a contraindication to HCR include the presence of severe lung disease precluding single-lung ventilation or patients with severe right ventricular dysfunction.

Technical contraindications include those with concerns about performing a good LIMA-to-LAD anastomosis. This includes a history of pericarditis, previous left thoracotomy or left chest wall surgery with extensive pleural adhesions, or damage to the LAD in previous cardiac surgery.

Lastly, there are patients in whom PCI is not feasible due to a variety of reasons, including diffuse and heavy calcification, small coronary arteries, or lack of vascular access. A comprehensive list of contraindications can be found in Table 12.2.

Table 12.2 Contraindications and reasoning for hybrid coronary revascularization

Contraindication	Rationale and description
Clinical factors and conditions	Hemodynamic instability
	Malignant ventricular arrhythmias
	Decompensated congestive heart failure or severely depressed ejection fraction
	History of chronic lung disease (FEv1 <50%) predicted or home oxygen dependence precluding intubation
	Coagulopathy (increasing risk of bleeding)
	History of pericarditis
	Prior left thoracotomy
Technical concerns about LIMA-to-LAD grafting	Unusable or previously used LIMA Previous thoracic surgery involving the left pleural space Left subclavian artery stenosis Chest wall irradiation Poor quality or diffusely diseased LAD
PCI related concerns	Risk of contrast-induced nephropathy Lesion characteristics indicative of a high predicted risk of restenosis Peripheral vascular disease precluding femoral, radial, or brachial access Dual antiplatelet intolerance

12.6 Setup of Heart Coronary Team

The performance of HCR depends on the maintenance and development of a collaborative coronary team. Although the original concept of a heart team developed during the early days of PCI, the contemporary heart team has mostly been devoted to structural heart cases in recent years. The coronary team should include a clinical cardiologist, heart failure specialist, interventional cardiologist, and cardiac surgeon. The elements of these coronary teams include multiple elements that should be common among centers seeking to provide optimal care for coronary artery disease patients. These include the following:

1. An understanding by participating healthcare providers (interventional cardiologists and cardiac surgeons) that medical management, PCI, and surgical revascularization play important roles in the care of patients with multivessel CAD. A collaborative coronary heart team precedes patient-centered comprehensive coronary care.
2. A shared recognition that being a good candidate for either multivessel PCI or surgical revascularization in a patient is not an indication to perform the procedure. Rather, only through a collaborative discussion of short- and long-term benefits of evidence-based guided medical therapy, PCI, traditional CABG, and HCR can we ensure that patients are assigned to the most suitable treatment option.
3. A comprehensive skill set that allows an institutional coronary team to provide cutting-edge care in coronary heart disease, including evidence-based medical therapy, multivessel PCI (with contemporary drug-eluting stents (DES), technical excellence, and routine use of fractional flow reserve), ability to perform CTO procedures, traditional and off-pump CABG (with multiple or all-arterial conduits, minimizing or avoiding aortic manipulation), and HCR (with minimally invasive sternal-sparing techniques, applied with minimal mortality and morbidity).
4. When the first three items above are achieved, the coronary heart team will collaboratively decide on which therapy is optimal for each individual patient, with the assurance that all members of the heart team will collectively benefit by maintaining their ethical obligation to provide the best care to each patient.

12.7 Timing of HCR Procedures

There are three possible timing strategies for hybrid revascularization, each with its inherent advantages and disadvantages.

1. CABG followed by PCI (two stage)
2. PCI followed by CABG (two stage)
3. Simultaneous CABG and PCI in a hybrid suite (one stage)

CABG Followed by PCI (Two Stages)
A strategy of first performing a CABG followed by PCI the next day, weeks, or a few months later has been shown to be the most common approach in HCR [10]. Benefits of this approach include assessment of the LIMA-LAD graft anastomosis which can be performed at the time of coronary angiography, prior to PCI. Typically, this is best accomplished from the left radial approach. After the LIMA graft is assessed, stent implantation of the remaining diseased segments is performed. This strategy facilitates full antiplatelet inhibition following CABG with no perioperative bleeding risk and provides a protected anterior wall, lowering procedural risks during PCI of non-LAD vessels. Should a problem be identified with the LIMA to LAD anastomosis, such as a severe stenosis, it can then be addressed by PCI. Some disadvantages of this approach include the risk of ischemia of non-LAD territories during the LIMA-to-LAD grafting and during the postoperative period. Of note, perianastomotic edema at the site of a LIMA to LAD anastomosis may lead to the appearance of a pseudo-stenosis at the distal anastomotic sites for days or weeks post-procedure. Generally, PCI of the distal LIMA-LAD anastomosis should be avoided unless there is TIMI (thrombolysis in myocardial infarction) flow grade 0–2 or ongoing ischemia, regardless of the severity of the stenosis [11].

PCI Followed by CABG (Two Stages)
In this approach, PCI is performed first, followed by CABG. This is also known as reverse HCR. It is preferred in the setting of acute coronary syndromes when the culprit lesion is in a non-LAD vessel, in the setting of LAD disease. Non-LAD arteries are stented first, and the LIMA-to-LAD is scheduled after 30 days, when oral antiplatelets can be withheld briefly. However, surgical procedures can sometimes invoke a systemic inflammatory response and promote platelet activation, increasing the risk of stent thrombosis, specifically after early interruption of dual antiplatelet therapy (DAPT) [12]. In patients with high risk of stent thrombosis, an alternative may include in-hospital admission 3–5 days before surgery, stopping oral antiplatelets, and bridging treatment with intravenous cangrelor [13]. Advantages of this approach include lower risks of ischemia during surgery and the possibility of performing grafting of the non-LAD arteries in the case of suboptimal PCI results.

Simultaneous CABG and PCI in a Hybrid Suite (One Stage)
This approach accounts for about 20% of all HCR procedures in the United States [14]. The increasing number of novel operating suites that provide true integration of fluoroscopic and surgical capabilities allows for complete hybrid revascularization in one session. This features state-of-the-art surgical and interventional equipment, usually starting with surgery first, followed by PCI. After performing a minimally invasive direct coronary artery bypass (MIDCAB)/totally endoscopic coronary artery bypass (TECAB) procedure, graft patency is verified, and PCI of other vessels are undertaken while the patient remains under general anesthesia. One major advantage of this approach is the immediate assessment of the LIMA-LAD graft anastomosis by angiography. Other advantages include reduced length of stay, hospital readmission rates between staged procedures, and reduced risk of lesion destabilization [15]. A major challenge is the balance between minimizing bleeding while preventing stent thrombosis. Additionally, patients with chronic kidney disease are exposed to the dual nephrotoxic insult of surgery and contrast.

12.8 Surgical Options and Results

The LIMA to LAD graft is the cornerstone of hybrid revascularization. Whatever method is used to perform this anastomosis, its integrity and full patency is the most important factor in the HCR strategy. The following are several important considerations:

12.8.1 MIDCAB

The minimally invasive direct coronary artery bypass (MIDCAB), also known as the sternal-sparing approach, is described as LIMA mobilization in an open fashion through a limited anterior or lateral thoracotomy incision in the fourth or fifth interspace. Rib retraction allows manual LIMA mobilization and anastomosis to the LAD on a beating heart [16]. Studies have shown that MIDCAB has similar long-term patency rates of LIMA graft with the traditional technique with a sternotomy. Perioperative morbidity and mortality are also low [17].

12.8.2 Off-Pump

Off-pump coronary artery bypass (OPCAB), sometimes referred to as the open sternotomy off-pump technique, was developed to avoid the complications of cardiopulmonary bypass. It uses LIMA mobilization through a limited sternotomy technique [15]. Whether performed through a sternotomy or through a left mini thoracotomy, a surgeon's ability to perform off-pump surgery is a key component in HCR.

12.8.3 Robotic Assistance

To avoid significant chest wall manipulation associated with MIDCAB and to improve postoperative pain control, robotic techniques have been developed. The development of robotic-enhanced minimally invasive direct coronary bypass (RECAB) allows endoscopic harvest of LIMA with a robot. This is performed through three port access sites introduced into the left chest. Using the da Vinci surgical platform (Intuitive Surgical, Sunnyvale, California), the LIMA is harvested either in a skeletonized or pedicled fashion. Next, a 3–5-cm thoracotomy is made over the LAD, and a hand-sewn anastomosis is performed on the beating heart. Studies show a high primary success rate with a patency graft rate of 95–100% with low perioperative morbidity and mortality [18, 19]. Advantages of the robot in this instance include the ability to harvest a longer LIMA, to simultaneously harvest a RIMA, if needed. Also, by opening the pericardium robotically, the surgical team is better able to identify the precise location of the thoracotomy.

The technique of robotic totally endoscopic coronary artery bypass (robotic TECAB) consists of LIMA mobilization and LAD arteriotomy and anastomosis with the robot [20]. In its early stages, the procedure was performed on the arrested heart, with intra-aortic balloon occlusion, but the beating-heart TECAB technique was later developed to avoid the use of CPB and to minimize the thoracotomy. Clinical freedom from graft failure was reported at 98.3% in 13 months in a retrospective study [21, 22].

12.8.4 Percutaneous Coronary Intervention (PCI)

Once the criterion for revascularization is met, PCI is performed with second- or third-generation drug-eluting stents (DES). Radial intervention is preferred to minimize vascular and bleeding complications. The duration of DAPT is dictated by individual patient's risks and current guidelines [23].

12.8.5 Quality Review

The evidence supporting HCR is shown in Table 12.3. HCR has been applied as a concept for approximately 20 years and provides an additional approach to revascularization for patients with multivessel CAD. The consensus is that it

Table 12.3 Evidence supporting the concept of hybrid coronary revascularization

Study (year)	Patients/controls (*n*)	HMR procedure	Surgical procedure	Timing	Follow-up	Authors' conclusions
Shen et al. (2013) [25]	141/141	MIDCAB	CABG or PCI	Simultaneous	3 years	Similar MACCE in HMR versus CABG, but increased versus PCI. HMR higher MACCE than CABG in high SYNTAX score and euroSCORE patients
Leacche et al. (2013)	80/301	OPCAB or CABG	OPCAB or CABG	Simultaneous	1 month	HMR a safe alternative to CABG increased repeat revascularization in HMR >33 SYNTAX score
Bachinsky et al. (2012) [24]	25/27	Robotic MIDCAB	OPCAB	Simultaneous	1 month	HMR feasible and safe
Hu et al. (2011)	104/104	MIDCAB	OPCAB	Simultaneous	1.5 years	HMR better 18-month clinical outcome (MACCE)
Halkos et al. (2011) [28]	147/588	MIDCAB	OPCAB	Staged	3.2 years	Similar rate of death and MACCE, revascularization increased in HMR
Halkos et al. (2011) [8]	27/81	MIDCAB	OPCAB	Staged	3.2 years	HMR is a safe and feasible in left main disease
Vassiliades et al. (2009) [38]	91/4175	MIDCAB	Endo-ACAB	Staged	3 years	HMR non inferior in 30-day MACCE and 3-year survival
Kon et al. (2008) [15]	15/30	MIDCAB	OPCAB	Simultaneous	1 year	Similar clinical results high patient satisfaction with HMR
Reicher et al. (2008) [39]	13/26	MIDCAB	OPCAB	Simultaneous	6 months	Similar safety and efficacy shorter hospital stay after HMR
de Cannière et al. (2001) [40]	20/20	MIDCAB	CABG	Mixed	2 years	Similar clinical results less perioperative morbidity
Kiaii (2008) [42]	58	RECAB		Simultaneous	1.8 year	HMR feasible and safe
Davidavicius (2005) [41]	20	RECAB		Mixed	19 month	HMR feasible and safe

remains safe and feasible. Despite its theoretical appeal, the number of clinical sites devoted to hybrid revascularization remains relatively low, and published data is limited.

12.8.6 HCR Versus Conventional Multivessel CABG

Bachinsky et al. published a prospective non-randomized study in 2012 that showed significant reductions in the number of blood transfusions and the length of stay associated with HCR ($p < 0.01$) [24]. HCR vs. CABG was associated with better outcomes at 3-year follow-up ($p = 0.003$) in the HCR + CABG (Shen et al.) observational study. Freedom from major adverse cardiac and cerebrovascular events (MACCE) after HCR was 93.6%, CABG was 86.5%, and PCI was 77.3% [25].

The POL-MIDES (Prospective Randomized Pilot Study Evaluating the Safety and Efficacy of Hybrid Revascularization in Multivessel Coronary Artery Disease) trial was a single-center, prospective randomized controlled trial comparing the feasibility of HCR in patients with multivessel coronary artery disease (MVCAD) to standard CABG [26]. A total of 200 consecutive patients with MCVAD involving the LAD and a critical lesion in at least 1 major non-LAD epicardial vessel amenable to both PCI and CABG were randomized in a 1:1 fashion to HMR ($n = 98$) (using MIDCAB and cobalt chromium EES) or conventional CABG ($n = 102$). Both groups had similar baseline demographic characteristics, risk factor profiles, and SYNTAX scores. The 5-year mortality rates between HCR and standard CABG (6.4% vs. 9.2%), myocardial infarction (4.3% vs. 7.2%), repeat revascularization (37.2% vs. 45.4%), and stroke (2.1% vs. 4.1%) were not statistically significant. This suggested that in patients with MCVCAD referred for surgical revascularization, HCR is safe and feasible. In 2020, Esteves et al. showed no difference in mortality or MACCE at 2 years, but in patients with high SYNTAX scores, there was a tendency for MACCE and increased revascularization in HCR arm compared to the CABG arm [27].

12.8.7 HCR Versus OPCAB

According to Halkos et al., HCR versus OPCAB was compared in patients with left main disease. Although MACCE rates were similar in both groups, HCR was associated with reduced blood transfusions and mechanical ventilation [28]. In 2016, Song et al. noted reductions in mechanical ventilation, chest tube drainage, and ICU length of stay in propensity-matched patients having simultaneous HCR versus OPCAB [29]. There was a 46% reduction of troponin I release after HCR compared to OPCAB in Harskamp et al., suggesting reduced myocardial injury with HCR [30]. Finally, Hage et al. demonstrated a reduced mortality over a long period of follow-up in patients that underwent single-stage HCR compared with OPCAB [31].

12.8.8 HCR Versus CABG Versus PCI

A study by Shen et al. sought to compare midterm clinical outcomes of one-step HCR with CABG and PCI for the treatment of MVCAD. One-step HCR incurred MACCE rate lower than that with PCI ($p < 0.001$) but similar to CABG ($p = 0.14$). HCR had numerically lower cumulative MACCE than either CABG or PCI across all three tertiles of the SYNTAX score. Specifically, the MACCE rate for patients in the high SYNTAX score tertile was significantly lower after HCR than after PCI ($p = 0.002$) but like that for CABG ($p = 0.36$) [25].

In addition, a recent prospective, single-center, open-label RCT by Ganyukov et al. was conducted from 2013 to 2017. One hundred fifty-five MVCAD patients were randomized into three groups on a 1:1:1 ratio. The groups were CABG (50), PCI (53), and HCR (52). MACCE and residual myocardial ischemia were similar across the three study arms at 12 months. This study provides no evidence for HCR benefit in patients in whom PCI, CABG, and HCR are equally feasible. However, the PCI arm observed significant reductions in hospital stay and major bleeding [32].

12.8.9 HCR Versus PCI

The National Institutes of Health (NIH) funded a multicenter, observational study to explore the characteristics and outcomes of patients undergoing clinically indicated HCR and multivessel PCI for hybrid-eligible coronary artery disease (defined as a proximal and/or mid LAD lesion plus at least one other non-LAD lesion).

Two hundred HCR and 98 multivessel PCI patients were enrolled at 11 sites over 18 months. The HCR approach included robotic ($n = 108$), MIDCAB ($n = 38$), robotic totally endoscopic ($n = 42$), and planned sternotomy ($n = 12$). At 12 and 18 months, event-free survival was similar between the two groups (hazard ratio: 1.06; 95% confidence interval: 0.66–1.69 and hazard ratio: 0.86; 95% confidence interval: 0.56–1.36), respectively (Table 12.4) [33].

12.8.10 Learning Curve

A successful minimally invasive/hybrid CABG program requires a well-trained team that is technically facile in all aspects of modern bypass

Table 12.4 Comparison of HCR versus multivessel PCI

	HCR (N = 200)		PCI with DES (n = 98)		
	n	Incidence rate per person-year	n	Incidence rate per person-year	HR (95% CI)
MACCE incidence at 30 days					
Any MACCE	6	0.393	2	0.264	2.658 (0.839–8.421)
Death	1	0.064	0	0	
Myocardial infarction	3	0.195	1	0.131	
Stroke	0	0	0	0	
Revascularization	4	0.26	1	0.131	
MACCE incidence at 12 months					
Any MACCE	23	0.143	10	0.119	1.063 (0.666–1.697)
Death	3	0.017	1	0.011	
Myocardial infarction	4	0.024	3	0.034	
Stroke	5	0.03	0	0	
Revascularization	14	0.085	8	0.094	
MACCE incidence through end of study					
Any MACCE		0.103	12	0.103	0.868 (0.556–1.355)
Death		0.012	2	0.016	
Myocardial infarction		0.017	3	0.024	
Stroke		0.021	0	0	
Revascularization		0.061	10	0.084	

Obtained with permission from Dr. John Puskas

surgery. This includes the ability to harvest skeletonized IMAs, to perform Y and T arterial grafts, and to perform sequential coronary anastomoses. In most cases, the main limiting step is adequate training and experience in off-pump CABG. A reasonable learning curve should include a progression from on-pump CABG to off-pump CABG in standard sternotomy cases. Once off-pump skills have been established, next would be the incorporation of a minimally invasive approach with off-pump anastomoses, via either a MIDCAB or Robotic assisted MIDCAB. Lastly, once that can be safely completed, one can purse a TECAB approach. Robotic cardiac surgery has been shown to be safe and feasible in dedicated centers. Cheng et al. analyzed the learning curve issues associated with TECAB using a stepwise approach by a single surgeon that performed >650 cases of different types of robotic cardiac cases at a single center from 2007 to 2013. During this time, 230 patients underwent robotic CABG on the beating heart, 90 of whom had successfully undergone beating heart TECAB using the da Vinci S/Si Surgical System without conversion to sternotomy. All of the beating heart TECAB procedures were completed using the following principles:

- Endoscopic LIMA harvesting
- Pericardiotomy and target vessel identification
- LIMA anastomosis to the target vessel

Perioperative outcomes were compared among the three quintiles, showing a significant decrease in operative time (P = 0.000), LITA harvesting time (P = 0.037), and anastomotic time (P = 0.000). A significant learning curve was observed for the operative time ($y(\text{min}) = 223 - 17 \times \ln(x)$; $r2 = 0.217$, $P = 0.000$); LITA harvesting time ($y(\text{min}) = 37 - 3 \times \ln(x)$; $r2 = 0.097$, $P = 0.003$); and LITA-left anterior descending artery anastomotic time ($y(\text{min}) = 18 - 2 \times \ln(x)$; $r2 = 0.298$, $P = 0.000$). No differences were found in the mean transit flow (P = 0.102) or perioperative complications among the three quintiles.

This study reports a steep learning curve with the first 18–20 patients. Apart from surgical errors and human factors, the slope precisely reflects the improvement in surgical performance of a dedicated cardiac surgery team. This is consistent with previous studies that have noted a reduction in LIMA takedown times. Additionally, the use of U-clips and stabilizers has reduced anastomotic times for LIMA-LAD in robotic TECABs.

In summary, LITA preparation without graft injury and anastomosis completion on the beating heart were the most demanding parts of TECAB. Given a LIMA to LAD anastomosis graft occlusion rate and anastomotic stenosis rate of 6% and >50%, respectively, attention to detail is necessary during TECAB procedure [34]. Interrupted anastomosis with U-clips can reduce the possibility of purse-stringing a continuous suture and help to manage the lack of tactile feedback associated with da Vinci surgery system. Large bites with U-clips from the outside of the incision of the target vessel is recommended to improve hemostasis [35].

12.9 Future Directions and Conclusion

The advantages of traditional sternotomy CABG mostly arise from the LIMA anastomosis to the LAD. However, it is a highly invasive procedure with increased risks of stroke and short-term morbidity compared to PCI [36]. HCR is a promising technique for the treatment of high-risk patients with CAD, retaining the benefit of LIMA anastomosis without comorbidities associated with traditional CABG. Furthermore, DES may provide superior long-term results compared with SVGs in the treatment of non-LAD lesions in many patients. It integrates the positive features of PCI and CABG.

The results of published HCR trials show low perioperative mortality, morbidity, and quick rehabilitation as well as acceptable outcomes. Ongoing technical refinements of advanced HCR offering multiple internal mammary arterial grafts done totally endoscopically remains promising [37]. The success of HCR depend on close collaboration between cardiac surgeons, interventional cardiologists and general cardiologist in a formal coronary team setting.

More complex multi-arterial left side grafting through minimally invasive approach (robotic BIMA or LIMA and radial) add more possibilities to extend the indications and use of HCR.

Despite the benefits of HCR, future studies should prove its cost-effectiveness, safety, and efficacy in RCTs.

References

1. Angelini GD, Wilde P, Salerno TA, Bosco G, Calafiore AM. Integrated left small thoracotomy and angioplasty for multivessel coronary artery revascularisation. Lancet. 1996;347(9003):757–8. https://doi.org/10.1016/s0140-6736(96)90107-5.
2. Fihn SD, Gardin JM, Abrams J, et al. 2012 ACCF/AHA/ACP/AATS/PCNA/SCAI/STS guideline for the diagnosis and management of patients with stable ischemic heart disease: a report of the American College of Cardiology Foundation/American Heart Association task force on practice guidelines, and the American College of Physicians, American Association for Thoracic Surgery, preventive cardiovascular nurses association, Society for Cardiovascular Angiography and Interventions, and Society of Thoracic Surgeons. J Am Coll Cardiol. 2012;60(24):e44–e164. https://doi.org/10.1016/j.jacc.2012.07.013.
3. Hillis LD, Smith PK, Anderson JL, et al. 2011 ACCF/AHA guideline for coronary artery bypass graft surgery. A report of the American College of Cardiology Foundation/American Heart Association task force on practice guidelines. Developed in collaboration with the American Association for Thoracic Surgery, Society of Cardiovascular Anesthesiologists, and Society of Thoracic Surgeons. J Am Coll Cardiol. 2011;58(24):e123–210. https://doi.org/10.1016/j.jacc.2011.08.009.
4. Mishra YK, Yadav J. Hybrid myocardial revascularization. Indian J Thorac Cardiovasc Surg. 2018;34(Suppl 3):310–20. https://doi.org/10.1007/s12055-018-0646-y.
5. Holzhey DM, Jacobs S, Mochalski M, et al. Seven-year follow-up after minimally invasive direct coronary artery bypass: experience with more than 1300 patients. Ann Thorac Surg. 2007;83(1):108–14. https://doi.org/10.1016/j.athoracsur.2006.08.029.
6. Harskamp RE, Bagai A, Halkos ME, et al. Clinical outcomes after hybrid coronary revascularization versus coronary artery bypass surgery: a meta-analysis of 1,190 patients. Am Heart J. 2014;167(4):585–92. https://doi.org/10.1016/j.ahj.2014.01.006.
7. Serruys PW, Morice MC, Kappetein AP, et al. Percutaneous coronary intervention versus coronary-artery bypass grafting for severe coronary artery disease [published correction appears in N Engl J Med. 2013 Feb 7;368(6):584]. N Engl J Med.

2009;360(10):961–72. https://doi.org/10.1056/NEJMoa0804626.
8. Halkos ME, Rab ST, Vassiliades TA, et al. Hybrid coronary revascularization versus off-pump coronary artery bypass for the treatment of left main coronary stenosis. Ann Thorac Surg. 2011;92(6):2155–60. https://doi.org/10.1016/j.athoracsur.2011.08.012.
9. Davierwala PM. Current outcomes of off-pump coronary artery bypass grafting: evidence from real world practice. J Thorac Dis. 2016;8(Suppl 10):S772–86. https://doi.org/10.21037/jtd.2016.10.102.
10. Lowenstern A, Wu J, Bradley SM, Fanaroff AC, Tcheng JE, Wang TY. Current landscape of hybrid revascularization: a report from the NCDR CathPCI registry. Am Heart J. 2019;215:167–77. https://doi.org/10.1016/j.ahj.2019.06.014.
11. Chen JP, Srivastava S. A vanishing lesion. JACC Cardiovasc Interv. 2010;3(3):360–1. https://doi.org/10.1016/j.jcin.2009.10.032.
12. Panoulas VF, Colombo A, Margonato A, Maisano F. Hybrid coronary revascularization: promising, but yet to take off. J Am Coll Cardiol. 2015;65(1):85–97. https://doi.org/10.1016/j.jacc.2014.04.093.
13. Khan A, Helton T, Forrest T, et al. Use of intravenous cangrelor/DAPT bridge therapy for post-PCi patients undergoing gastrointestinal surgery. J Am Coll Cardiol. 2019;73(9_Supplement_1):2670. https://doi.org/10.1016/S0735-1097(19)33276-0.
14. Harskamp RE, Brennan JM, Xian Y, et al. Practice patterns and clinical outcomes after hybrid coronary revascularization in the United States: an analysis from the society of thoracic surgeons adult cardiac database. Circulation. 2014;130:872–9.
15. Kon ZN, Brown EN, Tran R, et al. Simultaneous hybrid coronary revascularization reduces postoperative morbidity compared with results from conventional off-pump coronary artery bypass. J Thorac Cardiovasc Surg. 2008;135(2):367–75. https://doi.org/10.1016/j.jtcvs.2007.09.025. Epub 2007 Dec 26. PMID: 18242270; PMCID: PMC2962576.
16. Mack MJ, Acuff TE, Casimir-Ahn H, Lönn UJ, Jansen EW. Video-assisted coronary bypass grafting on the beating heart. Ann Thorac Surg. 1997;63(6 Suppl):S100–3. https://doi.org/10.1016/s0003-4975(97)00415-3.
17. Kettering K, Dapunt O, Baer FM. Minimally invasive direct coronary artery bypass grafting: a systematic review. J Cardiovasc Surg. 2004;45(3):255–64.
18. Subramanian VA, Patel NU, Patel NC, Loulmet DF. Robotic assisted multivessel minimally invasive direct coronary artery bypass with port-access stabilization and cardiac positioning: paving the way for outpatient coronary surgery? Ann Thorac Surg. 2005;79(5):1590–6. https://doi.org/10.1016/j.athoracsur.2004.10.067.
19. Derose JJ Jr, Balaram SK, Ro C, et al. Mid-term results and patient perceptions of robotically-assisted coronary artery bypass grafting. Interact Cardiovasc Thorac Surg. 2005;4(5):406–11. https://doi.org/10.1510/icvts.2004.103317.
20. Bonatti J, Schachner T, Bonaros N, Lehr EJ, Zimrin D, Griffith B. Robotically assisted totally. endoscopic coronary bypass surgery. Circulation. 2011;124:236–44.
21. Srivastava S, Gadasalli S, Agusala M, et al. Beating heart totally endoscopic coronary artery bypass. Ann Thorac Surg. 2010;89(6):1873–80. https://doi.org/10.1016/j.athoracsur.2010.03.014.
22. Puri R, Reed GW. Refining coronary stent platforms in the modern DES era: thinning, eluting, inhibiting, and absorbing. J Am Coll Cardiol. 2018;72(25):3298–300. https://doi.org/10.1016/j.jacc.2018.10.033.
23. Patel MR, Calhoon JH, Dehmer GJ, et al. ACC/AATS/AHA/ASE/ASNC/SCAI/SCCT/STS 2017 appropriate use criteria for coronary revascularization in patients with stable ischemic heart disease: a report of the American College of Cardiology appropriate use criteria task force, American Association for Thoracic Surgery, American Heart Association, American Society of Echocardiography, American Society of Nuclear Cardiology, Society for Cardiovascular Angiography and Interventions, Society of Cardiovascular Computed Tomography, and Society of Thoracic Surgeons [published correction appears in J Am Coll Cardiol. 2018 Apr 13]. J Am Coll Cardiol. 2017;69(17):2212–41. https://doi.org/10.1016/j.jacc.2017.02.001.
24. Bachinsky WB, Abdelsalam M, Boga G, Kiljanek L, Mumtaz M, McCarty C. Comparative study of same sitting hybrid coronary artery revascularization versus off-pump coronary artery bypass in multivessel coronary artery disease. J Interv Cardiol. 2012;25:460–8.
25. Shen L, Hu S, Wang H, et al. One-stop hybrid coronary revascularization versus coronary artery bypass grafting and percutaneous coronary intervention for the treatment of multivessel coronary artery disease: 3-year follow-up results from a single institution. J Am Coll Cardiol. 2013;61(25):2525–33. https://doi.org/10.1016/j.jacc.2013.04.007.
26. Gąsior M, Zembala MO, Tajstra M, et al. Hybrid revascularization for multivessel coronary artery disease. JACC Cardiovasc Interv. 2014;7(11):1277–83. https://doi.org/10.1016/j.jcin.2014.05.025.
27. Esteves V, Oliveira MAP, Feitosa FS, et al. Late clinical outcomes of myocardial hybrid revascularization versus coronary artery bypass grafting for complex triple-vessel disease: long-term follow-up of the randomized MERGING clinical trial. Catheter Cardiovasc Interv. 2021;97(2):259–64. https://doi.org/10.1002/ccd.28710.
28. Halkos ME, Vassiliades TA, Douglas JS, et al. Hybrid coronary revascularization versus off-pump coronary artery bypass grafting for the treatment of multivessel coronary artery disease. Ann Thorac Surg. 2011;92(5):1695–702. https://doi.org/10.1016/j.athoracsur.2011.05.090.

29. Song Z, Shen L, Zheng Z, et al. One-stop hybrid coronary revascularization versus off-pump coronary artery bypass in patients with diabetes mellitus. J Thorac Cardiovasc Surg. 2016;151:1695–701.
30. Harskamp RE, Abdelsalam M, Lopes RD, et al. Cardiac troponin release following hybrid coronary revascularization versus off-pump coronary artery bypass surgery. Interact Cardiovasc Thorac Surg. 2014;19(6):1008–12. https://doi.org/10.1093/icvts/ivu297.
31. Hage A, Giambruno V, Jones P, et al. Hybrid coronary revascularization versus off-pump coronary artery bypass grafting: comparative effectiveness analysis with long-term follow-up. J Am Heart Assoc. 2019;8(24):e014204. https://doi.org/10.1161/JAHA.119.014204.
32. Anyukov V, Kochergin N, Shilov A, et al. Randomized clinical trial of surgical vs. percutaneous vs. hybrid revascularization in multivessel coronary artery disease: residual myocardial ischemia and clinical outcomes at one year—Hybrid Coronary Revascularization Versus Stenting or Surgery (HREVS). J Interv Cardiol. 2020;2020:5458064.
33. Puskas JD, Halkos ME, DeRose JJ, Bagiella E, Miller MA, Overbey J, Bonatti J, Srinivas VS, Vesely M, Sutter F, Lynch J, Kirkwood K, Shapiro TA, Boudoulas KD, Crestanello J, Gehrig T, Smith P, Ragosta M, Hoff SJ, Zhao D, Gelijns AC, Szeto WY, Weisz G, Argenziano M, Vassiliades T, Liberman H, Matthai W, Ascheim DD. Hybrid coronary revascularization for the treatment of multivessel coronary artery disease: a multicenter observational study. J Am Coll Cardiol. 2016;68(4):356–65. https://doi.org/10.1016/j.jacc.2016.05.032. PMID: 27443431; PMCID: PMC5142519.
34. Moussa I, Oetgen M, Subramanian V, Kobayashi Y, Patel N, Moses J. Frequency of early occlusion and stenosis in bypass grafts after minimally invasive direct coronary arterial bypass surgery. Am J Cardiol. 2001;88(3):311–3. https://doi.org/10.1016/s0002-9149(01)01650-2.
35. Cheng N, Gao C, Yang M, Wu Y, Wang G, Xiao C. Analysis of the learning curve for beating heart, totally endoscopic, coronary artery bypass grafting. J Thorac Cardiovasc Surg. 2014;148(5):1832–6. https://doi.org/10.1016/j.jtcvs.2014.02.002.
36. Head SJ, Milojevic M, Taggart DP, Puskas JD. Current practice of state-of-the-art surgical coronary revascularization. Circulation. 2017;136:1331–45.
37. Balkhy HH, Kitahara H, Hirai T, Matsukage H, Nathan S. Residual SYNTAX score after advanced hybrid robotic totally endoscopic coronary revascularization. Ann Thorac Surg. 2020;109(6):1826–32. https://doi.org/10.1016/j.athoracsur.2019.09.011.
38. Vassiliades TA, Kilgo PD, Douglas JS, Babaliaros VC, Block PC, Samady H, Cates CU, Rab ST, Morris DC. Clinical outcomes after hybrid coronary revascularization versus off-pump coronary artery bypass: a prospective evaluation. Innovations (Phila). 2009;4(6):299–306. https://doi.org/10.1097/IMI.0b013e3181bbfa96. PMID: 22437225.
39. Reicher B, Poston RS, Mehra MR, Joshi A, Odonkor P, Kon Z, Reyes PA, Zimrin DA. Simultaneous "hybrid" percutaneous coronary intervention and minimally invasive surgical bypass grafting: feasibility, safety, and clinical outcomes. Am Heart J. 2008;155(4):661–7. https://doi.org/10.1016/j.ahj.2007.12.032. Epub 2008 Mar 5. PMID: 18371473; PMCID: PMC2636970.
40. de Cannière D, Jansens JL, Goldschmidt-Clermont P, Barvais L, Decroly P, Stoupel E. Combination of minimally invasive coronary bypass and percutaneous transluminal coronary angioplasty in the treatment of double-vessel coronary disease: Two-year follow-up of a new hybrid procedure compared with "on-pump" double bypass grafting. Am Heart J. 2001;142(4):563–70. https://doi.org/10.1067/mhj.2001.118466. PMID: 11579343.
41. Davidavicius G, Van Praet F, Mansour S, Casselman F, Bartunek J, Degrieck I, Wellens F, De Geest R, Vanermen H, Wijns W, De Bruyne B. Hybrid revascularization strategy: a pilot study on the association of robotically enhanced minimally invasive direct coronary artery bypass surgery and fractional-flow-reserve-guided percutaneous coronary intervention. Circulation. 2005 30;112(9 Suppl):I317–22. https://doi.org/10.1161/CIRCULATIONAHA.104.524264. PMID: 16159838.
42. Kiaii B, McClure RS, Stewart P, Rayman R, Swinamer SA, Suematsu Y, Fox S, Higgins J, Albion C, Kostuk WJ, Almond D, Sridhar K, Teefy P, Jablonsky G, Diamantouros P, Dobkowski WB, Jones P, Bainbridge D, Iglesias I, Murkin J, Cheng D, Novick RJ. Simultaneous integrated coronary artery revascularization with long-term angiographic follow-up. J Thorac Cardiovasc Surg. 2008;136(3):702–8. https://doi.org/10.1016/j.jtcvs.2008.02.081. PMID: 18805275.

13 The Emerging Concept of Hybrid Coronary Revascularization

Marco Coli, Stefano Rigattieri, Andrea Berni, and Giovanni Melina

13.1 Introduction

Coronary artery disease (CAD) is the foremost single cause of morbidity and mortality globally even if their prevalence continues to fall in the last decades in Western countries. This may be due both to improved primary and secondary preventive measures and to effective treatment of the acute phase. Many of these patients with multivessel CAD need a staged treatment of their disease following the acute phase either by percutaneous coronary intervention (PCI) or coronary artery bypass grafting (CABG), or both. In addition, the aging population, irrespective of additional bleeding risk criteria, warrant less intensive therapy [1]. This subgroup of patients, with a higher prevalence of comorbidities including CAD, needs specific revascularization strategies taking into account the bleeding risk related to such procedures. In this setting less invasive strategies including the use of advanced endoscopic and robotic approaches led to a new concept of hybrid coronary revascularization (HCR) for CAD. The rationale of HCR lies in the well-established survival benefit conferred by left internal mammary artery to left anterior descending coronary artery (LIMA-to-LAD) grafting combined with PCI to non-LAD coronary vessels using contemporary stent platforms. HCR can be performed with different strategies which may have some advantages both in terms of clinical outcomes and in the management of bleeding risk. One-stop HCR is performed simultaneously, starting with surgery followed by PCI. Two-stage HCR consists of two different procedures: in the standard two-stage HCR, surgery is followed by PCI after 1–2 months; in the reverse two-stage HCR, PCI is performed first. In this chapter we describe the different options and their possible clinical applications.

M. Coli (✉)
Department of Cardiac Surgery, Azienda Ospedaliero-Universitaria Sant'Andrea, Rome, Italy
e-mail: marco.coli@uniroma1.it

S. Rigattieri
Cardiology Unit, Sant'Andrea University Hospital, Rome, Italy
e-mail: srigattieri@ospedalesantandrea.it

A. Berni
Interventional Cardiology, Azienda Ospedaliero-Universitaria Sant'Andrea, Sapienza University of Rome, Rome, Italy
e-mail: andrea.berni@uniroma1.it

G. Melina
Department of Cardiac Surgery, Azienda Ospedaliero-Universitaria Sant'Andrea, Sapienza University of Rome, Rome, Italy
e-mail: giovanni.melina@uniroma1.it

B. Cortese, S. Rigattieri (eds.), *High Bleeding Risk Patients in Interventional Cardiology*,
https://doi.org/10.1007/978-3-031-87302-7_13

13.2 Hybrid Coronary Revascularization: Definition, Rationale, and Clinical Data

Hybrid coronary revascularization (HCR) is defined as the combination of coronary artery bypass grafting (CABG) and percutaneous coronary intervention (PCI) to treat multivessel coronary artery disease (CAD). The procedure aims to join the advantages of minimally invasive arterial revascularization with left internal mammary artery (LIMA) grafting to the left anterior descending (LAD) coronary artery with PCI for non-LAD territories. In patients with multivessel CAD, the aim of myocardial revascularization is to reduce the risk of mortality, myocardial infarction, residual ischemia, and chest pain. As reported in the most recent guidelines [2, 3], complete coronary revascularization (CR) achievement is associated with a substantial reduction in mortality and future coronary events. Therefore, CR of all significant coronary lesions has been proposed as the first priority in decision-making for myocardial revascularization between CABG and PCI [4, 5].

The rising interest in less invasive approaches coupled with the technological improvement could be applied to HCR in order to possibly achieve such results [6]. Specific subgroups of patients could benefit from a hybrid approach in order to reduce surgical injury and improve long-term outcomes by the well-established benefits of LIMA-to-LAD grafts [7, 8] and PCI to non-LAD coronary vessels using new stent platforms [9, 10]. Thus, improving alternative CABG strategies such as HCR could lead to better long-term outcomes compared to CABG in selected patients. The risk of complication [6] in PCI relates firstly to the complexity of the lesion (high SYNTAX score), whereas complications after CABG are due to the patient's noncardiac comorbidities. PCI has low risks of immediate complications [11], rapid recovery, and better long-term patency outcomes than vein grafts. Although recurrent events are significantly reduced with CABG thanks to LIMA to LAD graft, median sternotomy and ascending aorta manipulation may be related to the increased risk of stroke, atrial fibrillation, bleeding, infections, prolonged mechanical ventilation, and hospitalization [12]. The hybrid approach aims to join the advantages of both techniques with a minimally invasive LIMA harvesting, avoiding median sternotomy and aortic manipulation. Potential disadvantages may be the cost-effectiveness rates and the peri-procedural management of dual antiplatelet therapy (DAPT). The most relevant criteria to select patients suitable for HCR are summarized in Table 13.1.

Table 13.1 Selection criteria for HCR

Selection criteria for HCR
Multivessel coronary artery disease (MCAD) involving the left main or LAD with valid distal distribution and at least one non-LAD vessel amenable to PCI
SYNTAX score between 23 and 34
No contraindication to DAPT
Elevated likelihood to obtain complete revascularization
High-risk CABG
Left ventricle ejection fraction >30% (to prevent hypotension during CO2 insufflation)
Single-lung ventilation feasible
No history of prior irradiation/surgery of left chest wall
Low to moderate complexity of non-LAD coronary lesions (no chronic total occlusions or long, severely calcified lesions needing debulking)

13.2.1 LIMA to LAD Graft: A Survival Benefit

- CABG was introduced in 1968 and rapidly became the standard of care for CAD patients [13]. According to the current guidelines, CABG remains the treatment of choice for severe coronary artery disease including left main coronary artery, three-vessel disease, and proximal LAD. CABG is usually performed using the LIMA and saphenous vein grafts. The use of the LIMA graft to the LAD is the gold standard for coronary revascularization due to its excellent long-term patency and improved long-term outcomes [14], representing the cornerstone of CAD management worldwide [15]. Due to its characteristics, the LIMA is a unique conduit that has shown excellent results in terms of patency rates, survival, and event-free benefits when it is anastomosed to the LAD.

Graft patency rates are 93%, 88%, and 80% for internal thoracic arteries grafts and 78%, 65%, and 57% for saphenous veins grafts at 1, 5, and 10 years, respectively [16]. In a randomized study, the LIMA was found to be superior to saphenous vein graft to the LAD in terms of mortality, graft failure, myocardial infarction, need for graft PTCA, reoperation, and hospitalization [17]. The 10-year graft patency was 94.6% and 76.3% for LIMA and vein graft, respectively [17].

13.2.2 PCI Versus Vein Grafts: The Rationale for Completing the Revascularization with PCI

- In contemporary practice, approximately 95% of patients receive at least one saphenous vein graft (SVG) in addition to the LIMA graft [18]. Due to their macroscopic and microscopic features including endothelial response to the different systemic pressure load, vein grafts are at higher risk of early failure compared to arterial conduits. Furthermore, PCI reduces hospital stay, has low risks of immediate complications, and better long-term patency outcomes than vein grafts [11]. The patency rates for SVG vary widely in the literature, with estimates of 11–41% failure rate at less than 3 years, 19–33% failure rate at 5 to 10 years, and 39–61% at greater than 10-year follow-up [4, 5, 18, 19].
- Differently, new-generation DES lead to better clinical outcomes ensuring a reduced rate of restenosis after 1 and 5 years [7, 20]. The study by Nishiura et al. [2] has shown that the incidence rates of driven target lesion revascularization (cTLR) and target lesion revascularization (TLR) beyond 10 years after first generation sirolimus-eluting stent implantation were 16.4% and 36.8%, respectively. A randomized trial by Zocca et al. compared the 5-year outcomes after treating an all-comers population with newer-generation zotarolimus-eluting stents (ZES) and everolimus-eluting stents (EES). The 5-year incidence of target vessel failure (TVF) was 13.5%, and target vessel revascularization rate was 8% [3], confirming the improvement of long-term outcomes related to the new generation stent platforms.
- The high rate of venous graft occlusion observed in CABG patients and the decreasing rate of stent occlusion with PCI brings up the question to replace SVG with PCI [21].

13.2.3 Hybrid Coronary Revascularization: State of the Art

Multiple observational studies on HCR have been published, but there are some limitations due to the number of patients included, different hybrid approach, duration of follow-up, and inherent selection bias. The long-term efficacy of HCR versus conventional CABG (or multivessel PCI) still needs to be addressed in large-scale randomized clinical trials. Prospective randomized pilot study evaluating the safety and efficacy of standard two-stage HCR in the multivessel coronary artery disease (POLMIDES) [22] is the only randomized trial comparing HCR and conventional CABG. Since 2011, a total of 200 patients have been randomized (HCR group = 98, CABG group = 102). The early results suggest that HCR is feasible and safe in skilled hands, with 1- and 5-year outcomes noninferior to conventional CABG in low- to intermediate-risk patients with multivessel CAD. No differences in mortality, myocardial infarction (MI), repeat revascularization, or stroke were found at 1 and 5 years. LIMA to LAD graft patency rate was similar in both groups.

Numerous studies have demonstrated that HCR may offer benefits in short-term morbidity such as bleeding rate [23, 24].

However, the prevalence of the HCR as a revascularization technique between 2009 and 2016 is approximately 0.2% [25]. The use of HCR remains low, in part because of the lack of clinical evidence but also because of the practical limitations: logistics (simultaneous in hybrid operation room vs. two-stage); specific expertise, cooperation, and collaboration of surgical and interventional teams; and uncertain cost-effectiveness.

Due to the increasing ageing population with a higher prevalence of comorbidities, a growing number of patients at higher risk are facing appropriate treatment of multivessel CAD either by PCI or CABG [26]. In those patients, despite the anatomical indication, surgical revascularization may not be considered as the first choice due to the unavailability of grafts, calcifications of the proximal aorta, peripheral coronary stenoses, diffuse CAD, and patient's performance status. In such cases, HCR may play an important and complementary role in the treatment of multivessel coronary disease in the future [26].

Current AHA guidelines define HCR as a procedure with an unclear role as an alternative to multivessel PCI and with similar rates of death, MI, stroke, and revascularization compared with conventional CABG in small RCTs and propensity-matched observational studies [27]. According to ESC guidelines, HCR may be considered in specific patient subsets in experienced centers (class IIB LOE B) [28].

13.3 Surgical Protocols

Minimally invasive coronary surgical revascularization consists of the combination of minimal invasive LIMA harvesting and off-pump coronary artery bypass (OPCAB) grafting through a left thoracotomy avoiding the full sternal access.

13.3.1 LIMA Harvesting

A. *Direct Vision*

The patient is placed in a supine position with single-lung ventilation, and the left side of the chest is elevated at about 30–35 degrees. An anterolateral thoracotomy of 5–7 cm long is made in the fourth or fifth intercostal space (ICS) [29]. In men, the incision is made just below the left nipple, and in females at the level of the left breast fold. The intercostal retractor is placed [30]. The spreader's arm of the retractor eases the vision creating a tunnel toward the LIMA (Fig. 13.1) [31]. LIMA is then harvested in a pedicled or skeletonized fashion. The direct vision harvesting technique is similar to the one used in the median sternotomy approach. The disadvantages of this technique are related to the relatively small operative field, could be the difficulty of

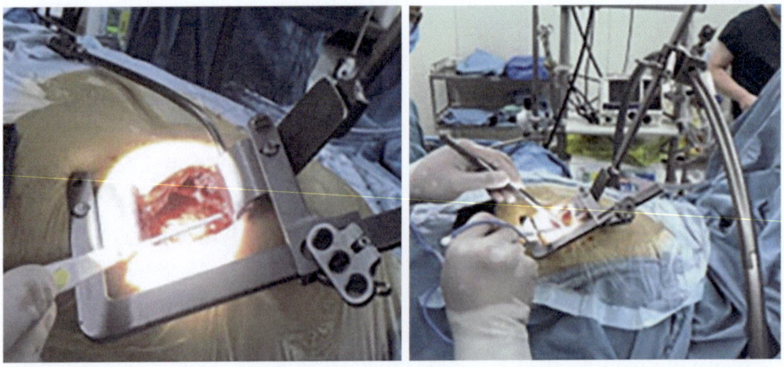

Fig. 13.1 Left thoracotomy LIMA harvesting

completing LIMA harvesting, the kinking of the graft, coronary steal syndrome, and the shortening of the graft. In addition, the use of the retractor could provoke postoperative pain and rib fractures [32].

B. *Thoracoscopic Approach*

The patient is positioned supine with a 30°-rotated decubitus toward the right side. The routine trocar arrangement is achieved by placing one 6-mm trocar at the level of the third–fourth ICS and other 6-mm trocar at the sixth–seventh ICS, on the anterior axillary line with 15-mm incisions [33]. These trocars are utilized for the endoscopic grasper and the harmonic scalpel, while the 11-mm trocar for the endoscopic camera is positioned in the fifth-sixth ICS at the level of the anterior axillary line. After the exclusion of the left lung, the first 11-mm trocar (for the endoscopic camera) is inserted, and CO2 insufflation is started. After inserting the endoscopic camera, the course of the LIMA can be assessed [31]. The LIMA is then harvested from the proximal to distal portion. The side branches are either clipped or coagulated. The distal end is trimmed between clips and cut after general heparinization. This technique allows complete harvesting of LIMA from the subclavian artery to the sixth intercostal branch reducing the risk of shortening of the graft and postoperative pain [34].

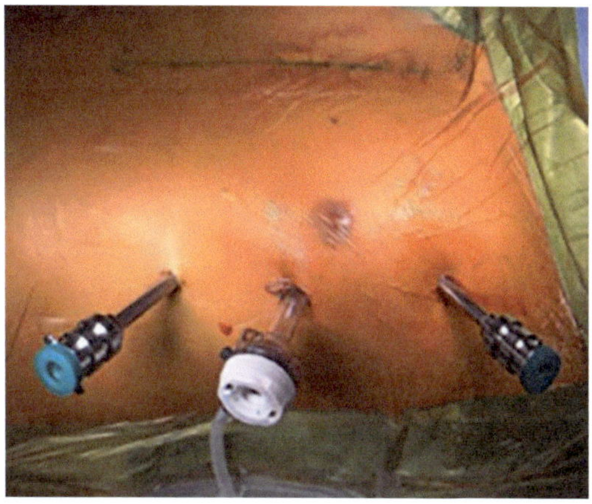

Fig. 13.2 Trocar placement

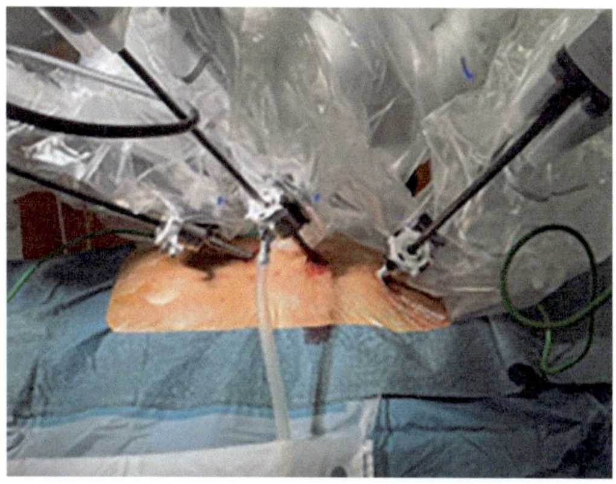

Fig. 13.3 Robot arms placement

C. *Robotic-Assisted*

Robotic-assisted cardiac surgery is the most advanced technology introduced in heart surgery. Robotic-assisted LIMA harvesting is also the less invasive procedure performed for LIMA takedown and coronary revascularization [31]. Da Vinci robotic system (Intuitive Surgical, Inc.) is commonly used for this purpose. The Da Vinci robotic cart which carries three or four robotic arms approaches the patient perpendicularly from the right side (Fig. 13.2) [35]. With the left lung deflated, a camera port is initially inserted in the fourth ICS on the anterior axillary line. Carbon dioxide is insufflated into the chest (6–10 mmHg). The robotic camera is used to inspect the thoracic cavity for adhesions and orient the insertion of the other two ports. The right arm port (8 mm) is inserted in the second ICS, and the left arm port (8 mm) is inserted in the sixth ICS (Figs. 13.3 and 13.4). For most part of the procedure, the left robotic arm is equipped with fine tissue De Bakey forceps, and the right robotic arm with a hook cautery. The camera provides a 10x magnification which leads to excellent visualization. The LIMA is then prepared in the standard fashion and LAD is assessed. The LIMA is exposed and harvested from the subclavian artery to the distal bifurcation (Fig. 13.5). The side branches are clipped with endoscopic clips. After heparinization, the distal extremity is partially incised to check the flow.

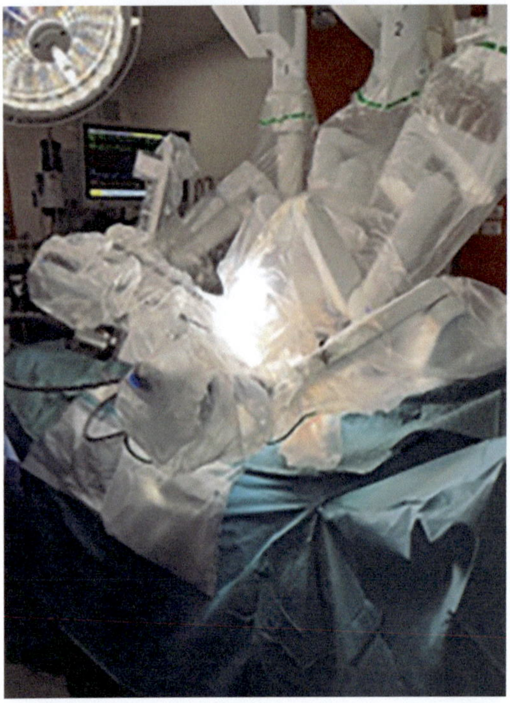

Fig. 13.4 Robot docking

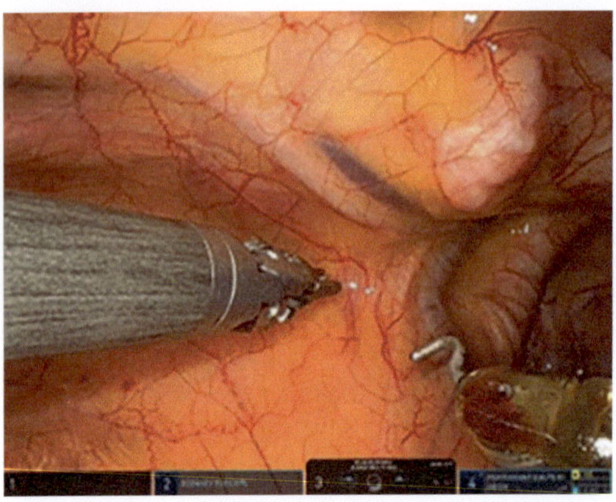

Fig. 13.5 Robotic harvesting of LIMA

Despite a learning curve, the robotic-assisted approach presents several advantages such as 10x magnification camera, elimination of physiological tremor of hands, large range of movements of robotic instrument, and small surgical incisions (Fig. 13.6) ensuring better results in order of harvesting time, vessel injury, and long-term graft patency compared with standard LIMA harvesting techniques [36].

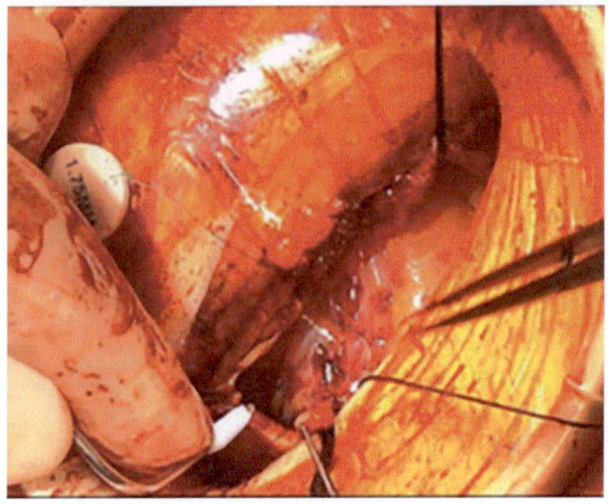

Fig. 13.6 Preparing LIMA-to-LAD anastomosis

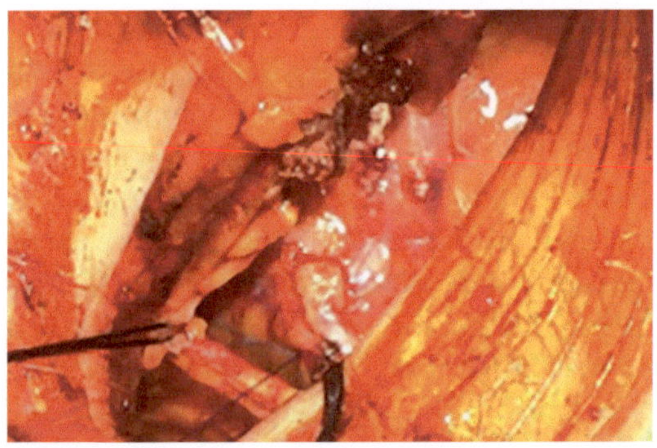

Fig. 13.7 LIMA-to-LAD anastomosis

13.3.2 LIMA to LAD Anastomosis

LIMA to LAD anastomosis is performed off-pump through a 3–5-cm left anterior mini-thoracotomy at the level of the fourth–fifth ICS. An epicardial stabilizer is placed through the sixth ICS incision, and the anastomosis is performed off pump. Once the site of anastomosis is identified, the LAD is incised longitudinally, and an appropriate shunt is placed avoiding bleeding and the likelihood of hemodynamic instability (Fig. 13.7) [37]. The direct anastomosis is performed using 7-0 or 8-0 Prolene running suture (Fig. 13.8). Totally endoscopic coronary artery bypass (TECAB) grafting is a technique that performs both LIMA harvest and LIMA to LAD anastomosis with an endoscopic approach. Four trocars are needed. The anastomosis is per-

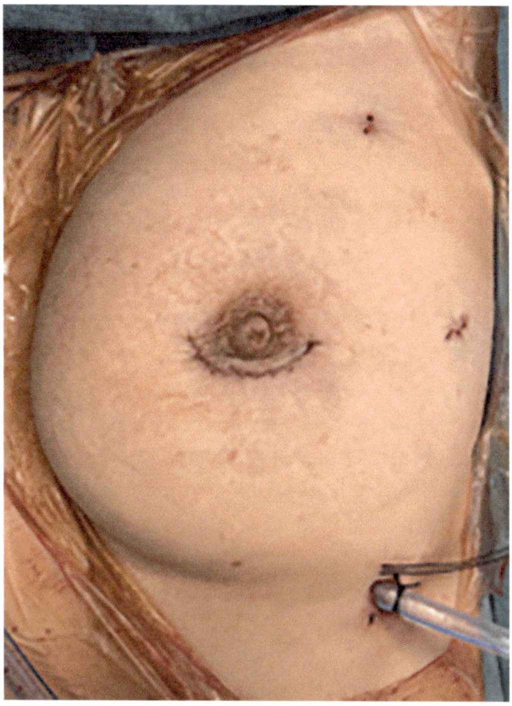

Fig. 13.8 Subareolar and trocar incisions

formed with a Prolene 8-0 running suture or with an automated anastomotic connector [38].

13.4 HCR Timing

Three possible timing strategies can be used: MIDCAB and PCI performed simultaneously (one stop) and MIDCAB first followed by PCI or MIDCAB following PCI (two steps) [39].

13.4.1 One Stop

One-stop HCR is performed in a hybrid suite, starting with surgery first, followed by PCI [7]. A significant advantage is the immediate assessment of the LIMA-LAD anastomosis with the angiography. After the closure of the thorax, the angiography is immediately performed to confirm patency of the LIMA-LAD graft, and then PCI is performed on non-LAD lesions through the femoral or radial artery [40]. Ceiling-mounted viewing screens are positioned and a floor-mounted C-arm is moved into position. Guidewire and stent selection are left to the discretion of the interventionist. Any major issue with the graft can be addressed. Also, the non-LAD PCI is performed with LAD territory already protected and with a surgical team at the bedside for any possible complication or unsuccessful PCI. Aspirin 100 mg/day is continued perioperatively. A loading dose of clopidogrel 600 mg is administered via a nasogastric tube after confirmation of LIMA-LAD graft patency. Activated clotting time >250 s is maintained. Hybrid suites are expensive and not universally available. In addition, minimizing bleeding while preventing stent thrombosis can be challenging. Several approaches have been suggested for DAPT use in this setting. The one-stop HCR approach counts for approximately 20% of all HCR procedures in the United States [37].

13.4.2 PCI After MIDCAB Procedure

The standard two-step HCR approach is defined as MIDCAB first followed by PCI. MIDCAB first is more common, followed by PCI usually after 1–2 months [21]. The LIMA-LAD anastomosis is rapidly assessed by angiography prior to PCI (Fig. 13.9). Severe anastomotic problems can be immediately assessed and eventually addressed via PCI [38]. Stent implantation of the non-LAD segments is performed. An advantage of this strategy could be the left ventricular protection that prior LIMA to LAD graft offers. DAPT may be given without the risk of mediastinal bleeding before PCI for the next 6–12 months [39]. Potentially, lesion instability in the waiting period between the CABG and PCI may require earlier, unplanned hospitalization. Two-step strategy does not require a hybrid operative room but requires two different admissions [40].

13.4.3 MIDCAB After PCI Procedure

Performing MIDCAB after PCI, known as reverse two-step HCR, may be considered in the setting of non-LAD acute coronary syndromes,

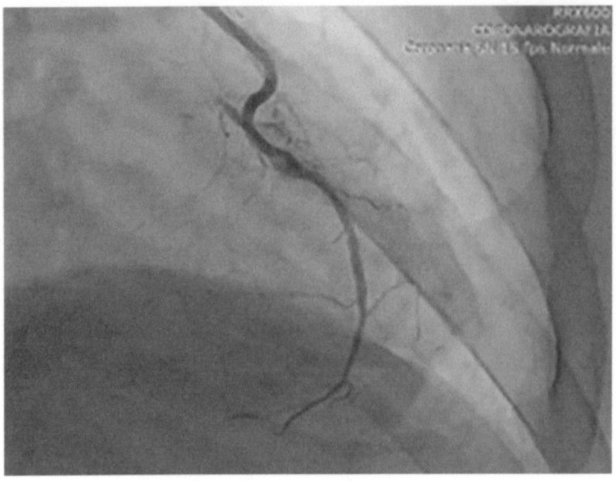

Fig. 13.9 LIMA-to-LAD graft, angiography assessment

where the culprit lesion is treated with PCI. In order to consider a hybrid approach, other non-LAD vessels may be treated by PCI and the LAD assessed for a staged MIDCAB. Despite the advantages, complex antiplatelet therapy management is required causing potentially higher risk of stent thrombosis and/or bleeding. In addition, LIMA to LAD graft is not evaluated. In situations that mandate the interruption of DAPT with a high risk of stent thrombosis, the continuous intravenous use of cangrelor, with an average half-life of 3–6 min as a bridge therapy, may provide a viable alternative [41].

13.5 HCR Versus Other Revascularization Techniques

13.5.1 HCR Versus Off-Pump Coronary Artery Bypass (OPCAB)

Halkos et al. [42] compared HCR versus OPCAB in patients with left main disease. HCR was associated with reduced blood transfusions and mechanical ventilation. MACCE rates were similar in both groups. Song et al. [43] noted reductions in chest tube drainage, mechanical ventilation, and intensive care unit stay in propensity-matched patients having one-stop HCR compared with OPCAB. Again, MACCE rates were similar in both groups. Harskamp et al. [44] reported a 46% reduction of troponin I release after HCR compared with OPCAB group, suggesting a reduced myocardial injury with HCR. Finally, Hage et al. [45] documented a trend of reduced mortality over a long-term follow-up in patients who underwent one-stop HCR compared with OPCAB.

13.5.2 HCR vs. PCI

The prospective, observational Hybrid [24] pilot study sponsored by the National Heart, Lung, and Blood Institute explored the feasibility and practices of HCR in patients with hybrid-eligible coronary anatomy at 11 clinical centers in North America. Unfortunately, the study was terminated early due to low enrollment rate. Two hundred ninety-eight patients were enrolled, including 200 treated with HCR and 98 treated with multivessel PCI with DES at the discretion of local cardiologists and surgeons. The HCR approach included RA-MIDCAB (n 108), TECAB (n 42), thoracoscopic MIDCAB (n 38), and planned full median sternotomy (n 12) approaches. Event-free survival was similar between the two groups at 12 months (HR: 1.06; 95% CI: 0.66 to 1.69) and at 18 months (HR: 0.86; 95% CI: 0.56 to 1.36).

13.6 The Role of Hybrid Coronary Revascularization in High-Bleeding-Risk Patients

According to ESC Guidelines, high-bleeding-risk patients are defined as BARC 3 or 5 bleeding risk of ≥4% at 1 year or a risk of an intracranial hemorrhage (ICH) of ≥1% at 1 year [46]. The 2017 ESC focused update on DAPT after PCI recommended (Class IIb, LOE A) that the use of risk scores such as the PRECISE-DAPT (Predicting Bleeding Complications In Patients Undergoing Stent Implantation and Subsequent Dual Anti Platelet Therapy) and DAPT scores may be considered to guide antiplatelet therapy after PCI [46, 47]. HCR may be an option for treating CAD of the subgroup of patients who are at higher risk of bleeding. The bleeding risk profile needs to be assessed in the three HCR techniques.

13.6.1 One-Stop HCR

In order to reduce perioperative bleeding risk, Gao et al. [48] proposed a modified antiplatelet protocol for one-stop HCR: aspirin 100 mg/day is continued until the procedure; ACT >250 is obtained before LIMA harvesting and maintained during the entire one-stop procedure; a loading dose of clopidogrel of 300 mg is administered through a nasogastric tube after the confirmation of LIMA graft patency. After PCI, protamine is administered in a non-totally antagonized dose, and clopidogrel is continued for 12 months with a 75-mg/day dose. In this prospective study, they observed that the degree of platelet inhibition obtained with the modified protocol, assessed by ADP-induced platelet aggregation, was similar to that observed in a cohort of patients undergoing PCI treated with the standard protocol at 2 h and 1 day after the operation [48]. Zhou et al. [49] compared the effects of HCR and OPCAB procedures on postoperative bleeding and renal injury. Although exposed to DAPT and heparin, less bleeding and fewer blood transfusions were observed in HCR patients compared with OPCAB patients. Interestingly, the rate of acute renal failure were also similar between groups despite the administration of contrast for PCI in HCR patients. In an observational study of Zhao et al. [50], coronary angiography in a hybrid suite was performed in two groups of patients, one undergoing CABG and the other undergoing CABG (mostly off-pump) plus PCI (hybrid group). Among the patients who underwent one-stop HCR, 60% had a preoperatively planned procedure, and 40% had a non-planned HCR based on intraoperative findings. Despite a 300-mg clopidogrel loading dose was given preoperatively to patients in the elective hybrid group, no differences in bleeding rate were observed compared with patients receiving clopidogrel through the nasogastric tube for unplanned PCI. Based on the potential hypercoagulability related to the platelet dysfunction that accompanies the extracorporeal circulation, the study of Halkos et al. [51] aimed to evaluate the bleeding risk of patients who underwent OPCAB. The group 1 and the group 2, to which DAPT was administered after 4 h from the procedure, showed similar results in terms of bleeding. These findings suggest that antiplatelet therapy timing is fundamental, and high-dose clopidogrel given after the surgical part of the procedure might have less effect on hemostasis. During the one-stop procedure, OPCAB could cause hypercoagulability and higher platelet activation in the early postoperative period, which lasts at least for several days [52]. Furthermore, considering at least 4 h from the administration to obtain maximal inhibition of platelet aggregation with clopidogrel, the management of the antiplatelet therapy and protamine reversal are crucial in order to reduce the risk of stent thrombosis. According to the studies of Kon et al. [53], Reicher et al. [54], and Bachinsky et al. [55], fewer blood transfusions were required after HCR procedure (versus off-pump CABG) despite higher ACT values and reduced platelet ADP response measured immediately after the end of the procedure. In fact, regional hypercoagulability was assessed measuring the trans-cardiac gradients of markers of thrombosis (F1.2 and activated factor XII) and inflammation (IL 8) showing a significant global reduction after HCR procedure [54]. The study of Vlot et al. detected and quantified platelet dysfunction during the one-stop approach with point-of-care (POC) multiple electrode aggregometry (MEA) to assess optimal patient coagulation management [56]. A linear relationship was shown between ADP-induced platelet aggregometry at baseline and postoperative blood loss ($r = -0.249$; $P = 0.015$). The study of Ding et al. [57] compared bleeding rate and renal function between one-stop HCR and OPCAB patients. Patients who underwent simultaneous HCR had significantly greater chest tube drainage on the day of the operation (492.7 ± 282.4 mL vs 441.0 ± 261.9 mL; $P = 0.023$), but no significant difference was documented in the total amount during the postoperative period (788.8 ± 458.9 mL vs 753.3 ± 409.8 mL; $P = 0.74$). The differences in re-exploration for bleeding (0.3% vs 1.6%; $P = 0.13$), blood transfusion (18.9% vs 16.4%; $P = 0.13$), acute kidney injury (23.3% vs 18.6%; $P = 0.53$), in-hospital major adverse cardiovascular, and cerebrovascular events (including all-cause death, myocardial infarction, stroke, and repeated revascularization) (2.5% vs 1.9%; $P = 0.67$) between the two groups did not reach statistical significance.

13.6.2 Standard Two-Step HCR Strategy

The standard two-step HCR may be the standard of choice for bleeding reduction, since surgery is performed in the absence of double antiplatelet therapy. In patients with stable coronary artery disease, the surgical stage is performed with single-antiplatelet therapy (SAPT) ensuring a lower rate of bleeding after the procedure. Protecting the left ventricle with LIMA to LAD graft leads to an improvement of cardiac function and reduces the likelihood of hemodynamic instability and acute event before the second, interventional, stage. DAPT is started the day before PCI avoiding bleeding related to surgery and ensuring an antiplatelet regimen equal to PCI alone. In our center the second stage is usually performed 1 month after surgery. According to the study of Lowenstern et al. [25], patients who underwent PCI and then CABG were more likely to have periprocedural myocardial infarction (3.9% vs. 1.2%, $p = 0.02$), HF (3.9% vs. 1.5%, $p = 0.04$), and bleeding (6.6% vs. 1.5%, $p < 0.001$) than patients who underwent CABG followed by PCI.

13.6.3 Reverse Two-Step HCR Strategy

Reverse two-step HCR likely represents the less suitable strategy for HBR patients due to the need for maintaining DAPT in the perioperative period. Balancing the risk of stent thrombosis and bleeding in these patients can be challenging. Furthermore, in clinical practice, these patients are not infrequent, usually being represented by patients presenting with an acute coronary syndrome on non-LAD territories [58]. There are three possible scenarios:

1. Deferring surgery after stopping DAPT
2. Performing MIDCAB on DAPT
3. Bridging P2Y12 blockers (clopidogrel, ticagrelor, prasugrel) with parenteral drugs

The first strategy should be preferred if clinically possible (stable patients without ongoing ischemia not controlled by medical therapy), and it is made even more attractive by the availability of several stent platforms in which a short-term DAPT therapy was proven to be effective and safe also in complex lesion [59, 60].

The second strategy should be discouraged, since it was reported to be associated to increased chest tube drainage and blood transfusions when clopidogrel was non-discontinued for at least 5 days even with the adoption of off-pump, sternal sparing, robotic-assisted MIDCAB [61].

The rationale of the third strategy is to safely interrupt oral P2Y12 blockers several days before surgery while giving intravenous antiplatelet agents. In this contest, the ideal drug should have similar pharmacodynamic action as oral antiplatelets as well as a short half-life, to be continued until the day of surgery. Cangrelor, a nonthienopyridine adenosine triphosphate analogue, is an intravenous (IV) antagonist of the P2Y12 receptor who presents these characteristics and was therefore compared to placebo in a pharmacodynamic, randomized controlled study, the BRIDGE trial [62]. In the cangrelor group platelet inhibition was significantly higher as compared to placebo, whereas no differences between groups were observed in CABG-related bleedings, although the study was not powered for clinical events. Glycoprotein IIb/IIIa receptor blockers represent a possible alternative to cangrelor but are limited by several factors including lack of selectivity for the P2Y12 receptor, long half-life, and need for dose-adjustment in the case of reduced renal function.

13.7 Conclusions

Hybrid coronary revascularization, combining off-pump, sternal sparing, robotic-assisted LIMA grafting to LAD territory, and PCI of non-LAD territories with contemporary DES platform needing short (30 days) DAPT, has the potential to minimize surgical trauma and bleeding especially in elderly and frail patients that represent a subgroup at higher bleeding risk independently from other criteria [1, 63]. Given the absence of evidence-based recommendation due to the lack of clinical trials, the choice of HCR and the specific timing strategy instead of multivessel PCI or CABG needs careful evaluation by the heart Team and the involvement of the patient.

Acknowledgments We are grateful to Dr. Emiliano M. Navarra for his unvaluable contribution to the development of robotic assisted MIDCAB in our center.

References

1. Valgimigli M, Landi A. Clopidogrel monotherapy for double-risk acute coronary syndrome. JAMA Cardiol. 2024;9(6):532–3. https://doi.org/10.1001/jamacardio.2024.0547. PMID: 38630487.
2. Nishiura N, Kubo S, Fujii C, Shima Y, Ikuta A, Osakada K, Tada T, Fuku Y, Tanaka H, Kadota K. Fifteen-year clinical outcomes after sirolimus-eluting stent implantation. Circ J. 2024;88(6):938–43. https://doi.org/10.1253/circj.CJ-23-0929. Epub 2024 Jan 24. PMID: 38267035.
3. Zocca P, Kok MM, Tandjung K, Danse PW, Jessurun GAJ, Hautvast RWM, van Houwelingen KG, Stoel MG, Schramm AR, Tjon Joe Gin RM, de Man FHAF, Hartmann M, Louwerenburg JHW, Linssen GCM, Löwik MM, Doggen CJM, von Birgelen C. 5-year outcome following randomized treatment of all-comers with zotarolimus-eluting resolute integrity and everolimus-eluting PROMUS element coronary stents: final report of the DUTCH PEERS (TWENTE II) trial. JACC Cardiovasc Interv. 2018;11(5):462–9. https://doi.org/10.1016/j.jcin.2017.11.031. PMID: 29519378.
4. Hess CN, Lopes RD, Gibson CM, Hager R, Wojdyla DM, Englum BR, Mack MJ, Califf RM, Kouchoukos NT, Peterson ED, Alexander JH. Saphenous vein graft failure after coronary artery bypass surgery: insights from PREVENT IV. Circulation. 2014;130(17):1445–51. https://doi.org/10.1161/CIRCULATIONAHA.113.008193. Epub 2014 Sep 26. PMID: 25261549; PMCID: PMC4206593.
5. Harskamp RE, Alexander JH, Schulte PJ, Brophy CM, Mack MJ, Peterson ED, Williams JB, Gibson CM, Califf RM, Kouchoukos NT, Harrington RA, Ferguson TB Jr, Lopes RD. Vein graft preservation solutions, patency, and outcomes after coronary artery bypass graft surgery: follow-up from the PREVENT IV randomized clinical trial. JAMA Surg. 2014;149(8):798–805. https://doi.org/10.1001/jamasurg.2014.87. Erratum in: JAMA Surg. 2014 Sep;149(9):961. PMID: 25073921; PMCID: PMC4332522.
6. Navarese EP, Tandjung K, Claessen B, Andreotti F, Kowalewski M, Kandzari DE, Kereiakes DJ, Waksman R, Mauri L, Meredith IT, Finn AV, Kim HS, Kubica J, Suryapranata H, Aprami TM, Di Pasquale G, von Birgelen C, Kedhi E. Safety and efficacy outcomes of first and second generation durable polymer drug eluting stents and biodegradable polymer biolimus eluting stents in clinical practice: comprehensive network meta-analysis. BMJ. 2013;347:f6530. https://doi.org/10.1136/bmj.f6530. PMID: 24196498; PMCID: PMC3819044.
7. Moreno PR, Stone GW, Gonzalez-Lengua CA, Puskas JD. The hybrid coronary approach for optimal revascularization: JACC review topic of the week. J Am Coll Cardiol. 2020;76(3):321–33. https://doi.org/10.1016/j.jacc.2020.04.078. PMID: 32674795.
8. Gabrylewicz B, Ochała A, Tendera M. Odległa obserwacja wydolności wysiłkowej i funkcji skurczowej lewej komory serca u pacjentów z choroba wieńcowa leczonych operacyjnie i zachowawczo [long-term observation of exercise capacity and left ventricular function in patients with coronary heart disease treated surgically and conservatively]. Wiad Lek. 2000;53(5–6):262–9. Polish. PMID: 10983380.
9. Bypass Angioplasty Revascularization Investigation (BARI) Investigators. Comparison of coronary bypass surgery with angioplasty in patients with multivessel disease. N Engl J Med. 1996;335(4):217–25. https://doi.org/10.1056/NEJM199607253350401. Erratum in: N Engl J Med 1997 Jan 9;336(2):147. PMID: 8657237.
10. BARI Investigators. The final 10-year follow-up results from the BARI randomized trial. J Am Coll Cardiol. 2007;49(15):1600–6. https://doi.org/10.1016/j.jacc.2006.11.048. Epub 2007 Apr 2. PMID: 17433949.
11. Stone GW, Kappetein AP, Sabik JF, Pocock SJ, Morice MC, Puskas J, Kandzari DE, Karmpaliotis D, Brown WM 3rd, Lembo NJ, Banning A, Merkely B, Horkay F, Boonstra PW, van Boven AJ, Ungi I, Bogáts G, Mansour S, Noiseux N, Sabaté M, Pomar J, Hickey M, Gershlick A, Buszman PE, Bochenek A, Schampaert E, Pagé P, Modolo R, Gregson J, Simonton CA, Mehran R, Kosmidou I, Généreux P, Crowley A, Dressler O, Serruys PW, EXCEL Trial Investigators. Five-year outcomes after PCI or CABG for left main coronary disease. N Engl J Med. 2019;381(19):1820–30. https://doi.org/10.1056/NEJMoa1909406. Epub 2019 Sep 28. Erratum in:

N Engl J Med. 2020 Mar 12;382(11):1078. PMID: 31562798.
12. Farkouh ME, Domanski M, Sleeper LA, Siami FS, Dangas G, Mack M, Yang M, Cohen DJ, Rosenberg Y, Solomon SD, Desai AS, Gersh BJ, Magnuson EA, Lansky A, Boineau R, Weinberger J, Ramanathan K, Sousa JE, Rankin J, Bhargava B, Buse J, Hueb W, Smith CR, Muratov V, Bansilal S, King S 3rd, Bertrand M, Fuster V, FREEDOM Trial Investigators. Strategies for multivessel revascularization in patients with diabetes. N Engl J Med. 2012;367(25):2375–84. https://doi.org/10.1056/NEJMoa1211585. Epub 2012 Nov 4. PMID: 23121323.
13. Serruys PW, Morice MC, Kappetein AP, Colombo A, Holmes DR, Mack MJ, Ståhle E, Feldman TE, van den Brand M, Bass EJ, Van Dyck N, Leadley K, Dawkins KD, Mohr FW, Investigators SYNTAX. Percutaneous coronary intervention versus coronary-artery bypass grafting for severe coronary artery disease. N Engl J Med. 2009;360(10):961–72. https://doi.org/10.1056/NEJMoa0804626. Epub 2009 Feb 18. Erratum in: N Engl J Med. 2013 Feb 7;368(6):584. PMID: 19228612.
14. Layton GR, Sinha S, Caputo M, Angelini GD, Fudulu DP, Zakkar M. Two decades of CABG in the UK: a propensity matched analysis of outcomes by conduit choice. J Clin Med. 2024;13(16):4717. https://doi.org/10.3390/jcm13164717. PMID: 39200859; PMCID: PMC11355931.
15. Loop FD, Lytle BW, Cosgrove DM, Stewart RW, Goormastic M, Williams GW, Golding LA, Gill CC, Taylor PC, Sheldon WC, et al. Influence of the internal-mammary-artery graft on 10-year survival and other cardiac events. N Engl J Med. 1986;314(1):1–6. https://doi.org/10.1056/NEJM198601023140101. PMID: 3484393.
16. Sabik JF 3rd, Lytle BW, Blackstone EH, Houghtaling PL, Cosgrove DM. Comparison of saphenous vein and internal thoracic artery graft patency by coronary system. Ann Thorac Surg. 2005;79(2):544–51. discussion 544–51. https://doi.org/10.1016/j.athoracsur.2004.07.047. PMID: 15680832.
17. Zeff RH, Kongtahworn C, Iannone LA, Gordon DF, Brown TM, Phillips SJ, Skinner JR, Spector M. Internal mammary artery versus saphenous vein graft to the left anterior descending coronary artery: prospective randomized study with 10-year follow-up. Ann Thorac Surg. 1988;45(5):533–6. https://doi.org/10.1016/s0003-4975(10)64526-2. PMID: 3259128.
18. Back L, Ladwiniec A. Saphenous vein graft failure: current challenges and a review of the contemporary percutaneous options for management. J Clin Med. 2023;12(22):7118. https://doi.org/10.3390/jcm12227118. PMID: 38002729; PMCID: PMC10672592.
19. Tranbaugh RF, Schwann TA, Swistel DG, Dimitrova KR, Al-Shaar L, Hoffman DM, Geller CM, Engoren M, Balaram SK, Puskas JD, Habib RH. Coronary artery bypass graft surgery using the radial artery, right internal thoracic artery, or saphenous vein as the second conduit. Ann Thorac Surg. 2017;104(2):553–9. https://doi.org/10.1016/j.athoracsur.2016.11.017. Epub 2017 Feb 16. PMID: 28215422.
20. Bangalore S. Response by Bangalore to letter regarding article, "newer-generation ultrathin strut drug-eluting stents versus older second-generation thicker strut drug-eluting stents for coronary artery disease: meta-analysis of randomized trials". Circulation. 2019;139(17):2083–4. https://doi.org/10.1161/CIRCULATIONAHA.119.039684. PMID: 31013134.
21. Leyvi G, Dabas A, Leff JD. Hybrid coronary revascularization – current state of the art. J Cardiothorac Vasc Anesth. 2019;33(12):3437–45. https://doi.org/10.1053/j.jvca.2019.08.047. Epub 2019 Sep 3. PMID: 31570244.
22. Tajstra M, Hrapkowicz T, Hawranek M, Filipiak K, Gierlotka M, Zembala M, Gąsior M, Zembala MO, POL-MIDES Study Investigators. Hybrid coronary revascularization in selected patients with multivessel disease: 5-year clinical outcomes of the prospective randomized pilot study. JACC Cardiovasc Interv. 2018;11(9):847–52. https://doi.org/10.1016/j.jcin.2018.01.271. Epub 2018 Apr 18. PMID: 29680218.
23. Willard R, Scheinerman J, Pupovac S, Patel NC. The current state of hybrid coronary revascularization. Ann Thorac Surg. 2024;118(2):318–28. https://doi.org/10.1016/j.athoracsur.2024.04.010. Epub 2024 Apr 25. PMID: 38677447.
24. Puskas JD, Halkos ME, DeRose JJ, Bagiella E, Miller MA, Overbey J, Bonatti J, Srinivas VS, Vesely M, Sutter F, Lynch J, Kirkwood K, Shapiro TA, Boudoulas KD, Crestanello J, Gehrig T, Smith P, Ragosta M, Hoff SJ, Zhao D, Gelijns AC, Szeto WY, Weisz G, Argenziano M, Vassiliades T, Liberman H, Matthai W, Ascheim DD. Hybrid coronary revascularization for the treatment of multivessel coronary artery disease: a multicenter observational study. J Am Coll Cardiol. 2016;68(4):356–65. https://doi.org/10.1016/j.jacc.2016.05.032. PMID: 27443431; PMCID: PMC5142519.
25. Lowenstern A, Wu J, Bradley SM, Fanaroff AC, Tcheng JE, Wang TY. Current landscape of hybrid revascularization: a report from the NCDR CathPCI registry. Am Heart J. 2019;215:167–77. https://doi.org/10.1016/j.ahj.2019.06.014. Epub 2019 Jun 28. PMID: 31349108; PMCID: PMC6753051.
26. Thielmann M, Bonaros N, Barbato E, Barili F, Folliguet T, Friedrich G, Gottardi R, Legutko J, Parolari A, Punjabi P, Sandner S, Suwalski P, Shehada SE, Wendt D, Czerny M, Muneretto C. Hybrid coronary revascularization: position paper of the European Society of Cardiology Working Group on cardiovascular surgery and European Association of Percutaneous Cardiovascular Interventions. Eur J Cardiothorac Surg. 2024;66(2):ezae271. https://doi.org/10.1093/ejcts/ezae271. PMID: 39142801.
27. Virani SS, Newby LK, Arnold SV, Bittner V, Brewer LC, Demeter SH, Dixon DL, Fearon WF, Hess B,

Johnson HM, Kazi DS, Kolte D, Kumbhani DJ, LoFaso J, Mahtta D, Mark DB, Minissian M, Navar AM, Patel AR, Piano MR, Rodriguez F, Talbot AW, Taqueti VR, Thomas RJ, van Diepen S, Wiggins B, Williams MS. AHA/ACC/ACCP/ASPC/NLA/PCNA guideline for the management of patients with chronic coronary disease: a report of the American Heart Association/American College of Cardiology Joint Committee on Clinical practice guidelines. Circulation. 2023;148(9):e9–e119. https://doi.org/10.1161/CIR.0000000000001168. Epub 2023 Jul 20. Erratum in: Circulation. 2023 Sep 26;148(13):e148. Erratum in: Circulation. 2023 Dec 5;148(23):e186. PMID: 37471501.

28. Neumann FJ, Sousa-Uva M, Ahlsson A, Alfonso F, Banning AP, Benedetto U, Byrne RA, Collet JP, Falk V, Head SJ, Jüni P, Kastrati A, Koller A, Kristensen SD, Niebauer J, Richter DJ, Seferovic PM, Sibbing D, Stefanini GG, Windecker S, Yadav R, Zembala MO, ESC Scientific Document Group. 2018 ESC/EACTS Guidelines on myocardial revascularization. Eur Heart J. 2019;40(2):87–165. https://doi.org/10.1093/eurheartj/ehy394. Erratum in: Eur Heart J. 2019 Oct 1;40(37):3096. PMID: 30165437.
29. Masroor M, Chen C, Zhou K, Fu X, Khan UZ, Zhao Y. Minimally invasive left internal mammary artery harvesting techniques during the learning curve are safe and achieve similar results as conventional LIMA harvesting techniques. J Cardiothorac Surg. 2022;17(1):203. https://doi.org/10.1186/s13019-022-01961-0. PMID: 36002863; PMCID: PMC9404583.
30. Boonstra PW, Grandjean JG, Mariani MA. Improved method for direct coronary grafting without CPB via anterolateral small thoracotomy. Ann Thorac Surg. 1997;63(2):567–9. https://doi.org/10.1016/s0003-4975(96)01024-7. PMID: 9033350.
31. Masroor M, Zhou K, Chen C, Fu X, Zhao Y. All we need to know about internal thoracic artery harvesting and preparation for myocardial revascularization: a systematic review. J Cardiothorac Surg. 2021;16(1):354. https://doi.org/10.1186/s13019-021-01733-2. PMID: 34961523; PMCID: PMC8711206.
32. Robin J, Bompard D, Tronc F, Beaune J, Wahid F, Champsaur G. Bilateral internal thoracic artery harvesting under robotic video-assistance. Surg Endosc. 2001;15(7):755–6. https://doi.org/10.1007/s004640010044. Epub 2001 Feb 6. PMID: 11591984.
33. Hrapkowicz T, Bisleri G. Endoscopic harvesting of the left internal mammary artery. Ann Cardiothorac Surg. 2013;2(4):565–9. https://doi.org/10.3978/j.issn.2225-319X.2013.07.11. PMID: 23977637; PMCID: PMC3741892.
34. Nataf P, Lima L, Regan M, Benarim S, Ramadan R, Pavie A, Gandjbakhch I. Thoracoscopic internal mammary artery harvesting: technical considerations. Ann Thorac Surg. 1997;63(6 Suppl):S104–6. https://doi.org/10.1016/s0003-4975(97)00420-7. PMID: 9203611.
35. Canale LS, Bonatti J. Mammary artery harvesting using the Da Vinci Si robotic system. Rev Bras Cir Cardiovasc. 2014;29(1):107–9. https://doi.org/10.5935/1678-9741.20140019. PMID: 24896171; PMCID: PMC4389484.
36. Oehlinger A, Bonaros N, Schachner T, Ruetzler E, Friedrich G, Laufer G, Bonatti J. Robotic endoscopic left internal mammary artery harvesting: what have we learned after 100 cases? Ann Thorac Surg. 2007;83(3):1030–4. https://doi.org/10.1016/j.athoracsur.2006.10.055. PMID: 17307454.
37. Mariani MA, Boonstra PW, Grandjean JG, van der Schans C, Dusseljee S, van Weert E. Minimally invasive coronary artery bypass grafting without cardiopulmonary bypass. Eur J Cardiothorac Surg. 1997;11(5):881–7. https://doi.org/10.1016/s1010-7940(97)01201-3. PMID: 9196304.
38. Bonatti J, Wallner S, Winkler B, Grabenwöger M. Robotic totally endoscopic coronary artery bypass grafting: current status and future prospects. Expert Rev Med Devices. 2020;17(1):33–40. https://doi.org/10.1080/17434440.2020.1704252. Epub 2020 Jan 9. PMID: 31829047.
39. Shen L, Hu S, Wang H, Xiong H, Zheng Z, Li L, Xu B, Yan H, Gao R. One-stop hybrid coronary revascularization versus coronary artery bypass grafting and percutaneous coronary intervention for the treatment of multivessel coronary artery disease: 3-year follow-up results from a single institution. J Am Coll Cardiol. 2013;61(25):2525–33. https://doi.org/10.1016/j.jacc.2013.04.007. Epub 2013 Apr 23. PMID: 23623906.
40. Adams C, Burns DJ, Chu MW, Jones PM, Shridar K, Teefy P, Kostuk WJ, Dobkowski WB, Romsa J, Kiaii B. Single-stage hybrid coronary revascularization with long-term follow-up. Eur J Cardiothorac Surg. 2014;45(3):438–42. discussion 442–3. https://doi.org/10.1093/ejcts/ezt390. Epub 2013 Aug 15. PMID: 23956269.
41. Gernhofer YK, Banks DA, Golts E, Pretorius V. Novel use of Cangrelor With heparin during cardiopulmonary bypass in patients with heparin-induced thrombocytopenia who require cardiovascular surgery: a case series. Semin Thorac Cardiovasc Surg. 2020;32(4):763–9. https://doi.org/10.1053/j.semtcvs.2019.10.002. Epub 2019 Oct 11. PMID: 31610233.
42. Halkos ME, Vassiliades TA, Douglas JS, Morris DC, Rab ST, Liberman HA, Samady H, Kilgo PD, Guyton RA, Puskas JD. Hybrid coronary revascularization versus off-pump coronary artery bypass grafting for the treatment of multivessel coronary artery disease. Ann Thorac Surg. 2011;92(5):1695–701. discussion 1701–2. https://doi.org/10.1016/j.athoracsur.2011.05.090. Epub 2011 Sep 21. PMID: 21939958.
43. Song Z, Shen L, Zheng Z, Xu B, Xiong H, Li L, Hu S. One-stop hybrid coronary revascularization versus off-pump coronary artery bypass in patients with diabetes mellitus. J Thorac Cardiovasc Surg.

2016;151(6):1695–1701.e1. https://doi.org/10.1016/j.jtcvs.2016.01.049. Epub 2016 Feb 13. PMID: 26969134.
44. Harskamp RE, Abdelsalam M, Lopes RD, Boga G, Hirji S, Krishnan M, Kiljanek L, Mumtaz M, Tijssen JG, McCarty C, de Winter RJ, Bachinsky WB. Cardiac troponin release following hybrid coronary revascularization versus off-pump coronary artery bypass surgery. Interact Cardiovasc Thorac Surg. 2014;19(6):1008–12. https://doi.org/10.1093/icvts/ivu297. Epub 2014 Sep 12. PMID: 25217621.
45. Hage A, Giambruno V, Jones P, Chu MW, Fox S, Teefy P, Lavi S, Bainbridge D, Harle C, Iglesias I, Dobkowski W, Kiaii B. Hybrid coronary revascularization versus off-pump coronary artery bypass grafting: comparative effectiveness analysis with long-term follow-up. J Am Heart Assoc. 2019;8(24):e014204. https://doi.org/10.1161/JAHA.119.014204. Epub 2019 Dec 12. PMID: 31826727; PMCID: PMC6951054.
46. Schäfer A, Bauersachs J. Fokussiertes update zur dualen Plättchenhemmung: ESC-Leitlinie 2017 [Focused update on dual antiplatelet treatment: ESC guidelines 2017]. Herz. 2017;42(8):739–45. German. https://doi.org/10.1007/s00059-017-4634-6. PMID: 29043405.
47. Costa F, van Klaveren D, James S, Heg D, Räber L, Feres F, Pilgrim T, Hong MK, Kim HS, Colombo A, Steg PG, Zanchin T, Palmerini T, Wallentin L, Bhatt DL, Stone GW, Windecker S, Steyerberg EW, Valgimigli M, PRECISE-DAPT Study Investigators. Derivation and validation of the predicting bleeding complications in patients undergoing stent implantation and subsequent dual antiplatelet therapy (PRECISE-DAPT) score: a pooled analysis of individual-patient datasets from clinical trials. Lancet. 2017;389(10073):1025–34. https://doi.org/10.1016/S0140-6736(17)30397-5. PMID: 28290994.
48. Gao P, Xiong H, Zheng Z, Li L, Gao R, Hu SS. Evaluation of antiplatelet effects of a modified protocol by platelet aggregation in patients undergoing "one-stop" hybrid coronary revascularization. Platelets. 2010;21(3):183–90. https://doi.org/10.3109/09537101003592700. PMID: 20201634.
49. Zhou S, Fang Z, Xiong H, Hu S, Xu B, Chen L, Wang W. Effect of one-stop hybrid coronary revascularization on postoperative renal function and bleeding: a comparison study with off-pump coronary artery bypass grafting surgery. J Thorac Cardiovasc Surg. 2014;147(5):1511–1516.e1. https://doi.org/10.1016/j.jtcvs.2013.05.026. Epub 2013 Jul 21. PMID: 23879931.
50. Zhao DX, Leacche M, Balaguer JM, Boudoulas KD, Damp JA, Greelish JP, Byrne JG, Writing Group of the Cardiac Surgery, Cardiac Anesthesiology, and Interventional Cardiology Groups at the Vanderbilt Heart and Vascular Institute, Ahmad RM, Ball SK, Cleator JH, Deegan RJ, Eagle SS, Fong PP, Fredi JL, Hoff SJ, Jennings HS 3rd, JA MP, Piana RN, Pretorius M, Robbins MA, Slosky DA, Thompson A. Routine intraoperative completion angiography after coronary artery bypass grafting and 1-stop hybrid revascularization results from a fully integrated hybrid catheterization laboratory/operating room. J Am Coll Cardiol. 2009;53(3):232–41. https://doi.org/10.1016/j.jacc.2008.10.011. PMID: 19147039.
51. Halkos ME, Cooper WA, Petersen R, Puskas JD, Lattouf OM, Craver JM, Guyton RA. Early administration of clopidogrel is safe after off-pump coronary artery bypass surgery. Ann Thorac Surg. 2006;81(3):815–9. https://doi.org/10.1016/j.athoracsur.2005.08.056. PMID: 16488678.
52. Bednar F, Osmancik P, Vanek T, Mocikova H, Jares M, Straka Z, Widimsky P. Platelet activity and aspirin efficacy after off-pump compared with on-pump coronary artery bypass surgery: results from the prospective randomised trial PRAGUE 11-Coronary Artery Bypass and REactivity of Thrombocytes (CABARET). J Thorac Cardiovasc Surg. 2008;136(4):1054–60. https://doi.org/10.1016/j.jtcvs.2008.03.052. Epub 2008 Jul 10. PMID: 18954649.
53. Kon ZN, Brown EN, Tran R, Joshi A, Reicher B, Grant MC, Kallam S, Burris N, Connerney I, Zimrin D, Poston RS. Simultaneous hybrid coronary revascularization reduces postoperative morbidity compared with results from conventional off-pump coronary artery bypass. J Thorac Cardiovasc Surg. 2008;135(2):367–75. https://doi.org/10.1016/j.jtcvs.2007.09.025. Epub 2007 Dec 26. PMID: 18242270; PMCID: PMC2962576.
54. Reicher B, Poston RS, Mehra MR, Joshi A, Odonkor P, Kon Z, Reyes PA, Zimrin DA. Simultaneous "hybrid" percutaneous coronary intervention and minimally invasive surgical bypass grafting: feasibility, safety, and clinical outcomes. Am Heart J. 2008;155(4):661–7. https://doi.org/10.1016/j.ahj.2007.12.032. Epub 2008 Mar 5. PMID: 18371473; PMCID: PMC2636970.
55. Bachinsky WB, Abdelsalam M, Boga G, Kiljanek L, Mumtaz M, McCarty C. Comparative study of same sitting hybrid coronary artery revascularization versus off-pump coronary artery bypass in multivessel coronary artery disease. J Interv Cardiol. 2012;25(5):460–8. https://doi.org/10.1111/j.1540--8183.2012.00752.x. Epub 2012 Jul 3. PMID: 22758203.
56. Vlot EA, Willemsen LM, Van Dongen EPA, Janssen PW, Hackeng CM, Kloppenburg GTL, Kelder JC, Ten Berg JM, Noordzij PG. Perioperative point of care platelet function testing and postoperative blood loss in high-risk cardiac surgery patients. Platelets. 2019;30(8):982–8. https://doi.org/10.1080/09537104.2018.1542123. Epub 2018 Nov 9. PMID: 30411659.
57. Ding T, Hu S, Qu J, Xiong H, Xu B, Wu Y, Shen L. Evaluation of the effect of simultaneous hybrid coronary revascularization on postoperative bleeding and renal function: a comparison study with minimally invasive direct off-pump coronary artery bypass grafting in patients with multivessel coronary artery disease. J Thorac Cardiovasc Surg. 2023;166(5):1446–1455.e4. https://doi.org/10.1016/j.jtcvs.2022.01.045. Epub 2022 Feb 8. PMID: 35272844.

58. Besola L, Colli A, De Caterina R. Coronary bypass surgery for multivessel disease after percutaneous coronary intervention in acute coronary syndromes: why, for whom, how early? Eur Heart J. 2024;26:ehae413. https://doi.org/10.1093/eurheartj/ehae413. Epub ahead of print. PMID: 39056269.
59. Kandzari DE, Kirtane AJ, Mehran R, Price MJ, Simon DI, Latib A, Kedhi E, Abizaid A, Worthley SG, Zaman A, Hudec M, Stoler R, Choi JW, Kanitkar M, Conradie A, Tam CF, Walton A, Gruberg L, Ando K, Lee LC, Lung TH, Windecker S, Stone GW. Clinical outcomes according to lesion complexity in high bleeding risk patients treated with 1-month dual antiplatelet therapy following PCI: analysis from the Onyx ONE clear study. Catheter Cardiovasc Interv. 2022;99(3):583–92. https://doi.org/10.1002/ccd.29939. Epub 2021 Sep 3. PMID: 34478233.
60. Valgimigli M, Smits PC, Frigoli E, Bongiovanni D, Tijssen J, Hovasse T, Mafragi A, Ruifrok WT, Karageorgiev D, Aminian A, Garducci S, Merkely B, Routledge H, Ando K, Diaz Fernandez JF, Cuisset T, Nesa Malik FT, Halabi M, Belle L, Din J, Beygui F, Abhyankar A, Reczuch K, Pedrazzini G, Heg D, Vranckx P, MASTER DAPT Investigators. Duration of antiplatelet therapy after complex percutaneous coronary intervention in patients at high bleeding risk: a MASTER DAPT trial sub-analysis. Eur Heart J. 2022;43(33):3100–14. https://doi.org/10.1093/eurheartj/ehac284. PMID: 35580836.
61. Daniel WT, Liberman HA, Kilgo P, Puskas JD, Vassiliades TA, Devireddy C, Jaber W, Guyton RA, Halkos ME. The impact of clopidogrel therapy on postoperative bleeding after robotic-assisted coronary artery bypass surgery. Eur J Cardiothorac Surg. 2014;46(1):e8–13. https://doi.org/10.1093/ejcts/ezu160. Epub 2014 Apr 8. PMID: 24713891.
62. Angiolillo DJ, Firstenberg MS, Price MJ, Tummala PE, Hutyra M, Welsby IJ, Voeltz MD, Chandna H, Ramaiah C, Brtko M, Cannon L, Dyke C, Liu T, Montalescot G, Manoukian SV, Prats J, Topol EJ, Investigators BRIDGE. Bridging antiplatelet therapy with cangrelor in patients undergoing cardiac surgery: a randomised controlled trial. JAMA. 2012;307(3):265–74. https://doi.org/10.1001/jama.2011.2002. PMID: 22253393; PMCID: PMC3774162.
63. Li Y, Li J, Wang B, Jing Q, Zeng Y, Hou A, Wang Z, Liu A, Zhang J, Zhang Y, Zhang P, Jiang D, Liu B, Fan J, Zhang J, Li L, Su G, Yang M, Jiang W, Qu P, Zeng H, Li L, Qiu M, Ru L, Chen S, Zhou Y, Qiao S, Stone GW, Angiolillo DJ, Han Y, OPT-BIRISK Investigators. Extended clopidogrel monotherapy vs DAPT in patients with acute coronary syndromes at high ischemic and bleeding risk: the OPT-BIRISK randomized clinical trial. JAMA Cardiol. 2024;9(6):523–31. https://doi.org/10.1001/jamacardio.2024.0534. PMID: 38630489; PMCID: PMC11024736.

Part III

Structural Heart Interventions in HBR Patients

14 Left Atrial Appendage Closure: From Randomized Trials to Contemporary Registries

Mohammed Alghammass, Rafey Feroze, Luis Augusto Palma Dallan, and Steven J. Filby

14.1 Introduction

Atrial fibrillation (AF) is the leading preventable cause of ischemic stroke and is associated with higher mortality when compared with stroke in non-AF patients [1]. Although oral anticoagulants are the standard therapeutic approach for stroke prevention in AF patients, many patients are unable to utilize these medications. Percutaneous left atrial appendage closure (LAAC) provides a non-pharmacologic alternative approach for stroke prevention. LAAC is a safe procedure that may be performed with a same-discharge strategy [2]. The WATCHMAN™ device (Boston Scientific Co., Fig. 14.1) and Amulet™ device (Abbott, Fig. 14.2) are United States Food and Drug Administration (FDA) approved for stroke prevention in patients with nonvalvular atrial fibrillation (NVAF) who have an appropriate rationale to seek an alternative to oral anticoagulation [3].

The morphology of the left atrial appendage (LAA) varies widely among individuals [4]. Pre-procedural imaging using cardiac computed tomography angiography (CTA) or transesophageal echocardiography (TEE) determines the choice and size of the device while intraprocedural imaging with intracardiac echocardiography (ICE) or TEE in conjunction with fluoroscopy guides device placement. Successful LAAC depends on appropriate interaction and apposition of the device with the LAA walls, ensuring adequate compression of the device and complete exclusion of all LAA lobes. LAAC is affected by various factors including LAA ostial diameter, LAA depth, morphology ("chicken wing," "cauliflower," "cactus," "windsock," etc.), septations, trabeculations, number of lobes, and orientation of the LAA body. Failure in device sizing or inadequate device positioning may result in peri-device leakage or even in device embolization [5].

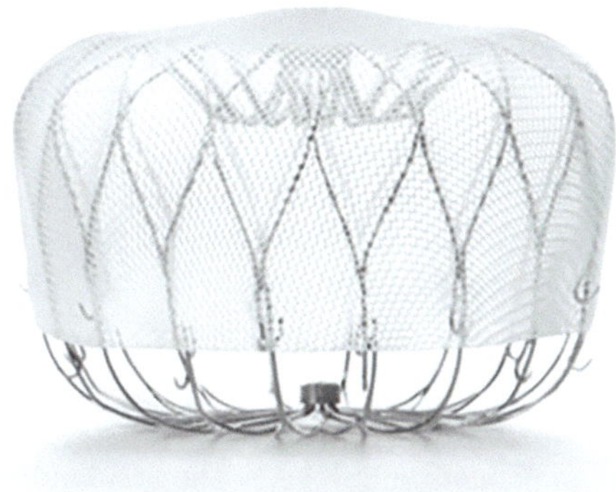

Fig. 14.1 WATCHMAN™ FLX device

M. Alghammass · R. Feroze · L. A. P. Dallan (✉)
S. J. Filby
Harrington Heart & Vascular Institute,
University Hospitals Cleveland, Cleveland, OH, USA

B. Cortese, S. Rigattieri (eds.), *High Bleeding Risk Patients in Interventional Cardiology*,
https://doi.org/10.1007/978-3-031-87302-7_14

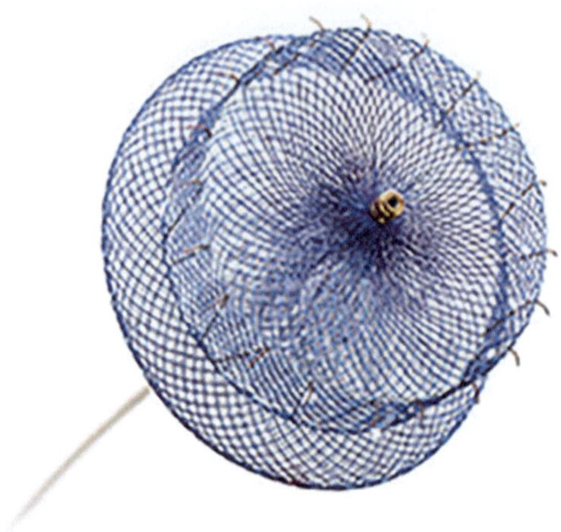

Fig. 14.2 Amplatzer™ Amulet™ LAA Occluder

14.2 Clinical Evidence for WATCHMAN

A large body of published evidence supports the WATCHMAN LAAC device's effectiveness and safety in patients with NVAF. The first landmark randomized trial was PROTECT AF, evaluating the WATCHMAN legacy device's efficacy and safety compared to warfarin for the prevention of stroke and systemic embolism in patients with NVAF [6]. This randomized, controlled multicenter trial of 707 patients evaluated primary efficacy endpoints for stroke and systemic embolism and cardiovascular death, along with primary safety endpoints for major bleeding and complications related to the procedure. In this study, the WATCHMAN legacy device met the criteria for non-inferiority at the primary efficacy endpoint measured against warfarin; these results were maintained at a 5-year follow-up. The PREVAIL trial, done with similar intention, was a randomized, prospective, multicenter study involving patients with NVAF who were eligible for warfarin therapy [7]. The trial met its primary safety endpoint, thus proving a supportive safety profile of WATCHMAN device's use; however, it did not meet the primary efficacy endpoint; therefore, non-inferiority was not established based on the results. This has been attributed to lower-than-expected event rate in the control group. A third randomized trial, the PRAGUE-17 trial, compared the efficacy and safety of the WATCHMAN device and the Amplatzer Amulet device versus direct oral anticoagulants in high-risk AF patients [8]. In the randomized non-inferiority trial, a total of 402 patients were enrolled for the primary efficacy endpoint evaluation, which included composite stroke, systemic embolism, cardiovascular death, major bleeding, or procedure- or device-related complications, with a mean follow-up duration of 20.8 months. PRAGUE-17 found that LAAC with either the WATCHMAN or Amulet devices was non-inferior to direct oral anticoagulant (DOAC) in preventing ischemic or bleeding events.

Not only has the use of WATCHMAN devices been shown to be safe and effective for stroke prevention in the aforementioned trials, but also extensive registry datasets including thousands of patients from the "real world" have also demonstrated that the WATCHMAN device is a safe alternative to DOAC, with lower procedural and in-hospital complications and a higher procedural success rate. Holmes and colleagues evaluated data in the CAP (Continued Access to PROTECT AF) and CAP2 (Continued Access to PREVAIL) registries, both of which provided additional data about the safety and efficacy of the WATCHMAN device [9]. In CAP, 566 patients versus 578 in CAP2 were included, and the reported average follow-up periods were 50.1 and 50.3 months, respectively. Both registries confirmed the initial findings of the PROTECT AF trial, demonstrating low rates for ischemic stroke and systemic embolism, in addition to a low complication rate associated with the device itself, which proved the reliability of the WATCHMAN device in preventing stroke in patients with NVAF over a longer follow-up period.

Furthermore, EWOLUTION was a 2-year prospective, multicenter follow-up study for assessing the safety and effectiveness of the WATCHMAN device in real-world settings [10]. This study included more than 1000 patients enrolled in the registry from 47 centers across 13 countries. A high procedural success rate was shown (98.5%), with low rates for ischemic stroke and bleeding. The *NCDR (National*

Cardiovascular Data Registry) registry analysis provided additional real-world dataset, which contributed to a considerably large amount of evidence supporting the WATCHMAN device in clinical practice [11]. This study comprised data from over 38,000 patients across 495 centers regarding procedural success rates, complication rates, and long-term outcomes in large and varied patient populations. Of particular note, the registry's principal findings included a procedural success rate of 98.3%. Moreover, the data also highlighted a very low complication rate with pericardial effusion requiring intervention (1.39%) and major bleeding events (1.25%), underpinning the safety in clinical practice.

Finally, the next-generation WATCHMAN FLX (Boston Scientific, Marlborough, MA) has been shown to be safer with higher procedural success compared with WATCHMAN 2.5. The device was investigated in the PINNACLE FLX trial, a prospective, single-arm, multicenter study including 400 patients with NVAF who were at an increased risk for stroke [12]. The primary goal of the trial to establish the safety and effectiveness of the WATCHMAN FLX device with advanced design attributes for advanced implantation and sealing of the LAA. Results demonstrated a high successful device implantation rate and a low primary safety event rate, establishing the WATCHMAN FLX device as safe and effective in stroke prevention for patients with NVAF. More recently, the data from SURPASS registry at 1 year were presented [13]. The registry which involves over 66,000 patients found that the device's real-world performance matched the positive results from recent clinical trials, with a 97.7% procedural success rate and low major procedural complication rates of 0.49% within 7 days of hospital discharge. The 1-year outcomes included an all-stroke rate of 1.6%, a major bleeding rate of 6.7%, and an 8.3% mortality rate, reflecting the high-risk patient population. WATCHMAN landmark trials and registry data are summarized in Table 14.1.

Table 14.1 Summary of WATCHMAN device landmark trials and registry data

Trial/registry	*N*	Follow-up period	Procedural success rate (%)	Overall procedural complication (defined by study)	Conclusion
PROTECT AF	707	3.8 years	88	8.70%	Landmark RCT demonstrating non-inferiority and superiority of WATCHMAN for the composite outcome of stroke, systemic embolism, and CV death compared to warfarin
PREVAIL	407	18 months	95.1	4.50%	Landmark RCT demonstrating non-inferiority of WATCHMAN compared to warfarin in prevention of ischemic stroke and systemic embolization
PRAGUE-17	402	20.8 months	96	4.50%	RCT for high-risk AF patients, LAAO was non-inferior to DOAC in preventing CV, neurologic, and bleeding events
CAP 1	566	50.1 months	94.3	4.20%	78% risk reduction in stroke with WATCHMAN
CAP 2	578	50.3 months	94.3	1.40%	69% risk reduction in stroke with WATCHMAN
EWOLUTION	1025	2 years	98.5	1.80%	WATCHMAN implantation provided 84% relative risk reduction in ischemic stroke
NCDR-LAAO	38,158	At least 4 years	98.1	2.16%	National WATCHMAN registry with various studies
PINNACLE FLX	400	24 months	98.8	0.50%	WATCHMAN FLX is associated with lower adverse events and more frequent LAA closure compared to first-generation WATCHMAN
SURPASS	66,894	Ongoing	97.6	0.49%- procedural adverse event rate within 7 days of hospital discharge	WATCHMAN FLX has high procedural success rate and low complication rate

Table 14.2 Summary of ongoing LAAO trials

Trial	Device used	Purpose of the study
OPTION	WATCHMAN FLX	Comparing safety and effectiveness of WATCHMAN FLX to OAC therapy post-ablation, aiming to expand indications for stroke risk reduction in NVAF patients
LAAOS-4	WATCHMAN FLX or FLX PRO	Investigating addition of WATCHMAN FLX or FLX PRO to long-term anticoagulation for high-risk NVAF patients to reduce ischemic stroke
CHAMPION-AF	WATCHMAN FLX	Assessing if WATCHMAN FLX is reasonable alternative NOACs in NVAF in patients eligible for NOACs
STROKE-CLOSE	Amplatzer AMULET	Evaluating efficacy in reducing the incidence of recurrent stroke, bleeding, and cardiovascular mortality in patient with NVAF and prior intracerebral hemorrhage
CATALYST	Amplatzer AMULET	Evaluating safety and effectiveness of Amplatzer Amulet compared to NOACs in NVAF patients
CLOSURE-AF	CE-mark approved LAA closure devices	Assessing safety and effectiveness in high-risk AF patients unsuitable for long-term anticoagulation therapy.

Other trials evaluating the WATCHMAN FLX safety and effectiveness are ongoing, including the OPTION trial, which will compare the use of WATCHMAN FLX LAAC device to oral anticoagulation (OAC) therapy in patients with atrial fibrillation post-ablation [14]. LAAOS-4 trial will investigate whether adding the WATCHMAN FLX device to long-term anticoagulation can help patients with NVAF who are at the highest residual risk for stroke [15]. Additionally, the CHAMPION-AF trial will compare the WATCHMAN FLX device with DOAC in patients with atrial fibrillation who are eligible for anticoagulation [16]. A summary of ongoing WATCHMAN FLX trials is shown in Table 14.2.

14.3 Clinical Evidence for the Amulet Device

The Amulet IDE trial was a pivotal study designed to evaluate the safety and effectiveness of the Amplatzer Amulet device in comparison to the device for LAAC in patients with NVAF [17]. This randomized trial enrolled 1878 patients with an average follow-up of 18 months. The results showed that the Amulet device was non-inferior to the WATCHMAN legacy device. Furthermore, The Global Amplatzer Amulet Observational Study was a large, prospective, multicenter registry with a follow-up period over 2 years [18]. It was designed to assess the real-world performance of the Amplatzer Amulet device and included 1088 patients from multiple centers worldwide, focusing on the procedural success, safety, and efficacy of the Amulet device. The primary endpoints were procedural success and rates of adverse events such as ischemic stroke, systemic embolism, major bleeding, and device-related complications. Results demonstrated a high procedural success rate of 99%, with low rates of ischemic stroke (2.7% per year), major bleeding (3.2% per year), and device-related complications.

The SWISS-APERO was a large open-label randomized clinical trial concluded in the period of 2018–2021 across eight European centers comparing AMULET with WATCHMAN [19]. The primary endpoint was the rate of LAA patency assessed by coronary computed tomography angiography (CCTA) at 45 days, which showed similar outcomes for both devices (Amulet 67.6% vs. WATCHMAN FLX 70%). Secondary endpoints revealed that the Amulet device had a lower rate of peri-device leaks (13.7%) compared to the WATCHMAN FLX (27.5%) at 45 days, indicating better sealing capacity for the Amulet. However, the Amulet device exhibited a higher rate of intra-device leaks (44.8% vs. 23% for

WATCHMAN). Procedural complications were more frequent with the Amulet device, which had a 9% complication rate compared to 2.7% for the WATCHMAN, primarily due to higher bleeding events (7.2% vs. 1.8%). Despite these procedural differences, the clinical outcomes at 13 months were similar, with comparable rates of cardiovascular death, stroke, and systemic embolism (Amulet 9.5% vs. WATCHMAN 10.2%). Another study analyzing the data from the ORIGINAL registry that includes 482 patients of whom 93 patients treated with the Amulet device found high successful implantation rate (97%), with an overall complication rate of 2.2%, similar to the WATCHMAN group (2.3%) [20].

The most recent publication that offers a thorough examination of the Amulet occluder's early post-approval results in the United States is the EMERGE study [21]. The study focused on patients who underwent implantation of the Amulet device between August 2021 and December 2022, utilizing data from the NCDR-LAAO Registry. The purpose of the 5499-patient study was to evaluate the device's effectiveness and safety in the real-world environment. Results showed a high implant success rate of 95.8% and a complete closure rate of 97.2% post-procedure, which decreased to 87.1% at 45 days. 2.9% of patients experienced major adverse events while they were in the hospital, and 5.7% experienced major bleeding after 45 days. Higher implant success and fewer pericardial effusions were observed with increasing operator experience.

The STROKE-CLOSE, CLOSURE-AF, and CATALYST trials are still ongoing and will be critical for expanding the understanding and applications of Amplatzer Amulet device, potentially offering more options and improved outcomes for patients with atrial fibrillation at risk of stroke [22–24]. A summary of ongoing Amplatzer Amulet device trials is shown in Table 14.2.

14.4 Future Perspectives

The field of LAAO continues to evolve with innovations to maximize the safety and effectiveness of the devices. The latest FDA-approved LAAO device is WATCHMAN FLX PRO. This new generation of WATCHMAN incorporates a fluoropolymer coating, a novel technology in LAAO devices, but known entity in the world of drug-eluting stent with existing literature demonstrating that such coating causes lower inflammatory and platelet adhesion, resulting in less thrombogenicity [25]. Saliba and colleagues tested the fluoropolymer-coated devices in vitro utilizing multi-experimental setups. Their results demonstrated that fluoropolymer-coated devices, when compared to WATCHMAN FLX, had higher percent area with albumin adsorption and lower percent area with platelet binding resulting in lesser platelet-activating surface [26]. In vivo experiments showed that the coated device had lesser inflammation and thrombosis with enhanced endothelia coverage. The study concluded that the WATCHMAN FLX PRO outperforms traditional devices in both thromboresistance and endothelial coverage which will contribute to reducing device-related thrombosis events and the need for prolonged anticoagulation therapy. As the WATCHMAN FLX PRO is now available in clinical practice, future studies will undoubtedly be done to examine the veracity of these preclinical findings.

14.5 Conclusions

Many randomized trials and multicenter registries over the past decade have supported the clinical use of LAAC, especially for the FDA-approved WATCHMAN and Amulet devices. Increased operator experience and widespread adoption of LAAC implantation techniques have seen improvements in safety, procedural, and clinical outcomes. It is important to highlight that the data available from RCTs involved earlier generation devices with less evolved implantation techniques. In addition, the patients of subsequent registry analyses often have more comorbidities than these landmark trials, and yet devices demonstrate superior safety and performance outcomes. The currently approved LAAC devices offer significant improvements compared to its predecessors and provide an excellent option for LAAC procedure. With the results of the CHAMPION-AF and CATALYST trials on the horizon, this therapy may be expanded to an even broader population of NVAF patients.

References

1. Saposnik G, Gladstone D, Raptis R, et al. Atrial fibrillation in ischemic stroke: predicting response to thrombolysis and clinical outcomes. Stroke. 2013;44(1):99–104. https://doi.org/10.1161/STROKEAHA.112.676551.
2. Dallan LAP, Bezerra HG, Cochet A, et al. Safety, efficacy, and cost-effectiveness of same-day discharge for left atrial appendage occlusion. J Invasive Cardiol. 2022;34(2):E124. PMID: 35100555.
3. Saw J, Holmes DR, Cavalcante JL, et al. SCAI/HRS expert consensus statement on transcatheter left atrial appendage closure. J Soc Cardiovasc Angiogr Interv. 2023;1(5):100577. https://doi.org/10.1016/j.jscai.2022.100577.
4. Naksuk N, Padmanabhan D, Yogeswaran V, et al. Left atrial appendage: embryology, anatomy, physiology, arrhythmia and therapeutic intervention. JACC Clin Electrophysiol. 2016;2(4):403–12. https://doi.org/10.1016/j.jacep.2016.06.006. Epub 2016 Aug 15. PMID: 29759858.
5. Korsholm K, Berti S, Iriart X, et al. Expert recommendations on cardiac computed tomography for planning transcatheter left atrial appendage occlusion. JACC Cardiovasc Interv. 2020;13(3):277–92. https://doi.org/10.1016/j.jcin.2019.08.054. Epub 2019 Oct 30. PMID: 31678086.
6. Reddy VY, Sievert H, Halperin J, et al. Percutaneous left atrial appendage closure vs warfarin for atrial fibrillation: a randomized clinical trial. JAMA. 2014;312(19):1988–98. https://doi.org/10.1001/jama.2014.15192. Erratum in: JAMA 2015 Mar 10;313(10):1061. PMID: 25399274.
7. Holmes DR Jr, Kar S, Price MJ, et al. Prospective randomized evaluation of the watchman left atrial appendage closure device in patients with atrial fibrillation versus long-term warfarin therapy: the PREVAIL trial. J Am Coll Cardiol. 2014;64(1):1–12. https://doi.org/10.1016/j.jacc.2014.04.029. Erratum in: J Am Coll Cardiol. 2014 Sep 16;64(11):1186. PMID: 24998121.
8. Osmancik P, Herman D, Neuzil P, et al. 4-Year outcomes after left atrial appendage closure versus nonwarfarin oral anticoagulation for atrial fibrillation. J Am Coll Cardiol. 2022;79(1):1–14. https://doi.org/10.1016/j.jacc.2021.10.023. Epub 2021 Nov 5. PMID: 34748929.
9. Holmes DR Jr, Reddy VY, Gordon NT, et al. Long-term safety and efficacy in continued access left atrial appendage closure registries. J Am Coll Cardiol. 2019;74(23):2878–89. https://doi.org/10.1016/j.jacc.2019.09.064. PMID: 31806131.
10. Boersma LV, Ince H, Kische S, et al. Efficacy and safety of left atrial appendage closure with WATCHMAN in patients with or without contraindication to oral anticoagulation: 1-year follow-up outcome data of the EWOLUTION trial. Heart Rhythm. 2017;14(9):1302–8. https://doi.org/10.1016/j.hrthm.2017.05.038. Epub 2017 May 31. PMID: 28577840.
11. Freeman JV, Varosy P, Price MJ, et al. The NCDR left atrial appendage occlusion registry. J Am Coll Cardiol. 2020;75(13):1503–18. https://doi.org/10.1016/j.jacc.2019.12.040. PMID: 32238316; PMCID: PMC7205034.
12. Kar S, Doshi SK, Sadhu A, et al. Primary outcome evaluation of a next-generation left atrial appendage closure device: results from the PINNACLE FLX trial. Circulation. 2021;143(18):1754–62. https://doi.org/10.1161/CIRCULATIONAHA.120.050117. Epub 2021 Apr 6. PMID: 33820423.
13. Torsello GF, Argyriou A, Stavroulakis K, et al. One-year results from the SURPASS observational registry of the CTAG stent-graft with the active control system. J Endovasc Ther. 2020;27(3):421–7. https://doi.org/10.1177/1526602820913007.
14. Wazni OM, Boersma L, Healey JS, et al. Comparison of anticoagulation with left atrial appendage closure after atrial fibrillation ablation: rationale and design of the OPTION randomized trial. Am Heart J. 2022;251:35–42. https://doi.org/10.1016/j.ahj.2022.05.003. Epub 2022 May 6. PMID: 35526570.
15. Available from https://clinicaltrials.gov/study/NCT05963698.
16. Kar S, Doshi SK, Alkhouli M, et al. Rationale and design of a randomized study comparing the Watchman FLX device to DOACs in patients with atrial fibrillation. Am Heart J. 2023;264:123–32. https://doi.org/10.1016/j.ahj.2023.05.022. Epub 2023 Jun 4. PMID: 37279840.
17. Lakkireddy D, Thaler D, Ellis CR, et al. Amplatzer amulet left atrial appendage occluder versus watchman device for stroke prophylaxis (Amulet IDE): a randomized, controlled trial. Circulation. 2021;144(19):1543–52. https://doi.org/10.1161/CIRCULATIONAHA.121.057063. Epub 2021 Aug 30. PMID: 34459659; PMCID: PMC8570346.
18. Hildick-Smith D, Diener HC, Schmidt B, et al. Rationale and design of a global registry to evaluate real-world clinical outcomes in patients with atrial fibrillation and high risk of stroke treated with left atrial appendage occlusion using the AMPLATZER amulet device-perspective of available/ongoing registries of catheter-based LAA occlusion. Catheter Cardiovasc Interv. 2018;91(3):540–7. https://doi.org/10.1002/ccd.27252. Epub 2017 Sep 1. PMID: 28862376.
19. Galea R, De Marco F, Meneveau N, et al. Amulet or watchman device for percutaneous left atrial

appendage closure: primary results of the SWISS-APERO randomized clinical trial. Circulation. 2022;145(10):724–38. https://doi.org/10.1161/CIRCULATIONAHA.121.057859.
20. Kretzler L, Mues C, Wunderlich C, et al. Short term outcome after left atrial appendage occlusion with the AMPLATZER Amulet and WATCHMAN device: results from the ORIGINAL registry (saxOnian RegIstry analyzinG and followINg left atrial Appendage cLosure). BMC Cardiovasc Disord. 2022;22(1):271. Published 2022 Jun 16. https://doi.org/10.1186/s12872-022-02708-4.
21. Alkhouli M, Freeman JV, Ellis CR, et al. First experience with Amulet in the United States: early insights from EMERGE LAA postapproval study. JACC Cardiovasc Interv. Published online January 19. 2024;17:422. https://doi.org/10.1016/j.jcin.2023.11.027.
22. Available from: https://clinicaltrials.gov/study/NCT02830152.
23. Available from: https://clinicaltrials.gov/study/NCT03463317.
24. Available from: https://clinicaltrials.gov/study/NCT04226547.
25. Sato Y, Jinnouchi H, Kolodgie FD, et al. Acute thrombogenicity of fluoropolymer coated stents versus competitive drug-eluting stents under single antiplatelet therapy. Int J Cardiol. 2021;338:42–9. https://doi.org/10.1016/j.ijcard.2021.06.034.
26. Saliba WI, Kawai K, Sato Y, et al. Enhanced thromboresistance and endothelialization of a novel fluoropolymer-coated left atrial appendage closure device. JACC Clin Electrophysiol. 2023;9(8 Pt 2):1555–67. https://doi.org/10.1016/j.jacep.2023.04.013.

15 Tips and Tricks for a Successful and Safe LAAO Procedure

Fabrizio Ugo, Ludovica Maltese, and Francesco Rametta

15.1 Introduction

Atrial fibrillation (AF) is a growing epidemic with a prevalence in the general population about 1% in different studies. It increases with age and reaches a prevalence of 9% in patients of age >80 years [1]. In 1978, the landmark Framingham study [2] demonstrated a fivefold increase in the incidence of ischaemic stroke among patients with non-valvular AF (NVAF) compared with patients without NVAF. Stroke is the most debilitating complication of AF, and its prevention is hence considered the cornerstone of AF management [3]. Autopsy series and transoesophageal echocardiography (TOE) examinations show that in patients with NVAF, >90% of thrombi observed come from the left atrial appendage (LAA) [4]. During past decades numerous stroke prevention strategies have been introduced, including the use of oral anticoagulation (OAC) and percutaneous left atrial appendage occlusion (LAAO) procedures. The newer direct OACs (DOACs) are largely used but carry high costs, despite the simplicity of administration about 30% of patients are nonadherent at 2 years [5], and there is a considerable group of patients who cannot tolerate them because of bleeding complications, cognitive impairment, fall risk, drug allergy or interactions, and renal dysfunction. Older patients often have unfavourable bleeding risk profiles for OAC, and one or more of these cited characteristics lead physicians to not prescribe or to discontinue OAC. This treatment gap has created an unmet clinical need for an effective and safe non-pharmacologic therapy for stroke prevention in patients with NVAF and has opened the way to LAA closure (LAAC) procedures either surgical or endovascular [6]. For percutaneous LAA occlusion, two main device designs have been used: "pacifiers" that are formed with a lobe and a disk and "plugs" with a single lobe design. It is also commercially available the LARIAT suture delivery device (SentreHEART, Inc., Redwood City, CA, USA) that is a system for ligating the LAA through a combined endovascular and epicardial approach. The main characteristics of the latest percutaneous LAAO devices are listed in Table 15.1.

The original version of the chapter has been revised. A correction to this chapter can be found at https://doi.org/10.1007/978-3-031-87302-7_27

F. Ugo · L. Maltese (✉) · F. Rametta
Cardiology Division, Sant'Andrea Hospital, Vercelli, Italy

B. Cortese, S. Rigattieri (eds.), *High Bleeding Risk Patients in Interventional Cardiology*, https://doi.org/10.1007/978-3-031-87302-7_15

Table 15.1 Left atrial appendage closure devices, main characteristics

Device	Manufacturer	Design	Sizes (mm)	Sheath (F)	Approval status
Watchman FLX	Boston Scientific	Single Lobe	5 sizes: 20, 24, 27, 31, 35	14	CE mark, FDA approved
Amulet	Abbott Vascular	Distal lobe and proximal disc	8 sizes: 16, 18, 20, 22, 25, 28, 31, 34	12–14 steerable (outer 19F)	CE mark, FDA approved
LAmbre	LifeTech	Distal lobe and proximal disc	11 sizes: 16, 18, 30, 22, 24, 26, 28, 30, 32, 34, 36	8–10	CE mark, FDA approved
WaveCrest	Biosense Webster	Single lobe	3 sizes: 22, 27, 32	12	CE mark
Occlutech	Occlutech International	Distal lobe and proximal disc	9 sizes: 15, 18, 21, 24, 27, 30, 33, 36, 39	12–14	CE mark
Ultraseal	Cardia	Distal lobe and proximal disc	9 sizes: 16, 18, 20, 22, 24, 26, 28, 30, 32	10–12	CE mark
Conformal	Conformal Medical	Single Lobe	2 sizes: regular, large	–	Under approval
Omega	Eclipse Medical	Distal lobe and proximal disc	9 sizes from 14 to 30	14	CE mark

15.2 Pre-procedural Aspects

Baseline pre-procedural imaging with TOE or cardiac computed tomography angiography (cardiac CT) is recommended before LAAC [7]. Pre-procedural TOE is the most commonly employed imaging modality. Some experienced centres perform the baseline TOE even the day of the LAAC procedure. This practice may be acceptable but should be discouraged with new programmes, because technical issues such as a lipomatous or aneurysmal septum, LAA thrombus, or atypical LAA size/morphology can be insurmountable for inexperienced operators.

Two-dimensional (2D) images of the LAA are recommended to be obtained at 0°, 45°, 90°, and 135° along the axis of the circumflex artery to identify the maximal width of the LAA landing zone [8] and depth dimensions must be obtained too. Three-dimensional (3D) TEE imaging of the LAA can provide improved accuracy for sizing measurements (Fig. 15.1). Description of septum and fossa ovalis in bicaval and short-axis view must be provided too.

Cardiac CT is an excellent 3D primary imaging tool for LAAC procedural planning and has a superior spatial resolution than TEE. In centres with availability and expertise, cardiac CT provides an optimal pre-procedural planning. The addition of 3D printing to assess how different devices/sizes can fit in individual patient anatomies may be helpful, especially with challenging anatomies. In Fig. 15.2 we show a 3D printing based on cardiac computed tomography scans, of a patient who had a previously closed patent foramen ovale (PFO) with a bulky septal occluder (STARflex™, NMT Medical, Boston, MA, USA). The procedure was simulated with a demo model, to check if it was possible to cross the interatrial septum (IS) behind the septal device [9].

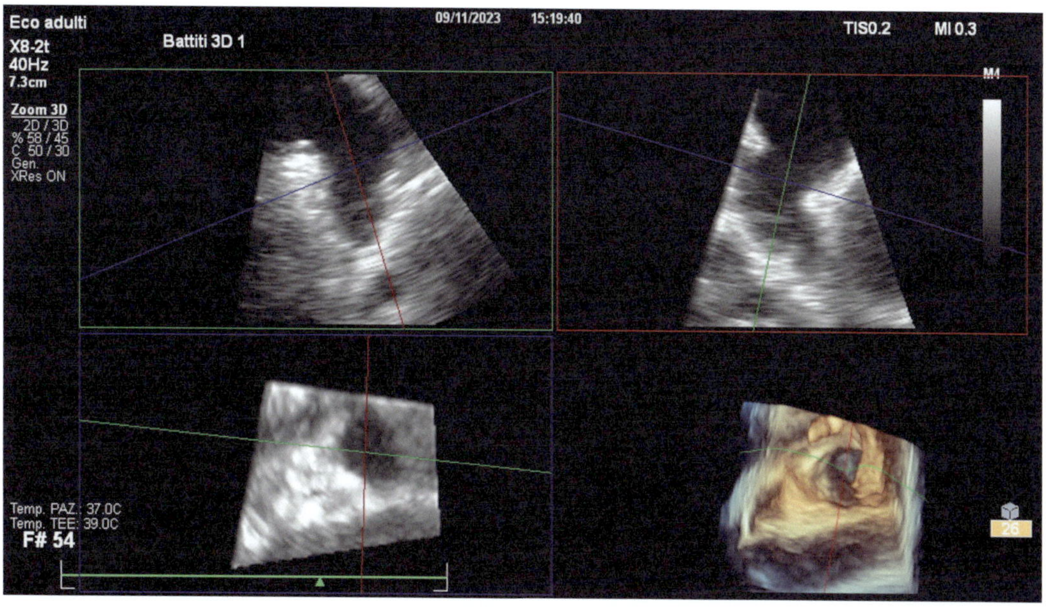

Fig. 15.1 Three-dimensional pre-procedural TOE imaging

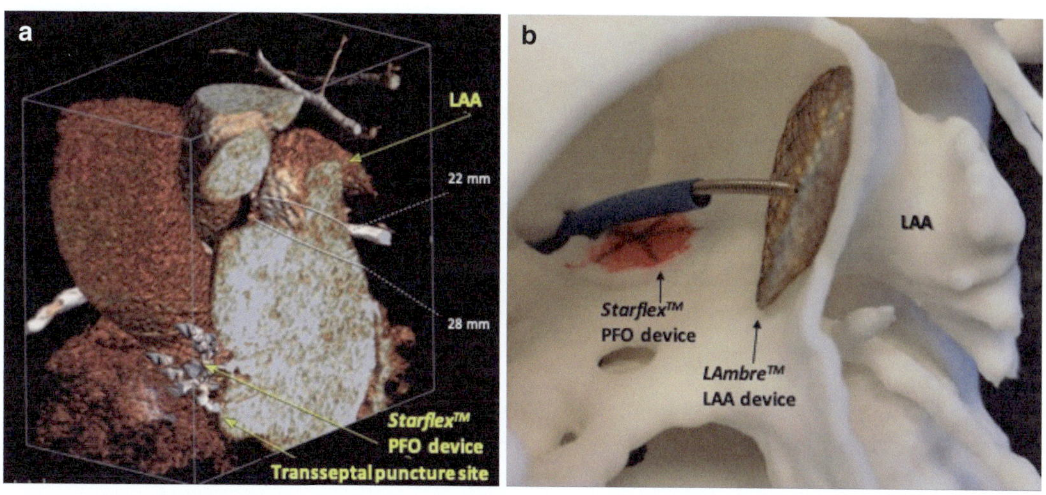

Fig. 15.2 (**a**) Cardiac CT. (**b**) Simulation of the procedure with the 3D model and a demo model of the selected device

15.3 Intraprocedural Aspects

15.3.1 Intraprocedural Imaging

Intraprocedural imaging guidance is strongly recommended for all LAAC procedures. This tool helps in every single step: guidance of transseptal puncture (TSP); evaluation of origin, morphology, and axis of LAA; presence of intra-appendage thrombi; visualization of device implantation, stability, compression, and peridevice leaks (PDLs); and monitoring for pericardial effusion. Fluoroscopy alone without imaging is not recommended and should be avoided [7]. TOE guidance with standardized views as described above has been the traditional intraprocedural imaging modality for LAAC. Intracardiac echocardiography (ICE) is an evolving imaging modality to guide LAAC [10, 11]. For LAAC procedural guidance, the ICE probe needs to be placed in the left atrium (LA). This can be performed through a separate transseptal puncture or through the same puncture used for LAAC device delivery sheath. ICE views (with probe in the LA in the retroflex, supramitral, and left upper pulmonary vein positions) that simulate standard TOE views may be achievable. Anyway, when using ICE, baseline pre-procedural imaging with cardiac CT or TOE is recommended to provide detailed information regarding LAA morphology.

Balancing pros and cons, TOE gives higher imaging definition and is familiar to most cardiologists but on the other side has some critical drawbacks. First, it often requires the logistic presence of an anaesthesiologist (although specific protocols have been developed to warrant deep sedation managed by the interventionist) and of an echocardiographer, while ICE probe is generally handled by the interventional cardiologist performing the procedure. Second, TOE needs general anaesthesia (with the above-described exception), which may be harmful for fragile patients, and endotracheal intubation may contribute to complications, such as injuries and bleeding of gastrooesophageal and respiratory tract, laryngospasm, and bronchospasm requiring additional intervention and prolonged hospitalization. Last, interference with fluoroscopy may represent a limit for TOE. On the opposite, ICE probe has higher expenses and a longer learning curve for the operators that needs to be considered. Alternatives to TOE in patients who cannot undergo general anaesthesia or have oropharyngeal abnormalities are ICE used via oesophageal route (ICE-TOE or "Contarini Technique") [12] or the microTOE system (S8–3t, Philips Healthcare). As a matter of fact, an ICE probe has an 8-F diameter (around 2.66 mm), the TOE probe a diameter of about 1.5 cm, while the head of the microTOE has a width, height, and length of 16 × 12 × 40 mm (Fig. 15.3). Small studies have demonstrated that during LAAC in adults, microTOE is feasible for procedural guidance. It offers comparable image quality with a much wider field of view than ICE and a slightly reduced but sufficient image quality and comparable accuracy as standard TEE [13]. Comparisons between TOE and microTOE images are shown in Fig. 15.4. For difficult procedures/anatomies or learning physicians, standard TOE guidance remains the preferred procedural imaging choice.

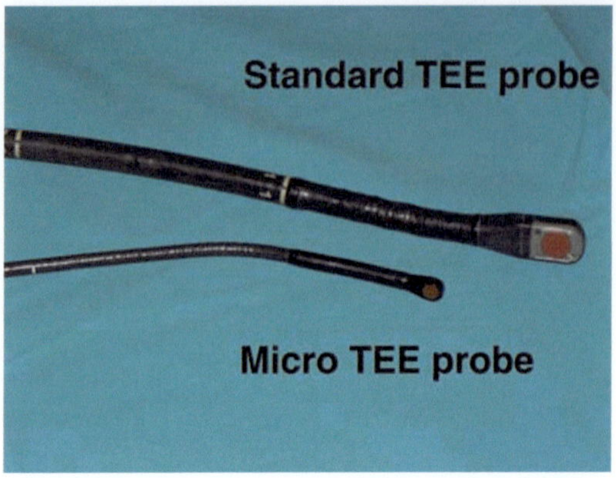

Fig. 15.3 Comparison between TOE and microTOE dimensions

15.3.2 Vascular Access Management and Pressure Monitoring

The LAAC procedure is generally performed through the right or left femoral vein. Ultrasound guidance can be helpful and is strongly recommended for vein cannulation and avoidance of bleeding complications. Intravenous antibiotic prophylaxis is administered once prior to the procedure, with the choice of antibiotic depending on the institutional preference and allergy history of the patient. At the end of the procedure, haemostasis can be achieved through manual compression, suture-mediated closure, or figure-of-8 suture, in accordance with operator comfort. Administration of protamine may be considered if haemostasis is not achieved. For procedures performed under general anaesthesia, it is also advisable to use two pressure transducer lines, one for continuous invasive arterial pressure monitoring (e.g. radial artery cannulation with a 5-F sheath) and the second to monitor the trans-

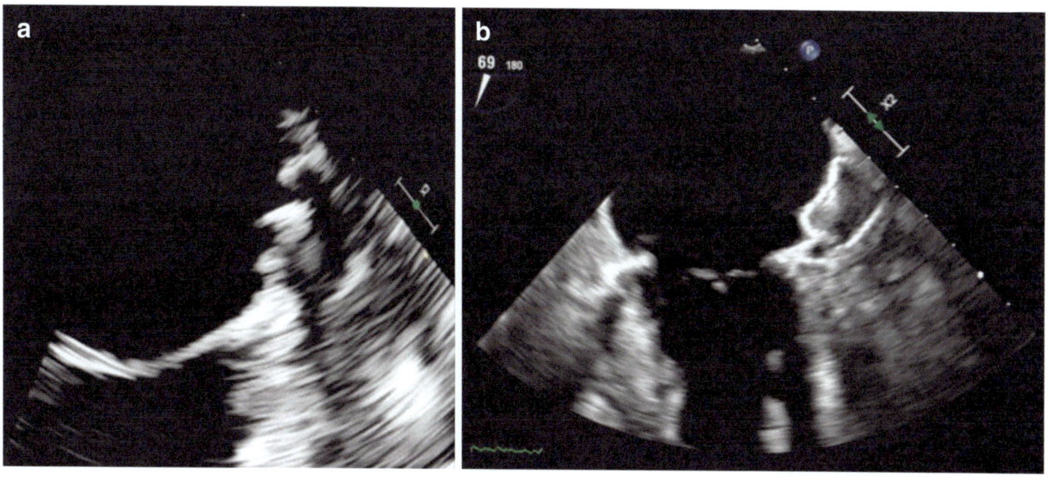

Fig. 15.4 Watchman implantation guided by microTOE (**a**) and TOE (**b**)

septal puncture (TSP) and determine LA pressure. A LA pressure >12 mmHg suggests a state of maximal filling of the LAA and ensures that maximal dimensions are obtained, avoiding underestimation of device size, which can lead to PDL or embolization [14].

15.3.3 Transseptal Puncture

For a successful TSP, it is important to start from anatomical considerations. The anatomic interatrial septum (IS) is the entire area interposed between the two atria and should be distinguished from the "true" IS, which is only the area that can be crossed without going into the extracardiac space: it accounts for only approximately 20% of the total septal area and anatomically corresponds to the fossa ovalis [15]. TSP can be in most cases performed with traditional transseptal systems composed by a sheath and a needle. The Brockenbrough (BRK) needle has an arrow-shaped proximal handle to define needle orientation and a stylet inside the lumen to prevent friction while advancing it into the sheath. The standard BRK needle (St. Jude Medical, St. Paul, MN, USA) has a 19° angle between the distal curved part and the needle shaft, whereas the BRK-1 (St. Jude Medical) is characterized by a 53° angle curvature. In adults with enlarged left atria, a condition usually encountered in patients with AF, the BRK-1 needle may be preferable, although the needle curve can be hand shaped. Several sheaths with a dilator protruding beyond the sheath tip can be used with BRK needles. Nowadays, the most common sheaths are the Mullins sheath and the Swartz™ Braided Superior Left (SL) (St. Jude Medical), both of which are available with different bores (8–12 Fr) and different curvatures according to atrial size. In general, SL sheaths are preferred because they have more pushability and torquability compared to the Mullins sheath and a curvature that points directly at the superior left pulmonary vein, whereas the Mullins sheath has an ideal curve to reach the mitral valve [16].

For TSP, we usually rely on fluoroscopic monitoring, echo monitoring and pressure monitoring. Once the fossa ovalis is engaged (we can follow "the fall" on both fluoroscopy and echocardiophy), tenting and puncture location should be confirmed by echocardiographic imaging (TOE/ICE/microTOE). X-plane imaging allows simultaneous visualization of both bicaval and mid-oesophageal short-axis views, to clarify inferior–superior and anterior–posterior orientation, respectively (Fig. 15.5). Most appendages are directed anteriorly and superiorly; therefore, an inferior–posterior puncture is desired in most cases. In more unusual LAAs that have a lateral or posterior orientation (e.g. reverse chicken-wing configuration), the puncture site may be better in the mid fossa to anterior, rather than posterior [17]. During TSP, we may

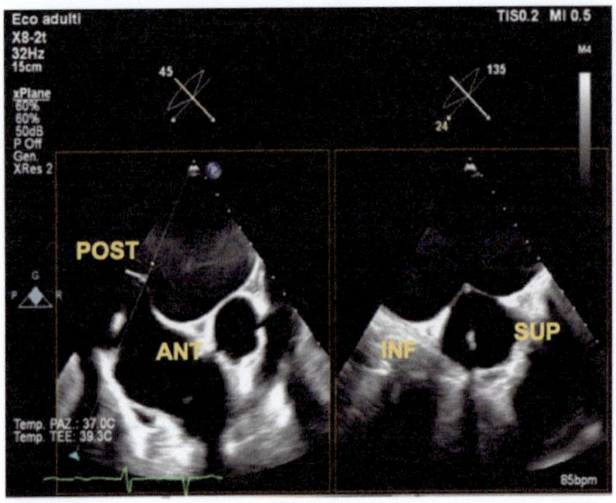

Fig. 15.5 X-plane of bicaval and short-axis views during tenting and transseptal puncture, to clarify inferior–superior and anterior–posterior orientation

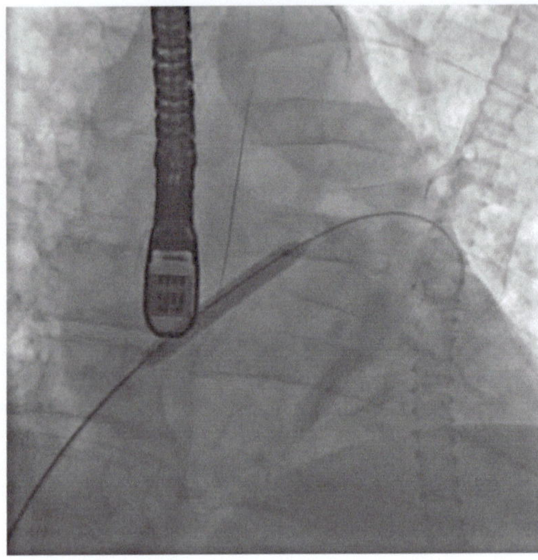

Fig. 15.6 Septal septostomy with a peripheral balloon for crossing a difficult hyper-elastic septum

encounter challenging septa/situations. In case of floppy/hypermobile or fibrotic septa, puncture may be difficult. In these cases, alternative solutions to augment the support and enhance puncture success are to advance through the BRK needle the stylet, the back-end of a 0.014-inch wire or a dedicated wire (e.g. SafeSept®; Pressure Products Medical Supplies, San Pedro, CA, USA). The use of energy is another option, either by a dedicated radiofrequency (RF) catheter (e.g. Baylis Medical, Burlington, MA, USA) or by touching the proximal end of the BRK needle with an electrosurgical knife. It is important to remember to administer heparin (80–100 units/kg) before or upon transseptal crossing for a target-activated clotting time (ACT) of >250 s. The timing of heparin administration varies according to the operator. Our strategy is to administer 2000 units of heparin at the beginning of the procedure, immediately after cannulation of femoral venous access, and the remaining dose after TSP. Regardless of strategy, it is of great importance to achieve a therapeutic ACT level as soon as possible after transseptal crossing because of the low flow state in the left atrium and thrombogenicity of the equipment (sheath, wires, and device).

15.3.4 LAA Engagement and Closure

The first step for a successful LAA engagement and closure is choosing the right delivery sheath. Commercially available devices come with the manufacturer's delivery sheath. They vary in width (from 10 to 14 F), and usually the fixed single or double curve shapes are sufficient to provide coaxial orientation with the LAA; otherwise there are also available steerable sheaths. Once TSP is completed, the delivery sheath is introduced into the left atrium (LA) by anchoring a stiff support wire in the left upper pulmonary vein. If difficulty is encountered introducing the device delivery sheath into the LA, one can predilate the atrial septum by performing atrial septostomy using a 5.0-mm or larger balloon (Fig. 15.6). Once in the LA, the delivery sheath should be carefully deaired and flushed. Recommendations for inexperienced operators are to advance the device delivery sheath into the LAA over a 5- to 6-F pigtail catheter; but when we have a good alignment between TSP and LAA axis and a good reliance on echo, we can skip this step and introduce, carefully, directly the delivery sheath into LAA. At this point, in patients without significant kidney disease and in whom the goal of LA pressure ≥12 mmHg is achieved, we perform at least two contrast cineangiography: right anterior oblique/caudal projection that approximately corresponds to 135° mid-oesophageal TEE view and right oblique/cranial that corresponds to 45° TEE view (Fig. 15.7). In this way we can compare TEE and fluoroscopic measures

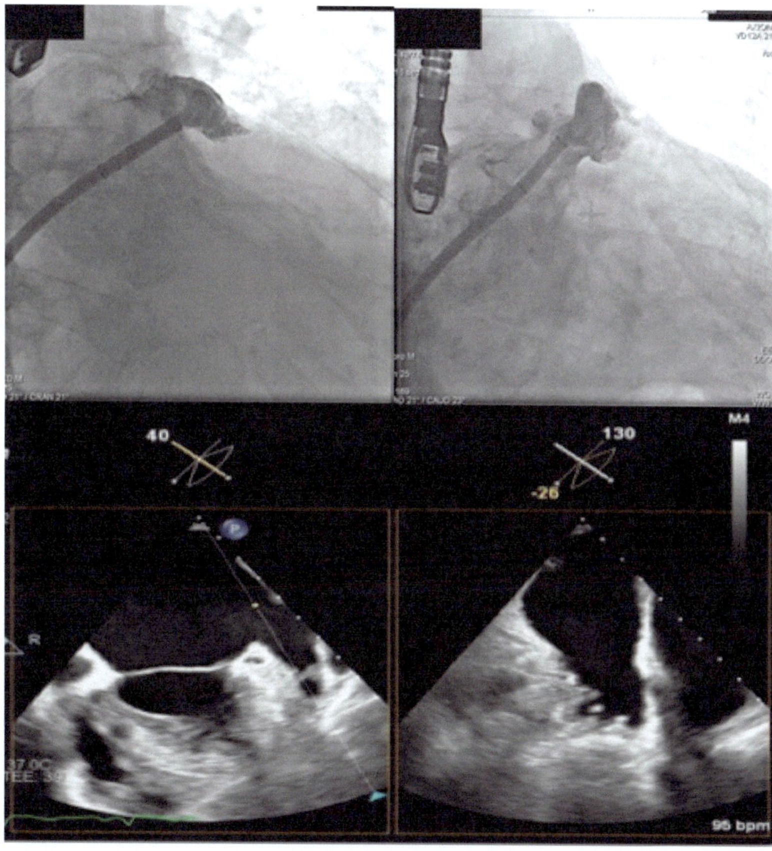

Fig. 15.7 Comparison between TOE and fluoroscopy. On the left a RAO cranial projection that corresponds to TOE short-axis view and on the right a RAO caudal that corresponds to 135° view

and avoid over or undersizing. In the case of patients with kidney disease, an ultrasound-only-guided procedure can be carried out without fluoroscopy and contrast dye use [18].

The device can then be released, according to manufacturer's instructions and operators should observe established criteria to ensure proper positioning before device release. Care should be taken to sizing, anchoring, positioning within the LAA, compression, and absence of significant PDLs.

15.4 Tips for a Satisfying LAAC: Not Just Close It *But Close It Well*

From a theoretical point of view, LAA can be grouped into four morphologies: windsock, chicken wing, cauliflower, and cactus. The practical reality, however, is completely different, and LAAs have such a variety of shapes, sizes, and directions that make it difficult to standardize them. Thus, when approaching this procedure, it is important to consider multiple parameters in order to optimize it. In addition to the morphology, it is also necessary to take into consideration: axis of the body of the LAA with respect to the ostium and to the TSP, depth of the main lobe, length of the Coumadin ridge, presence of proximal recess, calibre mismatch between ostium and landing zone, presence of bioprosthetic mitral valve, thrombosis, multilobed LAA, and allergies. Despite all the variables mentioned, most closures can be satisfactorily performed with any of the many devices commercially available, whether with or without disc, with some exceptions. In our opinion in fact, three are the main features that must lead us to choose a single lobe (e.g. Watchman) device: a prominent pulmonary (or Coumadin) ridge (PR), a low and close to the mitral valve LAA origin, and presence of mitral valve bio-

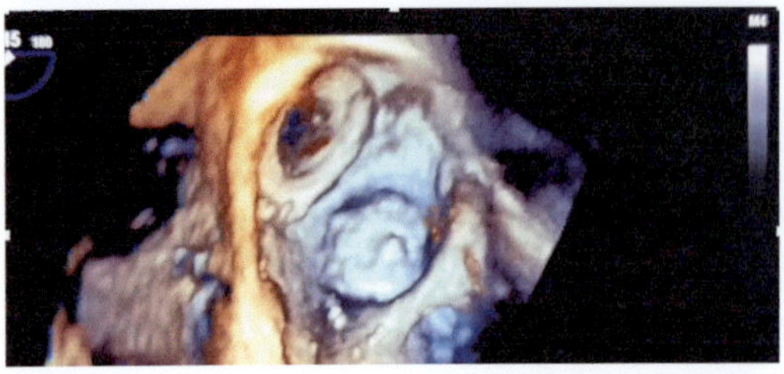

Fig. 15.8 In presence of mitral bioprosthesis is advisable to choose a device without disc in order to avoid interferences with the structure of the bio-prosthesis. In this case LAAC was performed with a Watchman device

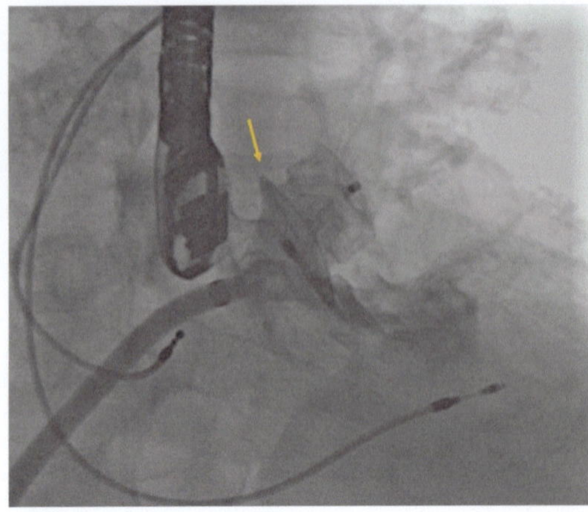

Fig. 15.9 LAA with a prominent pulmonary ridge closed with an Amulet device in a deep position, the arrow shows the point where the disc imprints LAA wall and can provoke late erosion

prosthesis (Fig. 15.8). In anatomies with long and prominent PR, it is desirable to avoid deep implants and devices with the disk. In case a pacifier is chosen, the disk should preferably be pulled over the edge of the ridge. Infact deep implants could favour DRT, and a disk prolapsed in the body of the LAA can lead to late wall erosion, a rare but already described complication. Areas of flow recirculation at low velocities could indicate potential regions at risk of thrombus formation, and their localization depends on the patient's LA anatomy and the LAAO device's final deployment. A study that analysed haemodynamic flow of LAA and LA combining cardiac CT and ultrasounds revealed the device upper region with an uncovered pulmonary ridge as the preferred area for eddies and flow stagnation [19]. This finding was consistent with the literature available on pulmonary ridge uncovering and a higher risk of DRT [20, 21]. According to this study, covering the pulmonary ridge, which is often not possible due to anatomical constraints, would only be critical if blood flow velocities are not high enough. In Fig. 15.9 we show a case of an appendage with a prominent pulmonary ridge closed with an Amulet device in a deep position, which can theoretically lead to a risk of late erosion by the disc, while in Fig. 15.10 a LAmbre device is recaptured and repositioned more proximally to optimize LAA sealing. Figure 15.11 shows a case of DRT after a deep implant at the 45-day TOE evaluation.

Features that instead favour two-element devices such as Amulet or LAmbre are short landing zone (as it is sometimes encountered in chicken-wing configuration), presence of proximal recess, calibre mismatch between the ostium and landing zone, and multilobed LAAs. In the last two situations, closure with special devices where lobe and disc have different dimensions is advisable (Fig. 15.12). The "sandwich technique" is used in chicken-wing LAA with short landing zone and consists in deploying the lobe deeper and in parallel with the wing segment, thereby "sandwiching" the too short landing zone and ostium between the lobe and the disc. Table 15.2 summarizes LAA features to consider for selection of the closure device.

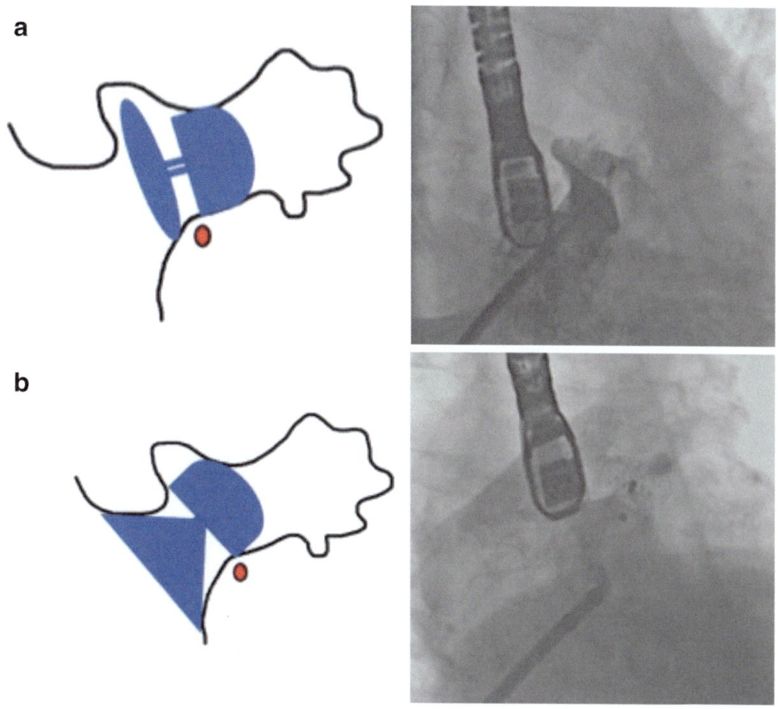

Fig. 15.10 (**a**) LAAO with the disc in the proximal recess. (**b**) Device pulled out to make the disc cover the proximal recess

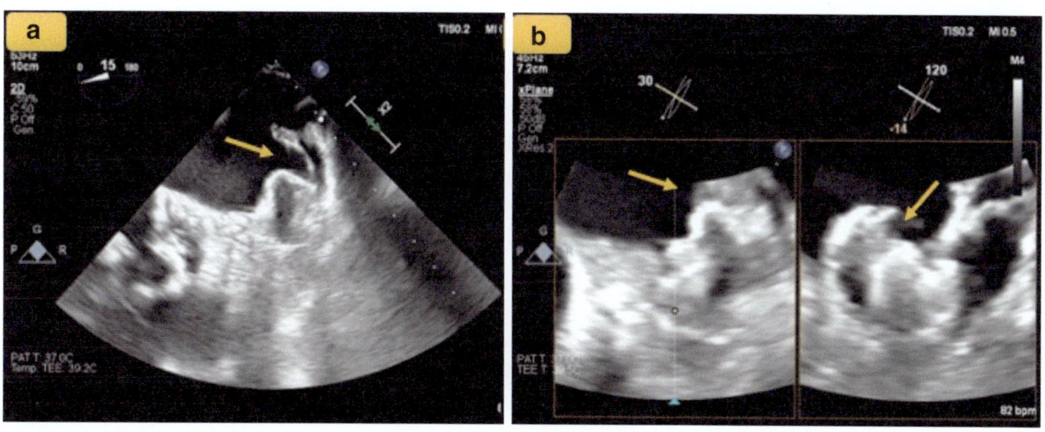

Fig. 15.11 (**a**) Deep implant with uncovered proximal recess. (**b**) DRT at 90-day follow-up (arrows)

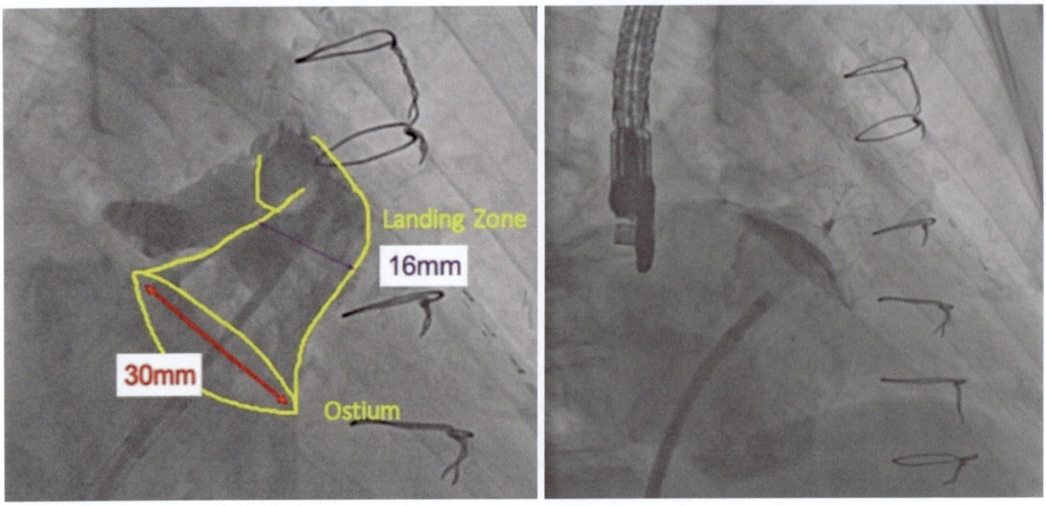

Fig. 15.12 Implantation of LAmbre special device 22–34 mm for a reverse chicken-wing LAA with calibre mismatch between ostium and landing zone

Table 15.2 Features to consider for selection of LAA closure device

	Type of device	
Features	Single lobe	Distal lobe + proximal disc
Prominent pulmonary ridge	+	–
Origin of LAA close to the mitral valve	+	–
Mitral valve bioprosthesis	+	–
Short landing zone (chicken-wing configuration)	–	+
Proximal recess	–	+
Calibre mismatch between ostium and landing zone	–	+
Multilobed	–	+
Thrombosis	+/–	+

15.5 Thrombotic Appendages

The management of patients with atrial fibrillation referred for LAAC who are found to have LAA thrombus is challenging. Previously the presence of left atrial thrombus was considered an absolute contraindication to LAAC, and patients with LAA thrombosis were excluded from randomized trials (e.g. the PROTECT AF trial [22]), but in the last years, data from case reports and case series have suggested the feasibility of LAAC in this context [23].

Thrombotic appendages are better closed with the "no-touch" technique than with standard deployment techniques. The no-touch technique involves the avoidance of either contrast injections or guidewire and catheter manipulation within the LAA. The procedure is totally echo-guided, the device is loaded with the delivery sheath in the left superior pulmonary vein, and then it is partially unsheathed into its atraumatic "ball" structure in the left atrium and in the end the device is completely opened while advancing in the LAA, sealing it. The procedure, therefore, is performed without engaging the LAA with the delivery sheath and is feasible with devices with and without disc [24].

Embolic protection devices (EPDs) can be used at the operator's discretion but are highly recommendable in case of thrombus.

So far, published experience with cerebral protection devices (CPDs) in LAAO is limited [25, 26]. They vary in the mechanism for protection, access site and delivery sheath size, and provide a partial or complete supra-aortic trunk

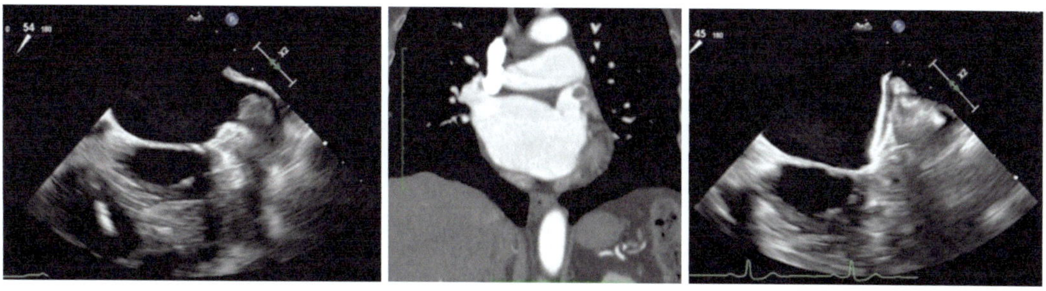

Fig. 15.13 On the left a huge thrombotic formation protruding in LAA ostium; in the centre pre-procedural CT reconstruction; on the right LAA closure procedure

coverage. Among them the most established system is the Sentinel Cerebral Protection Device (Boston Scientific, Marlborough, MA), which is a capture device consisting of two filter baskets within a single 6-F delivery catheter placed percutaneously from the right radial artery over a 0.014-in. guidewire. The filters are positioned in the brachiocephalic and the left common carotid arteries before the intervention and are removed afterwards; the left subclavian artery is left unprotected [27]. The second most studied device is the TriGuard 3 system (Venus Medtech, Inc.). This device covers all three supra-aortic vessels with an over-the-wire design via an 8-F femoral sheath [27]. CPDs are successful in preventing dreadful complications like embolic stroke; anyway embolic events can occur despite the use of these devices, as these filters do not prevent embolization in coronary, renal, mesenteric, and femoral arteries. Since non-cerebral embolization may be easier to manage percutaneously or surgically and the need of further extra-arterial vascular accesses and the prolonged procedure duration may increase periprocedural adverse events in such a fragile and complex patient population, non-cerebral EPDs are not routinely used. In Fig. 15.13 we show a case of a huge thrombus protruding in the neck of the LAA. In this case where embolization was likely, three embolic protection devices were placed in the right coronary artery (RCA), supra-aortic trunks, and superior mesenteric artery. LAA was closed with a pacifier device and a "touch & push" technique, which consists in opening the device while advancing inside the LAA, pushing down the thrombus, and closing the LAA orifice with the disk.

15.6 Detection of Complications

For a safe LAAC procedure, all the implanters must be skilled in the recognition and treatment of procedural complications and be attentive to the details necessary to prevent such events. Contemporary clinical data suggest that serious complication rates and pericardial effusions/tamponade have dropped significantly since the first trials (e.g. PROTECT-AF [22]) and now are well <2%. We can divide complications in periprocedural complications and late complications. Periprocedural complications are death (<0.2%), stroke (<0.2%), systemic embolism (rare), pericardial tamponade (~1%), device embolization (~0.2%), and vascular complications [7]. Between late complications we must recognize late pericardial effusion/tamponade (~1%), peridevice leak, device-related thrombosis (3–5%), late device migration/embolization (infrequent), device erosion (rare), and iatrogenic atrial septal defects (rare to require intervention) [7]. PDLs are believed to be significant if >5 mm. For small leaks (<5 mm), data suggest that they can be associated with a slightly higher rate of stroke, TIA, and systemic embolism over 1 year [28, 29], but their treatment is not well established; instead for PDLs >5 mm current practice is generally to continue OAC. Case reports and small case series have demonstrated the feasibility of closing leaks using interventional approaches including placement of occlusion or plug devices or coiling, but stronger data are still lacking.

15.7 Post-procedural Aspects

Performing transthoracic echocardiography (TTE) prior to discharge to exclude pericardial effusion or device embolization is recommended. In the follow-up TOE or cardiac CT, preferably using the same pre-procedural imaging is recommended at 45–90 days after LAAC for device surveillance and to assess for PDL and DRT; in fact the majority of DRT (64%) is diagnosed ≤180 days following procedural implant [21].

Post-procedural antithrombotic therapy will be discussed elsewhere and is highly variable and tailored on patients' characteristics and indication to LAAC.

References

1. Go AS, Hylek EM, Phillips KA, Chang Y, Henault LE, Selby JV, et al. Prevalence of diagnosed atrial fibrillation in adults: national implications for rhythm management and stroke prevention: the AnTicoagulation and Risk Factors In Atrial Fibrillation (ATRIA) Study. JAMA. 2001;285(18):2370–5.
2. Wolf PA, Dawber TR, Emerson Thomas H Jr, Kannel WB. Epidemiologic assessment of chronic atrial fibrillation and risk of stroke. Neurology. 1978;28(10):973.
3. Alkhouli M, Friedman PA. Ischemic stroke risk in patients with nonvalvular atrial fibrillation: JACC review topic of the week. J Am Coll Cardiol. 2019;74(24):3050–65.
4. Johnson WD, Ganjoo AK, Stone CD, Srivyas RC, Howard M. The left atrial appendage: our most lethal human attachment! Surgical implications. Eur J Cardiothorac Surg. 2000;17(6):718–22.
5. Martinez C, Katholing A, Wallenhorst C, Freedman SB. Therapy persistence in newly diagnosed non-valvular atrial fibrillation treated with warfarin or NOAC. Thromb Haemost. 2016;115(01):31–9.
6. Franchin L, Piroli F, Demola P, Mantovani F, Iannaccone M, Manfredi R, et al. Efficacy and safety of left atrial appendage closure compared with oral anticoagulation in atrial fibrillation: a meta-analysis of randomized controlled trials and propensity-matched studies. Front Cardiovasc Med. 2023;10:1212161.
7. Saw J, Holmes DR, Cavalcante JL, Freeman JV, Goldsweig AM, Kavinsky CJ, et al. SCAI/HRS expert consensus statement on transcatheter left atrial appendage closure. J Soc Cardiovasc Angiogr Interv. 2023;2(3):100577.
8. Wang DD, Forbes TJ, Lee JC, Eng MH. Echocardiographic imaging for left atrial appendage occlusion: transesophageal echocardiography and intracardiac echocardiographic imaging. Interv Cardiol Clin. 2018;7(2):219–28.
9. Matta M, Maltese L, Ugo F, Di Ruocco MV, Rametta F. Feasibility and safety of left atrial appendage closure in a patient with previous foramen ovale occlusion: a case report. Eur Heart J Case Rep. 2021;5(3):ytab113.
10. Alkhouli M, Chaker Z, Alqahtani F, Raslan S, Raybuck B. Outcomes of routine intracardiac echocardiography to guide left atrial appendage occlusion. JACC Clin Electrophysiol. 2020;6(4):393–400.
11. Berti S, Pastormerlo LE, Santoro G, Brscic E, Montorfano M, Vignali L, et al. Intracardiac versus transesophageal echocardiographic guidance for left atrial appendage occlusion: the LAAO Italian Multicenter Registry. JACC Cardiovasc Interv. 2018;11(11):1086–92.
12. Laterra G, Artale C, Sacchetta G, Contarini M. Intracardiac echocardiography probe via oesophageal to guide percutaneous left atrial appendage closure procedure: a case series. Eur Heart J Case Rep. 2023;7(6):ytad261.
13. Nijenhuis VJ, Alipour A, Wunderlich NC, Rensing BJWM, Gijsbers G, Ten Berg JM, et al. Feasibility of multiplane microtransoesophageal echocardiographic guidance in structural heart disease transcatheter interventions in adults. Neth Heart J. 2017;25(12):669–74.
14. Glikson M, Wolff R, Hindricks G, Mandrola J, Camm JA, Lip YHG, et al. EHRA/EAPCI expert consensus statement on catheter-based left atrial appendage occlusion—an update. EuroIntervention. 2020;15(13):1133.
15. Almendarez M, Alvarez-Velasco R, Pascual I, Alperi A, Moris C, Avanzas P. Transseptal puncture: review of anatomy, techniques, complications and challenges, a critical view. Int J Cardiol. 2022;351:32–8.
16. Russo G, Taramasso M, Maisano F. Transseptal puncture: procedural guidance, challenging situations and management of complications. EuroIntervention. 2021;17(9):720–7.
17. Fukutomi M, Fuchs A, Bieliauskas G, Wong I, Kofoed FG, Søndergaard L, et al. Computed tomography-based selection of transseptal puncture site for percutaneous left atrial appendage closure. EuroIntervention. 2022;17(17):e1435–44.
18. Abdirashid M, Ugo F, Matta M, Cavallino C, Maltese L, Reale D, et al. LAA closure in pre-dialytic and dialytic patients: a case report and mini review of literature. Nephrol Renal Dis. 2021;6:1–3.
19. Mill J, Agudelo V, Li CH, Noailly J, Freixa X, Camara O, et al. Patient-specific flow simulation analysis to predict device-related thrombosis in left atrial appendage occluders. REC Interv Cardiol. 2021;3:278–85.
20. Freixa X, Cepas-Guillén P, Flores-Umanzor E, Regueiro A, Sanchis L, Fernandez-Valledor A, et al. Pulmonary ridge coverage and device-related

thrombosis after left atrial appendage occlusion. EuroIntervention. 2021;16(15):e1288–94.
21. Simard T, Jung RG, Lehenbauer K, Piayda K, Pracoń R, Jackson GG, et al. Predictors of device-related thrombus following percutaneous left atrial appendage occlusion. J Am Coll Cardiol. 2021;78(4):297–313.
22. Reddy VY, Holmes D, Doshi SK, Neuzil P, Kar S. Safety of percutaneous left atrial appendage closure: results from the Watchman Left Atrial Appendage System for Embolic Protection in Patients with AF (PROTECT AF) clinical trial and the Continued Access Registry. Circulation. 2011;123(4):417–24.
23. Sharma SP, Cheng J, Turagam MK, Gopinathannair R, Horton R, Lam YY, et al. Feasibility of left atrial appendage occlusion in left atrial appendage thrombus: a systematic review. JACC Clin Electrophysiol. 2020;6(4):414–24.
24. Jalal Z, Iriart X, Dinet ML, Selly JB, Tafer N, Renou P, et al. Extending percutaneous left atrial appendage closure indications using the AMPLATZER™ Cardiac Plug device in patients with persistent left atrial appendage thrombus: the thrombus trapping technique. Arch Cardiovasc Dis. 2016;109(12):659–66.
25. Boccuzzi GG, Montabone A, D'Ascenzo F, Colombo F, Ugo F, Muraglia S, et al. Cerebral protection in left atrial appendage closure in the presence of appendage thrombosis. Catheter Cardiovasc Interv. 2021;97(3):511–5.
26. Tarantini G, D'Amico G, Latib A, Montorfano M, Mazzone P, Fassini G, et al. Percutaneous left atrial appendage occlusion in patients with atrial fibrillation and left appendage thrombus: feasibility, safety and clinical efficacy. EuroIntervention. 2018;13(13):1595–602.
27. Haussig S, Linke A, Mangner N. Cerebral protection devices during transcatheter interventions: indications, benefits, and limitations. Curr Cardiol Rep. 2020;22(9):96.
28. Alkhouli M, Du C, Killu A, Simard T, Noseworthy PA, Friedman PA, et al. Clinical impact of residual leaks following left atrial appendage occlusion: insights from the NCDR LAAO Registry. JACC Clin Electrophysiol. 2022;8(6):766–78.
29. Lazar L, Sanchez-Jimenez EF, Cortese B. Efficacy and safety of a dedicated left atrial appendage occlusion protocol. Cardiovasc Revasc Med. 2022;42:64–6.

Transradial Balloon Aortic Valvuloplasty

16

Carlo Tumscitz, Paolo Cataldo, and Matteo Tebaldi

16.1 Introduction

The combination of an aging population and earlier diagnosis has led to an increased number of patients with aortic stenosis, especially frail ones. In addition, with increasing survival, the likelihood of developing multiple comorbidities, including chronic kidney disease, heart failure, peripheral artery disease, anemia, coronary artery disease, and atrial fibrillation, increases [1, 2].

The high prevalence of comorbidities, higher frailty score, low BMI, concurrent use of anticoagulant, and antiplatelet medications are predictors of vascular and bleeding complications during interventional procedures [3].

Balloon aortic valvuloplasty (BAV) offers a simple therapeutic option for addressing severe aortic stenosis, alleviating symptoms by mechanically widening the constricted valve using an inflated balloon. Originally pioneered by Alain Cribier in 1985, BAV predates the introduction of transcatheter aortic valve implantation (TAVI) by nearly two decades [4].

While historically performed primarily via the common femoral artery with a greater than 10 French (Fr) vascular access, alternative approaches such as antegrade through the femoral vein or trans-septal routes have been explored but remain less common due to their increased complexity.

Despite the very high mid-term risk of restenosis, the procedure still represents a valuable tool for the management of aortic stenosis. Currently, clinical guidelines reserve BAV for hemodynamically unstable patients or those needing urgent noncardiac surgery [5]. Nevertheless, BAV offers significant short-term symptomatic relief with reduced procedural complexity compared to TAVI or surgical valve replacement. This makes it a valuable option for improving the health status of patients undergoing TAVI or surgical aortic valve replacement (SAVR), particularly when futility risks are significant. Consequently, despite the recent exponential rise in TAVI procedures, there has been an unexpected rise in BAV use [6]. Importantly, for patients deemed unsuitable for TAVI due to futility concerns, BAV can deliver a substantial enhancement in the quality of life.

Simplifying the BAV technique to mitigate vascular complications compared to conventional methods can enhance its use, especially among patients at high risk of bleeding. Traditionally reliant on large-bore femoral access, newer approaches such as radial BAV have emerged, offering a short learning curve and enhanced fea-

C. Tumscitz (✉)
Cardiology Unit, Azienda Ospedaliero-Universitaria di Cona, Ferrara, Italy

P. Cataldo · M. Tebaldi
Cardiology Unit, "Degli Infermi" Hospital, Faenza, Italy
e-mail: tblmtt@unife.it

B. Cortese, S. Rigattieri (eds.), *High Bleeding Risk Patients in Interventional Cardiology*,
https://doi.org/10.1007/978-3-031-87302-7_16

sibility. Advances in balloon technology have further widened the applicability of radial BAV; indeed, distal radial BAV has demonstrated comparable success rates and efficacy as compared to conventional radial BAV while potentially reducing the incidence of radial artery occlusion, a crucial consideration for patients requiring future transcatheter interventions.

16.2 How to Perform Radial BAV

A practical, step-by-step guide is provided for conducting radial or distal radial access balloon aortic valvuloplasty (rBAV or drBAV), highlighting its potential advantages in mitigating bleeding risk. The use of radial access brings several of advantages such as faster hemostasis, reduced nursing staff time, increased comfort and ergonomics for both the patient and the operator, and, in case of drBAV, preservation of the proximal forearm's radial segment for future intervention and possibly lower radiation doses due to arm positioning on the pelvis. Materials required closely resemble those for traditional femoral BAV, with some variations based on operator preference.

A. *Radial or Distal Radial Access*: Obtain distal radial access in both arms using a 5- or 6-Fr sheath. Heparin administration precedes the procedure to minimize clotting risks, with attention given to extremely obese patients who may require adjusted dosages. While single radial access BAV is feasible, limitations exist, underscoring the importance of considering alternative access if necessary.
B. *Aortic Valve Crossing*: Various catheters can facilitate aortic valve crossing from radial access points, with careful attention to pressure monitoring and gradient calculations. Utilizing appropriate catheters enhances procedural efficiency and accuracy (Figs. 16.1 and 16.2).
C. *Large Sheath Insertion*: Transitioning from 6 Fr to larger sheath sizes compatible with chosen balloons requires precision to minimize discomfort and complications. Low-profile balloons recently allow to deliver a 20-mm balloon through a 8-Fr sheath, allowing good efficacy in a wide population and reducing severe complications and safer outcomes (Table 16.1 and Fig. 16.3).
D. *Aortic Valve Dilation*: Preparation and inflation of the dilation balloon catheter demand meticulous air removal to avoid embolism in case of rupture. Rapid pacing is often

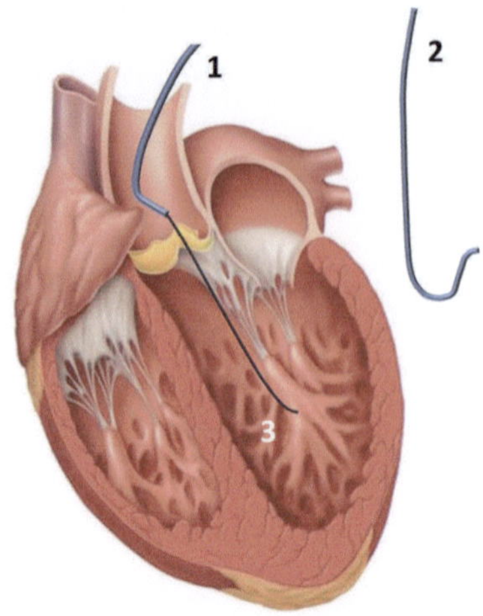

Fig. 16.1 Aortic valve crossing (1) JR catheters are the first choice because they better orientate toward aortic valve from right radial. (2) Alternatively, an AL catheter can be used. (3) A 0.035″ straight wire is used to cross the aortic valve

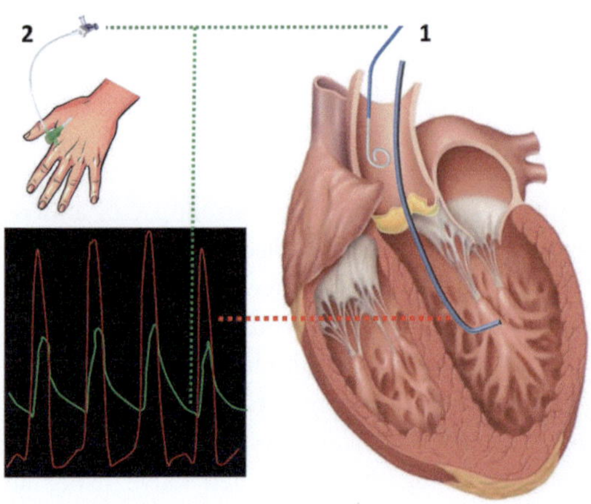

Fig. 16.2 Gradients calculation. (1) Aortic pressure can be measured at the ascending aorta with a catheter advanced through the contralateral access. (2) Pressure monitoring through contralateral radial sheath's side port has the same accuracy

Table 16.1 Sheath compatibility for balloon dilations catheters commonly used in radial balloon aortic valvuloplasty

	8 Fr (mm)	9 Fr (mm)	10 Fr (mm)
Cristal (Balt, France)	18–22	23	25
VACSII (Osypka, Germany)	18–20–22	24	–
Valver (Balton, Poland)	18–20	23	25
ThyshakII (NuMed, United States)	18–20–22	23–24–25	–

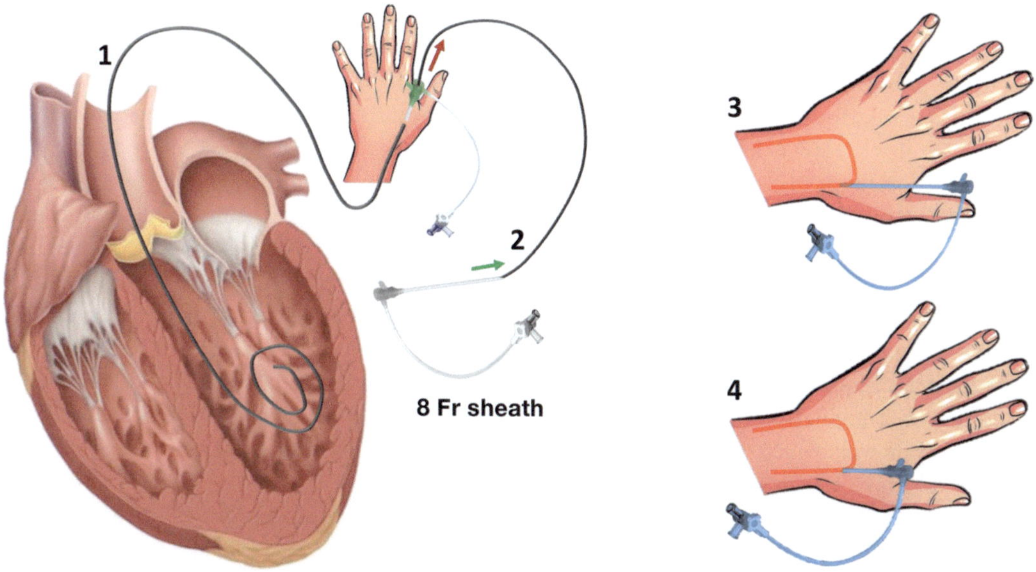

Fig. 16.3 Large sheath insertion. (1) An extra stiff 0.035″ wire is advanced to the left ventricle. (2) Once the stiff wire is in the left ventricle, the 5- to 6-Fr radial sheath is exchanged for an 8-Fr sheath. (3) Regular 11-cm-long sheath. (4) 5.5-cm sheath

used for stabilization during inflations. Alternatively, central vein access for pacing can be avoided by using a wire connected to the stiff wire in the left ventricle and the subcutaneous tissue through a small needle (Fig. 16.4).

E. *Balloon Retrieval*: Careful balloon aspiration after dilatation reduces the risk of balloon entrapment allowing better crossing profile. Collaboration between two operators performing the push-and-pull maneuver maintains wire position and facilitates fester withdrawal, minimizing patient discomfort.

F. *Hemostasis*: Achieving effective hemostasis is crucial, particularly in mitigating the risk of radial artery occlusion. While closure devices are optional, meticulous attention to hemostasis ensures favorable patient outcomes.

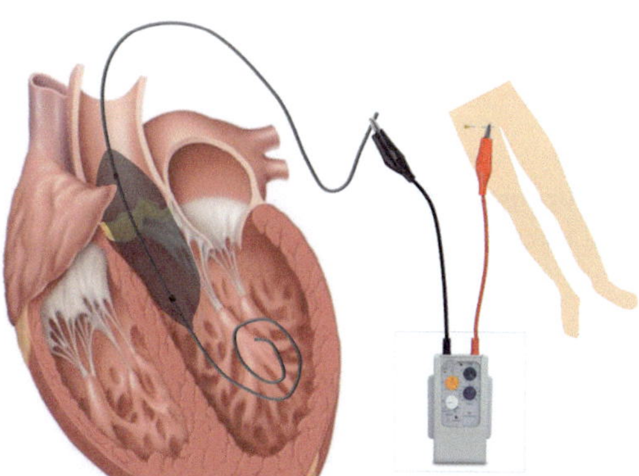

Fig. 16.4 Aortic valve dilation. Pacing through the 0.035″ wire reduces the risk of perforation and simplifies the technique. It consists of an alligator clip style cable with one end (anode + red) connected to the subcutaneous tissue through a small needle, and the other end (cathode, black) connected to the 0.035″ wire a few centimeters proximal to the balloon catheter end

16.3 Special Consideration and Complications

Challenges can arise, especially in elderly patients, particularly due to vessel tortuosity. Using double radial access permits a shift to contralateral radial access avoiding femoral puncture in most cases. Nevertheless, crossover to femoral access occurs in 5% of instances and can be caused by a bilateral tortuosity, impossibility to obtain any access from two arms, and vessel calcifications that prevent balloon advancement (such as Monckeberg disease).

Special attention must be taken during balloon withdrawal when the "push-and-pull" maneuver should be performed by two operators, and additional sedation may be required. In the case of balloon rupture during radial BAV, especially if the burst caused a circular cut of the balloon surface, there is a high risk of balloon entrapment during withdrawal, which necessitates surgical removal (Fig. 16.5). This rare event occurred in only one case (0.3%) of the largest multicenter prospective study [7]. The same study reported one case (0.3%) of subclavian dissection, which was treated conservatively and had no clinical sequelae. Other problems included a forearm hematoma (0.9%). As a result, any ruptures that occur during inflation require special attention.

Temporary hypotension and bradycardia may be a result of a vagal response, but persistent hypotension requires prompt assessment. Different causes, such as acute severe aortic insufficiency, pump failure due to worsened systolic function, cardiac tamponade, aortic annular rupture, coronary occlusion or dissection, and rhythm disturbances, should be excluded or promptly treated.

16.4 Discussion

The widely adopted practice, refined by the introduction of TAVI, of echo-guided puncture, coupled with the use of smaller vascular sheaths, lower-profile balloons, and vascular closure devices, has reduced access site complications compared to the early cases of BAV. However, vascular complications still remain the most frequent drawback of transcatheter procedures for aortic stenosis [8].

In recent years, radial balloon aortic valvuloplasty (rBAV or drBAV) has emerged as a promising approach in the management of severe aortic stenosis, demonstrating safety and efficacy profiles. Radial access, after initial training, is relatively straightforward to perform. It does not require dedicated closure devices, and if complications arise, they are generally less severe compared to those associated with femoral access like noncompressible bleeding events (particularly retroperitoneal bleeding) or the risk of developing pseudoaneurysm. Additionally, it enhances patient comfort post-procedure, promoting early ambulation.

Current literature highlights the applicability of radial BAV across various patients, with a particular emphasis on its safety in the elderly population. Studies addressing the elderly cohort

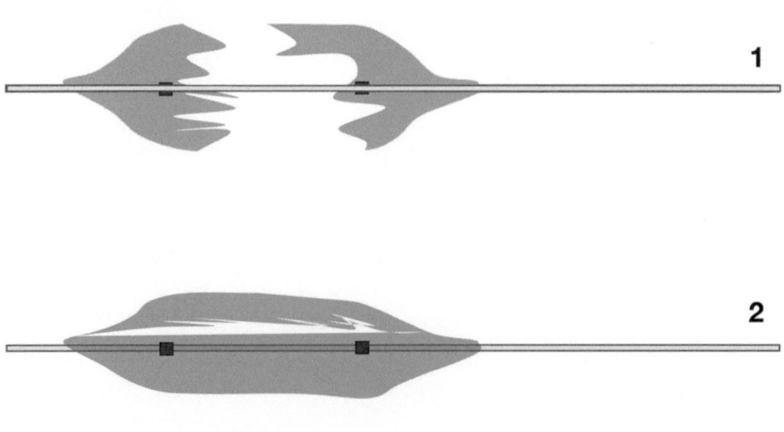

Fig. 16.5 Balloon rupture. (1) Transverse rupture: high risk of balloon entrapment (2) Longitudinal rupture: low risk of balloon entrapment

consistently report favorable outcomes, attesting to the procedure's feasibility and efficacy.

Data from the SOFTLY II [7], a multicenter Italian prospective registry that included 330 patients undergoing radial BAV, show excellent results in terms of success rate. In the elderly population, BAV was also associated with a significant improvement in frailty, as measured by three different scales. The results from SOFTLY II were also verified in a single-center retrospective study from Argentina [9], which included 24 younger patients, showing a success rate of 91% (defined as invasive peak gradient reduction of at least 30%). Another study, the DR-BAV, explored the efficacy of mini distal radial balloon aortic valvuloplasty, showing good technical, hemodynamic, and clinical success matched with no major complication and bleeding. Furthermore, at the echocardiographic follow-up, the radial artery was patent in 94% of the patients [10].

Summarizing this evidence, radial BAV or distal radial BAV may be beneficial in different settings such as:

- Multimorbid patients, as a bridge to decision, mitigating the risk of bleeding while improving functional status
- Patients suitable for TAVI or SAVR, particularly when futility risks are significant
- Patients who need noncardiac surgery prioritizing the best treatment
- Palliation in patients excluded from intervention

Further studies with a randomized, multicenter design will hopefully confirm this hypothesis in a larger population.

References

1. Osnabrugge RLJ, Mylotte D, Head SJ, Van Mieghem NM, Nkomo VT, LeReun CM, Bogers AJJC, Piazza N, Kappetein AP. Aortic stenosis in the elderly: disease prevalence and number of candidates for transcatheter aortic valve replacement: a meta-analysis and modeling study. J Am Coll Cardiol. 2013;62:1002–12.
2. Divo MJ, Martinez CH, Mannino DM. Ageing and the epidemiology of multimorbidity. Eur Respir J. 2014;44:1055–68.
3. Van Mieghem NM, Tchetche D, Chieffo A, et al. Incidence, predictors, and implications of access site complications with transfemoral transcatheter aortic valve implantation. Am J Cardiol. 2012;110:1361–7.
4. Cribier A, Savin T, Saoudi N, Rocha P, Berland J, Letac B. Percutaneous transluminal valvuloplasty of acquired aortic stenosis in elderly patients: an alternative to valve replacement? Lancet. 1986;1:63–7.
5. Otto CM, Nishimura RA, Bonow RO, et al. 2020 ACC/AHA guideline for the management of patients with valvular heart disease: executive summary: a report of the American College of Cardiology/American Heart Association Joint Committee on Clinical Practice Guidelines. Circulation. 2021;143:e35–71.
6. Alkhouli M, Zack CJ, Sarraf M, et al. Morbidity and mortality associated with balloon aortic valvuloplasty: a national perspective. Circ Cardiovasc Interv. 2017;10:e004481.
7. Tumscitz C, Di Cesare A, Balducelli M, et al. Safety, efficacy and impact on frailty of mini-invasive radial balloon aortic valvuloplasty. Heart. 2021;107:874–80.
8. Eltchaninoff H, Durand E, Borz B, et al. Balloon aortic valvuloplasty in the era of transcatheter aortic valve replacement: acute and long-term outcomes. Am Heart J. 2014;167:235–40.
9. Medina DE, Chazal HA, Seropian IM, Romeo F, Chiabrando JG, Valle Raleigh J, Berrocal DH, Agatiello CR. Balloon aortic valvuloplasty through the novel transradial technique. Minerva Cardiol Angiol. 2021;69:458–63.
10. Achim A, Szűcsborus T, Sasi V, Nagy F, Jambrik Z, Nemes A, Varga A, Homorodean C, Bertrand OF, Ruzsa Z. Safety and feasibility of distal radial balloon aortic valvuloplasty: the DR-BAV study. JACC Cardiovasc Interv. 2022;15:679–81.

17 Minimalistic TAVI Setup in High Bleeding Risk Patients

Myriam Akodad, Matteo Casenghi,
and Thierry Lefèvre

"Simplification is the ultimate sophistication."

–Leonardo Da Vinci

Abbreviations

GA	General anaesthesia
HBR	High bleeding risk
MSCT	Multi-slice computational tomography
TAVI	Transcatheter aortic valve Implantation
THV	Transcatheter heart valve
TOE	Transoesophageal echocardiography
VR	Virtual reality

17.1 Introduction

Although TAVI indications have recently been extended to include lower-risk patients, the vast majority of patients currently undergoing TAVI are elderly patients with significant comorbidities [1]. Indeed, around 20–25% of TAVI patients have associated atrial fibrillation and chronic kidney disease (Table 17.1), placing them at HBR [2, 3]. The initial idea of Professor Cribier when developing TAVI was to be able to offer an interventional cardiology procedure for patients who could not undergo conventional surgery. Thus, the first-in-human procedure was performed successfully in April 2002, in the catheterization laboratory, under conscious sedation in a highly comorbid patient with cardiogenic shock [4]. Moreover, considering the high bleeding and vascular complications risks associated with the main access inserted throughout an arterial access, the first procedure was performed via the femoral vein using a transseptal access.

Since the last two decades, TAVI procedure was dramatically simplified from the procedural planning to the procedure itself as well as the hospital pathway with early discharge (Fig. 17.1). Simplification was allowed by increased operators' experience, lower profile sheaths, improved devices and very active research leading to a drastic reduction in complications [5, 6]. Nowadays, the routine TAVI procedure is performed in the catheterization laboratory and includes conscious sedation, ultrasound-guided percutaneous femoral arterial access, secondary radial access, direct THV implantation, pacing on the left ventricle wire, low volume of contrast

M. Akodad · T. Lefèvre (✉)
Institut Cardiovasculaire Paris Sud, Hôpital Privé Jacques Cartier, Ramsay Santé, Massy, France
e-mail: t.lefevre@icps.com.fr

M. Casenghi
Department of Cardiology, Sant'Andrea Hospital, Sapienza University of Rome, Rome, Italy

B. Cortese, S. Rigattieri (eds.), *High Bleeding Risk Patients in Interventional Cardiology*,
https://doi.org/10.1007/978-3-031-87302-7_17

Table 17.1 Evolution of the TAVI population

Surgical risk	High	Intermediate	Low
Valve used	*Sapien*	*Sapien XT/Corevalve-Evolut R*	*Sapien 3/Corevalve-Evolut R-Pro*
Pacemaker implantation	3.8%	8.5/25.9%	6.6/17.4%
Atrial fibrillation	8.6%	9.1/12.9%	5.0/7.7%
Vascular complications	11%	7.9/6.0%	2.2/3.8%
Disabling stroke	3.8%	3.2/1.2%	0/0.5%
Mortality	6.6%	3.9/2.2%	0.4/0.5%
Aortic regurgitation > grade 2	12.2%	3.7/3.5%	0.8/4.3%
Acute kidney injury	4.1%	1.3/1.7%	0.4/0.9%
Reiintervention	4.6%	0.4/0.9%	0/0.4%
Major bleedings	9.3%	10.4/12.2%	3.6/2.4%
Coronary occlusion	NK	0.4/0.2%	0.2/0.9%

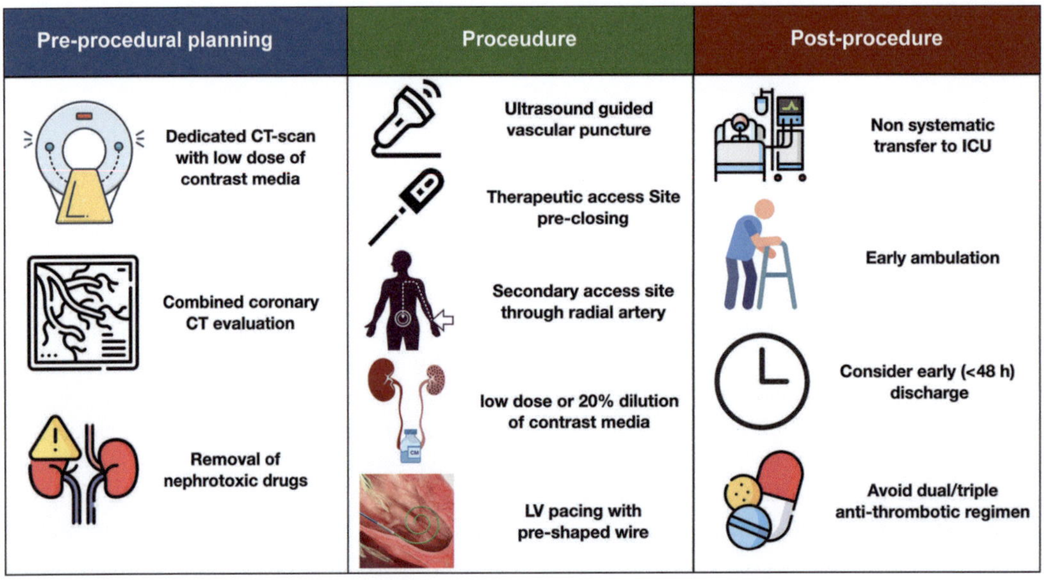

Fig. 17.1 Main elements of TAVI simplification

media, early ambulation and discharge, and simplification of the procedural and post-procedural antithrombotic treatment.

This chapter presents why and how TAVI procedure should be simplified in all patients even more in HBR patients.

17.2 Why Should TAVI Procedure Be Simplified?

The initial aim of TAVI procedure was to offer a minimally invasive aortic valve intervention for patients deemed at prohibitive risk for conventional surgery. Despite a first procedure performed under light sedation and local anaesthesia in 2002 [4], the initial experience of TAVI was developed under general anaesthesia (GA) in the majority of centres, to allow in particular the use of transoesophageal echocardiography (TOE) which was used in routine for valve sizing, THV positioning and assessment of paravalvular leak [7–9]. GA was also associated with better stability of the deployment of the prosthesis and better comfort for patients and operators [7–9]. Since the advent of MSCT scan for valve selection and sizing, TOE in now only performed in limited cases and GA is therefore not necessary. GA is

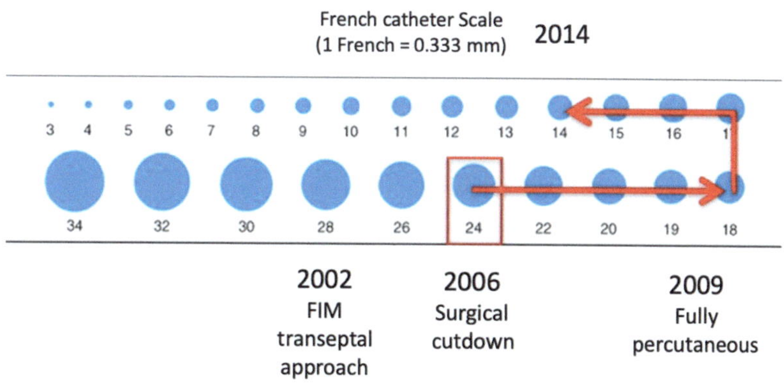

Fig. 17.2 Evolution of sheath size for TAVI implantation

more invasive and often combined with excessive monitoring including urinary catheterization, central venous line and arterial catheter and increasing the duration of the procedure and may potentially be associated with a risk of iatrogenesis and in particular with a risk of infection. Additionally, several registries report an increased risk of haemodynamic instability, lung infections, late identification of complications, major bleeding and longer length of hospital stay compared to conscious sedation. Furthermore, a potential stroke might not be diagnosed early with GA and appropriate management might be delayed [7–9].

Thus, local anaesthesia in transfemoral TAVI associated with light sedation has gradually supplanted GA in the majority of centres in France and worldwide [7–10]. This less invasive approach is feasible in the vast majority of cases and has been shown to be safe. GA and local anaesthesia are similar in terms of mortality, surgical conversion, major vascular and bleeding complications as well as stroke, but catecholamine and transfusion requirements are less frequent in patients under local anaesthesia, as hospitalization and intensive care unit lengths of stay [9, 11, 12]. Conversion from local to general anaesthesia is necessary only in a small number of patients (2–6%) due to procedural complications or haemodynamic instability. Only one randomized trial compared brain desaturation between the two approaches and found no difference [12]. The minimalist approach is performed using the transfemoral access in the majority of cases and in few cases using the transcarotid or transsubclavian approach. Indeed, the "percutaneous" transfemoral approach with the advent of dedicated closure systems has largely supplanted the initially "surgical" cut-down approach since 2009 [13–16]. This evolution of practices is largely linked to the better profile of the catheters and the reduction in the size of the introducers going from 24 French in the initial experience of TAVI to 14 French (Fig. 17.2) with the latest generations of prostheses [17].

Finally, the aim of simplifying TAVI is mainly to improve safety and allow for rapid recovery of the patients, especially in the elderly where fast recovery is crucial. Additionally, TAVI simplification is associated with early discharge and reduces costs and staff workload without compromising patients' safety.

17.3 How Was TAVI Procedure Simplified?

Beside GA and percutaneous approach, each TAVI step was progressively simplified over the years, from hybrid room to catheterization laboratory, from femoral to radial secondary access, from right ventricular to left ventricular wire pacing, from systematic predilatation to direct THV implant in the majority of cases and from systematic intensive coronary care unit to early discharge.

Hybrid room for TAVI procedure has been shown to be associated with increased procedure duration and increased risk of infection [18].

Table 17.2 TRA as an alternative vascular access for TAVI

	Femoral	Radial	*p* value
Patients (*n*)	194	217	–
Age (years)	83.5 ± 7.6	82.5 ± 6.2	NS
Euroscore (%)	15.4 ± 10.2	16.2 ± 10.7	NS
Secondary access site complication (%)	24.2	0	<0.001
Peripheral disease (%)	13.4	14.3	NS
Bleeding complications (%)	17.0	9.2	0.026
Major bleeding (%)	7.7	4.2	0.142
Vascular complications (%)	18.0	9.7	0.01
Major vascular complications (%)	3.6	1.8	0.362
Major stroke (%)	4.6	0.5	0.008
30-day death (%)	4.1	3.3	0.793

Thus, catheterization laboratory might be safer for TAVI and allow for simplified setup.

Pre-procedural vascular screening allows to safely select the most appropriate vascular access and to anticipate for potential complications. Ultrasound-guided femoral puncture and pre-closing are now the gold standard for transfemoral TAVI and have shown to dramatically decrease the incidence of major vascular complications and may be associated with a shorter hospitalization length of stay [19].

Another approach to limit vascular complications is the increasingly frequent use of radial access as a contralateral approach. Indeed, although vascular complications have decreased considerably over time, a third of these complications still occur at the level of the contralateral femoral access [20]. The selection of a radial access as a secondary approach then appears to be attractive in order to reduce vascular complications and has been described previously [19–22]. In the literature, the radial secondary approach in TAVI has been shown to be feasible and safe (Tables 17.2, 17.3, 17.4, and 17.5) with reduced vascular complications during percutaneous interventions and TAVI procedures [19–22].

Additionally, with increased operators' experience, management of VC from the radial access improved over the years with specific sheaths and balloon. We developed a peripheral radial kit in order to be able to manage femoral or iliac complications: long 110 cm sheath 6 or 7 French, long 400 cm guidewires, special 260 cm wire for the treatment of femoral or iliac occlusion and over the wire balloons (5–12 mm in diameter) with long sheath (180–200 cm). For stenting, Self-expandable, balloon-expandable and covered stents compatible through 6- or 7-French sheath are available with a long shaft (120–150 cm).

Table 17.3 The first 1072 TAVI Pts with transradial contralateral approach

Patients characteristics	
Age (years)	82 + 4
Male (*n*, %)	547 (51%)
Body mass index (mean)	28.2
Diabetes mellitus (*n*, %)	316 (29.5%)
Hypertension (*n*, %)	826 (77.1%)
Atrial fibrillation (*n*, %)	307 (28.6%)
Previous stroke (*n*, %)	61 (5.7%)
Peripheral vascular disease (*n*, %)	109 (10.2%)
Carotid artery disease (*n*, %)	90 (8.4%)
Chronic kidney disease (*n*, %)	289 (27.0%)
Chronic dialysis (*n*, %)	22 (2.1%)

Data prospectively collected at Institut Cardiovaculaire Paris Sud

Table 17.4 The first 1072 TAVI Pts with transradial contralateral approach

Procedure	*n* (%)
Radial approach success	98%
Sapien	559 (52.1%)
Acurate Neo	50 (4.7%)
Evolut-R	325 (30.3%)
Evolut-Pro	138 (12.9%)
Cerebral protection device	2 (0.1%)
Ilio-femoral predilatation	15 (1.4%)

Data prospectively collected at Institut Cardiovaculaire Paris Sud

Table 17.5 The first 1072 TAVI Pts with transradial contralateral approach

Complications	*N* (%)
In-hospital death	13 (1.2%)
Tamponade	15 (1.4%)
Annulus rupture	3 (0.3%)
Cardiac surgery	6 (0.6%)
Transfusion	20 (1.9%)
Infectious disease	22 (2.%)
Disabling stroke	8 (0.7%)

In few cases, a femoral cross-over approach may be necessary, particularly if a large stent graft implantation is required.

TAVI work-up from the radial access might also help to anticipate any challenging radial access. Radial access is particularly of interest in HBR patients to limit vascular complications and major bleeding from the secondary access [23].

During the TAVI procedure, rapid ventricular pacing is mandatory for balloon-expandable valves in order to induce transient severe hypotension necessary during valve deployment, thus avoiding embolization of the prosthesis. In the initial TAVI experience, rapid pacing was performed through the right ventricle temporary pacing by venous access [6]. However, this technique can be challenging with anatomical variations and can lead to increased X-ray exposure as well as specific complications. Indeed, venous puncture may be associated with the occurrence of vascular complications such as hematoma, arteriovenous fistula or thrombosis. Similarly, placement of the lead in the right ventricle may be associated with a risk of perforation and tamponade [6]. Recently, rapid ventricular pacing through the left ventricle wire has been described (Fig. 17.3) with the aim of simplifying the procedure by removing additional vascular access during TAVI [5, 6, 24]. This approach was efficient and allowed to reduce the procedure time with a low complication rate in a randomized trial [24]. However, in patients with a high risk of conduction disorder including right bundle branch block on baseline ECG, a right ventricle temporary pacing remains necessary and may be left in place if required. New wires have been proposed to offer left ventricular pacing using dedicated stimulation wire as well as pressure assessment.

During the initial experience of TAVI, balloon predilatation was systematic to allow passage of the prosthesis and optimize its deployment. However, performing TAVI without predilatation was first described in 2011 by Grübe et al. [25–27] and has been shown to be feasible in non-randomized studies with both self-expandable and balloon-expandable valves. With current-generation devices having a better crossing profile and systematic use of MSCT for valve selection and sizing, predilatation with a balloon does not seem essential before implantation of the THV. This “direct TAVI” approach has been adopted by many centres in more than 80% of cases [28]. In addition, predilatation could have some disadvantages such as an increased risk of cerebral embolization, paravalvular leak and instability of the THV during deployment. Furthermore, the occurrence of a massive aortic regurgitation after predilatation (1–2% of cases) that is poorly tolerated haemodynamically is avoided [25–28]. Thus, “direct TAVI” is the current trend with the aim of simplifying the procedure with two randomized trials which demonstrated non-inferiority with the self-expanding and the balloon-expandable valves [29, 30]. However, predilatation may sometimes be considered in cases of severely calcified aortic stenosis to reduce the risk of THV under-expansion and in patients with severe aortic or iliofemoral tortuosity with vertical aortic annulus to avoid THV crossing failure.

As chronic kidney disease is frequently observed in patients undergoing TAVI, additional simplified setup may be to prevent acute kidney injury following TAVI. Prevention is the cornerstone in chronic kidney disease, and careful hydration as well as removal of nephrotoxic medications may be useful in patients with severe aortic stenosis. Pre-TAVI MSCT is crucial to determine coplanar views to allow THV implantation and reduce contrast injection during the index TAVI procedure. To reduce MSCT-induced nephropathy, dedicated MSCT protocols with very low-contrast media volumes (<55 cc) have been proven to be feasible for imaging of TAVI

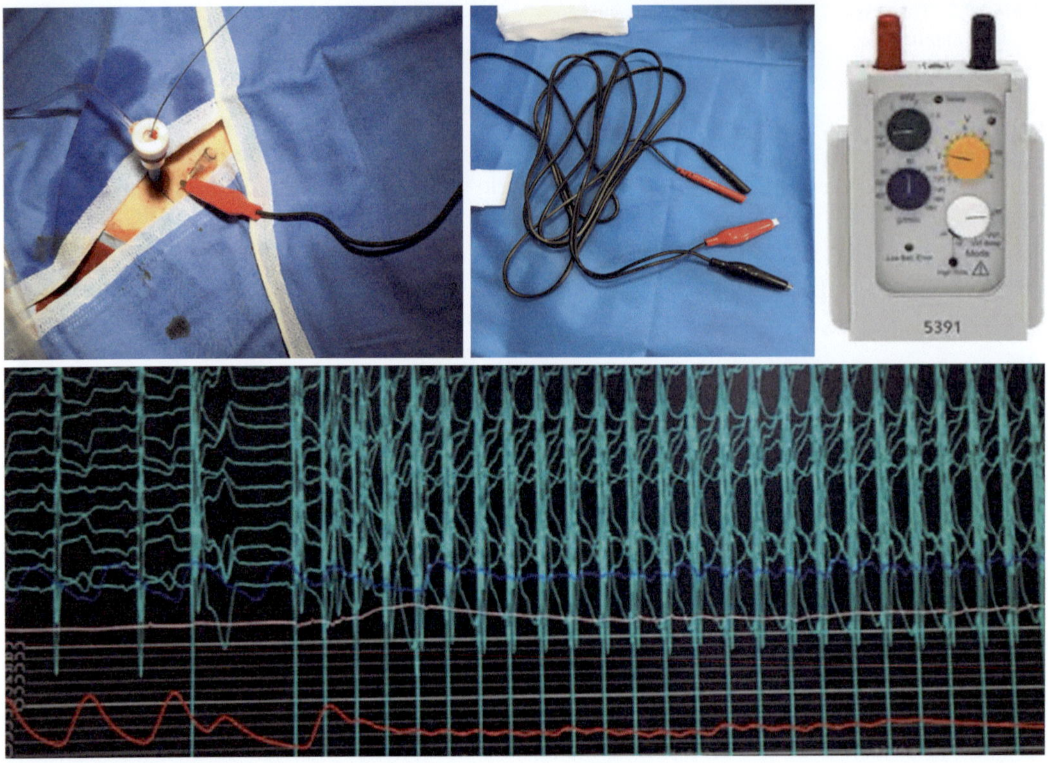

Fig. 17.3 Rapid pacing using the left ventricular wire using maximal energy and low detection

candidates [31]. Additionally, combined coronary MSCT can be useful to avoid additional contrast injection with coronary angiogram required during TAVI work-up [32]. During the procedure, the amount of contrast can be drastically decreased also using a 20% contrast dilution with saline without compromising imaging quality. Following the procedure, close monitoring may be necessary to ensure that renal function remains stable.

TAVI simplification is necessary in the contemporary TAVI area and allows to aim for post-procedural simplification in selected patients.

17.4 Post-procedure Simplification

Another aspect of TAVI simplification concerns post-procedural care. Nonsystematic transfer to cardiology intensive care unit has been shown to be feasible and safe, after rigorous evaluation and 2-hour monitoring in the recovery room, in selected patients with low risk of complications [33, 34]. Indeed, one of the risks to anticipate is the risk of delayed conduction disorder. In the study by Toggweiller et al. [35], at least 30% of patients with a normal baseline Electrocardiogramm (EKG) and no conductive disorder after TAVI could be referred immediately to a conventional unit with zero risk of delayed conductive disorder. This approach fits perfectly into minimalist management and better risk stratification could improve the selection of patients who can benefit from this approach.

Early discharge has been evaluated in the literature demonstrating the safety of this approach in patients hospitalized less than 48 hours [36–38]. Indeed, the median length of hospitalization was 1 day in the early discharge group, with no difference between early discharge and discharge after 48 hours in terms of mortality, stroke and readmission at 1 month. A "minimalist" TAVI procedure predicted early discharge in this study with local anaesthesia, less balloon predilatation and less invasive monitoring. Thus, this approach is considered even before the procedure by selecting upstream the patients who can benefit from this approach according to the risk profile (comorbidities) and the presence or not of a family circle as previously described [39]. Early mobilization has been shown also to be associated with next-day discharge which is routinely performed in many centres.

With the extension of TAVI to lower-risk patients, shortened hospitalization length of stay remains a priority objective, requiring rigorous selection of patients and reflection on downstream structures.

Post-procedural antithrombotic treatment has also been simplified over the years in these HBR patients, from the initial dual antiplatelet regimen to the current monotherapy which is currently recommended as the default strategy for patients without previous indication for anticoagulant and no antiplatelet treatment in patients who are already on anticoagulant treatment [40], except recent stent implantation.

TAVI simplification has already been routinely adopted in experienced centres with a low complication rate, shorter procedure time, better patient comfort, reduced costs and staff workload. However, careful patient selection and accurate complication risk stratification are keys to ensuring the safety of this minimalist approach.

17.5 How Far Can We Go in TAVI Simplification?

Although local anaesthesia alone is routinely performed, periprocedural anxiety and pain remain a concern. Virtual reality (VR) using specific glasses allows distraction that can modulate pain and anxiety. A recent randomized study assessed VR for pain and anxiety reduction in 117 patients undergoing transfemoral TAVI. Post-interventional anxiety scores (STAI-S) and the perceived duration of the procedure were significantly lower in the VR group compared with the standard of care group. VR may be a useful tool to decrease anxiety in selected patients undergoing minimalistic TAVI [41].

Distal radial access has been rapidly adopted by many centres for coronary interventions and is associated with high rate of success and low complication rates. More recently, distal radial access as the secondary access during TAVI has been evaluated in 41 patients with no radial access complications, 100% puncture success and no emergent transfemoral secondary access. Around a half of main femoral access vascular complications were resolved through distal radial access [42]. Thus, distal radial approach for secondary access in TAVI appears safe and may represent a step forward in TAVI simplification.

Next-day discharge is part of TAVI simplification and has been shown to be safe and effective in selected patients [43]. More recently, same-day discharge has been proposed in highly selected patients, especially during the COVID-19 pandemic to regulate patients' flow. In the multicentre registry published by Barker et al., same-day discharge was feasible and safe in highly selected patients at low risk of adverse events, especially at low risk of conduction disorder [44].

17.6 Conclusion

TAVI procedure has been drastically simplified over the years at each step, from procedural planning to patient discharge. Although TAVI indications shifted towards lower-risk patients with less comorbidities, elderly patients with HBR remain one of the targeted TAVI populations and may benefit even more from TAVI simplification. More simplification is expected in the future and may help to improve outcomes by decreasing vascular complications by the use of radial access, systematic LV wire pacing with dedicated wires and same-day safe discharge in selected patients.

Conflict of Interest Myriam Akodad has nothing to disclose.

Matteo Casenghi has nothing to disclose.

Thierry Lefèvre received minor fees from Abbott, Edwards and Boston scientific.

References

1. Vahanian A, Beyersdorf F, Praz F, et al. 2021 ESC/EACTS Guidelines for the management of valvular heart disease. Eur J Cardiothorac Surg. 2021;60(4):727–800.
2. Okuno T, Hagemeyer D, Brugger N, et al. Valvular and nonvalvular atrial fibrillation in patients undergoing transcatheter aortic valve replacement. JACC Cardiovasc Interv. 2020;13(18):2124–33. https://doi.org/10.1016/j.jcin.2020.05.049.
3. Crimi G, De Marzo V, De Marco F, et al. Acute kidney injury after transcatheter aortic valve replacement mediates the effect of chronic kidney disease. J Am Heart Assoc. 2022;11(19):e024589. https://doi.org/10.1161/JAHA.121.024589.
4. Cribier A, Eltchaninoff H, Bash A, Borenstein N, Tron C, Bauer F, et al. Percutaneous transcatheter implantation of an aortic valve prosthesis for calcific aortic stenosis: first human case description. Circulation. 2002;106(24):3006.
5. Akodad M, Lefèvre T. TAVI: simplification is the ultimate sophistication. Front Cardiovasc Med. 2018;5:96. https://doi.org/10.3389/fcvm.2018.00096.
6. Leclercq F, Meunier PA, Gandet T, et al. Simplified TAVR procedure: how far is it possible to go? J Clin Med. 2022;11(10):2793. https://doi.org/10.3390/jcm11102793.
7. Villablanca PA, Mohananey D, Nikolic K, Bangalore S, Slovut DP, Mathew V, et al. Comparison of local versus general anesthesia in patients undergoing transcatheter aortic valve replacement: a meta-analysis. Catheter Cardiovasc Interv. 2017;91:330.
8. Maas EHA, Pieters BMA, Van de Velde M, Rex S. General or local anesthesia for TAVI? A systematic review of the literature and meta-analysis. Curr Pharm Des. 2016;22(13):1868–78.
9. Ehret C, Rossaint R, Foldenauer AC, Stoppe C, Stevanovic A, Dohms K, et al. Is local anaesthesia a favourable approach for transcatheter aortic valve implantation? A systematic review and meta-analysis comparing local and general anaesthesia. BMJ Open. 2017;7(9):e016321.
10. Auffret V, Lefevre T, Van Belle E, et al. Temporal trends in transcatheter aortic valve replacement in France: FRANCE 2 to FRANCE TAVI. J Am Coll Cardiol. 2017;70(1):42–55. https://doi.org/10.1016/j.jacc.2017.04.053.
11. Yamamoto M, Meguro K, Mouillet G, Bergoend E, Monin J-L, Lim P, et al. Effect of local anesthetic management with conscious sedation in patients undergoing transcatheter aortic valve implantation. Am J Cardiol. 2013;111(1):94–9.
12. Mayr NP, Hapfelmeier A, Martin K, Kurz A, van der Starre P, Babik B, et al. Comparison of sedation and general anaesthesia for transcatheter aortic valve implantation on cerebral oxygen saturation and neurocognitive outcome†. Br J Anaesth. 2016;116(1):90–9.
13. Kadakia MB, Herrmann HC, Desai ND, Fox Z, Ogbara J, Anwaruddin S, et al. Factors associated with vascular complications in patients undergoing balloon-expandable transfemoral transcatheter aortic valve replacement via open versus percutaneous approaches. Circ Cardiovasc Interv. 2014;7(4):570–6.
14. Barbash IM, Barbanti M, Webb J, Molina-Martin De Nicolas J, Abramowitz Y, Latib A, et al. Comparison of vascular closure devices for access site closure after transfemoral aortic valve implantation. Eur Heart J. 2015;36(47):3370–9.
15. Leclercq F, Akodad M, Macia J-C, Gandet T, Lattuca B, Schmutz L, et al. Vascular complications and bleeding after transfemoral transcatheter aortic valve implantation performed through open surgical access. Am J Cardiol. 2015;116(9):1399–404.
16. Toggweiler S, Gurvitch R, Leipsic J, Wood DA, Willson AB, Binder RK, et al. Percutaneous aortic valve replacement: vascular outcomes with a fully percutaneous procedure. J Am Coll Cardiol. 2012;59(2):113–8.
17. Webb J, Gerosa G, Lefèvre T, Leipsic J, Spence M, Thomas M, et al. Multicenter evaluation of a next-generation balloon-expandable transcatheter aortic valve. J Am Coll Cardiol. 2014;64(21):2235–43.
18. Spaziano M, Lefèvre T, Romano M, et al. Transcatheter aortic valve replacement in the catheterization laboratory versus hybrid operating room: insights from the FRANCE TAVI registry. JACC Cardiovasc Interv. 2018;11(21):2195–203. https://doi.org/10.1016/j.jcin.2018.06.043.
19. Dato I, Burzotta F, Trani C, Crea F, Ussia GP. Percutaneous management of vascular access in transfemoral transcatheter aortic valve implantation. World J Cardiol. 2014;6(8):836–46.
20. Allende R, Urena M, Cordoba JG, Ribeiro HB, Amat-Santos I, DeLarochellière R, et al. Impact of the use of transradial versus transfemoral approach as secondary access in transcatheter aortic valve implantation procedures. Am J Cardiol. 2014;114(11):1729–34.
21. Curran H, Chieffo A, Buchanan GL, Bernelli C, Montorfano M, Maisano F, et al. A comparison of the femoral and radial crossover techniques for vascular access management in transcatheter aortic valve implantation: the Milan experience. Catheter Cardiovasc Interv. 2014;83(1):156–61.
22. Jolly SS, Amlani S, Hamon M, Yusuf S, Mehta SR. Radial versus femoral access for coronary angiography or intervention and the impact on major bleeding and ischemic events: a systematic review and meta-analysis of randomized trials. Am Heart J. 2009;157(1):132–40.
23. Fernandez-Lopez L, Chevalier B, Lefèvre T, et al. Implementation of the transradial approach as an alternative vascular access for transcatheter aortic valve replacement guidance: experience from a high-volume center. Catheter Cardiovasc Interv. 2019;93(7):1367–73. https://doi.org/10.1002/ccd.28024.

24. Faurie B, Abdellaoui M, Wautot F, Staat P, Champagnac D, Wintzer-Wehekind J, et al. Rapid pacing using the left ventricular guidewire: reviving an old technique to simplify BAV and TAVI procedures. Catheter Cardiovasc Interv. 2016;88(6):988–93.
25. Grube E, Naber C, Abizaid A, Sousa E, Mendiz O, Lemos P, et al. Feasibility of transcatheter aortic valve implantation without balloon pre-dilation: a pilot study. JACC Cardiovasc Interv. 2011;4(7):751–7.
26. Fiorina C, Maffeo D, Curello S, Lipartiti F, Chizzola G, D'Aloia A, et al. Direct transcatheter aortic valve implantation with self-expandable bioprosthesis: feasibility and safety. Cardiovasc Revasc Med. 2014;15(4):200–3.
27. Spaziano M, Sawaya F, Chevalier B, Roy A, Neylon A, Garot P, et al. Comparison of systematic predilation, selective predilation, and direct transcatheter aortic valve implantation with the SAPIEN S3 valve. Can J Cardiol. 2017;33(2):260–8.
28. Deharo P, Jaussaud N, Grisoli D, Camus O, Resseguier N, Le Breton H, et al. Impact of direct transcatheter aortic valve replacement without balloon aortic valvuloplasty on procedural and clinical outcomes: insights from the FRANCE TAVI registry. JACC Cardiovasc Interv. 2018;11(19):1956–65.
29. Toutouzas K, Benetos G, Voudris V, Drakopoulou M, Stathogiannis K, Latsios G, Synetos A, Antonopoulos A, Kosmas E, Iakovou I, et al. Predilatation versus no pre-dilatation for implantation of a self-expanding valve in all comers undergoing TAVR: the DIRECT trial. JACC Cardiovasc Interv. 2019;12:767–77.
30. Leclercq F, Robert P, Akodad M, Macia J-C, Gandet T, Delseny D, Chettouh M, Schmutz L, Robert G, Levy G, et al. Prior balloon valvuloplasty versus direct transcatheter aortic valve replacement: results from the DIRECTAVI trial. JACC Cardiovasc Interv. 2020;13:594–602.
31. Spagnolo P, Giglio M, Di Marco D, et al. Feasibility of ultra-low contrast 64-slice computed tomography angiography before transcatheter aortic valve implantation: a real-world experience. Eur Heart J Cardiovasc Imaging. 2016;17(1):24–33.
32. Gohmann RF, Pawelka K, Seitz P, et al. Combined cCTA and TAVR planning for ruling out significant CAD: added value of ML-based CT-FFR. JACC Cardiovasc Imaging. 2022;15(3):476–86. https://doi.org/10.1016/j.jcmg.2021.09.013.
33. Leclercq F, Iemmi A, Lattuca B, et al. Feasibility and safety of transcatheter aortic valve implantation performed without intensive care unit admission. Am J Cardiol. 2016;118(1):99–106. https://doi.org/10.1016/j.amjcard.2016.04.019.
34. Akodad M, Aldhaheri E, Marin G, et al. Transcatheter aortic valve replacement performed with selective telemetry monitoring: a prospective study. Int J Cardiol. 2021;330:158. https://doi.org/10.1016/j.ijcard.2021.02.028.
35. Toggweiler S, Stortecky S, Holy E, Zuk K, Cuculi F, Nietlispach F, et al. The electrocardiogram after transcatheter aortic valve replacement determines the risk for post-procedural high-degree AV block and the need for telemetry monitoring. JACC Cardiovasc Interv. 2016;9(12):1269–76.
36. Barbanti M, Capranzano P, Ohno Y, Attizzani GF, Gulino S, Immè S, et al. Early discharge after transfemoral transcatheter aortic valve implantation. Heart. 2015;101(18):1485–90.
37. Barbanti M, Baan J, Spence MS, Iacovelli F, Martinelli GL, Saia F, et al. Feasibility and safety of early discharge after transfemoral transcatheter aortic valve implantation – rationale and design of the FAST-TAVI registry. BMC Cardiovasc Disord. 2017;17(1):259.
38. Barbanti M, van Mourik MS, Spence MS, Icovelli F, Martinelli GL, Muir DF, et al. Optimising patient discharge management after transfemoral transcatheter aortic valve implantation: the multicentre European FAST-TAVI trial. EuroIntervention. 2019;15(2):147–54.
39. Durand E, Eltchaninoff H, Canville A, Bouhzam N, Godin M, Tron C, et al. Feasibility and safety of early discharge after transfemoral transcatheter aortic valve implantation with the Edwards SAPIEN-XT prosthesis. Am J Cardiol. 2015;115(8):1116–22.
40. Hindi MN, Akodad M, Nestelberger T, Sathananthan J. Antithrombotic therapy after transcatheter aortic valve replacement: an overview. Struct Heart. 2022;6(5):100085. https://doi.org/10.1016/j.shj.2022.100085.
41. Lind A, Ahsan M, Totzeck M, et al. Virtual reality-assisted distraction during transcatheter aortic valve implantation under local anaesthesia: a randomised study. Int J Cardiol. 2023;387:131130. https://doi.org/10.1016/j.ijcard.2023.131130.
42. Achim A, Szűcsborus T, Sasi V, et al. Distal radial secondary access for transcatheter aortic valve implantation: the minimalistic approach. Cardiovasc Revasc Med. 2022;40:152–7. https://doi.org/10.1016/j.carrev.2021.11.021.
43. Wood DA, Lauck SB, Cairns JA, Humphries KH, Cook R, Welsh R, et al. The vancouver 3M (multidisciplinary, multimodality, but minimalist) clinical pathway facilitates safe next-day discharge home at low-, medium-, and high-volume transfemoral transcatheter aortic valve replacement centers: the 3M TAVR study. JACC Cardiovasc Interv. 2019;12(5):459–69.
44. Barker M, Sathananthan J, Perdoncin E, et al. Same-day discharge post-transcatheter aortic valve replacement during the COVID-19 pandemic: the multicenter PROTECT TAVR study. JACC Cardiovasc Interv. 2022;15(6):590–8. https://doi.org/10.1016/j.jcin.2021.12.046.

Part IV

Antithrombotic Therapy in HBR Patients

18 Intravenous Antiplatelet Drugs

Marco Frazzetto, Julia Tirelli, Stefano Rigattieri, and Bernardo Cortese

18.1 Introduction/Preamble

Platelet activation and aggregation have a crucial role in the development of atherosclerosis and thrombotic events [1]. This underscores the paramount importance of antiplatelet therapy for the treatment of coronary artery disease, especially in patients undergoing percutaneous coronary intervention (PCI) [2]. In this setting, thrombotic events such as early stent thrombosis, leading to acute myocardial infarction (MI), are related to high morbidity and mortality [3]. Nevertheless, a personalized balance between thrombotic and hemorrhagic risk in the management of antiplatelet therapy is essential to avoid catastrophic sequelae.

M. Frazzetto
University Hospitals Harrington Heart & Vascular Institute Cleveland, Cleveland, OH, USA

J. Tirelli
Faculdade de Medicina de Jundiai – Hospital São Vicente de Paula, Jundiai, São Paulo, Brazil

S. Rigattieri
Cardiology Unit, Sant'Andrea University Hospital, Rome, Italy

B. Cortese (✉)
University Hospitals Harrington Heart & Vascular Institute, Cleveland, OH, USA

Fondazione Ricerca e Innovazione Cardiovascolare, Milan, Italy

DCB Academy, Milan, Italy

To date, numerous antiplatelet drugs with different molecular targets are currently available. Among these, the only intravenous (I.V.) agents available are aspirin, the $P2Y_{12}$ inhibitor cangrelor, and the three glycoprotein IIb/IIIa receptor inhibitors (GPIs), abciximab, eptifibatide, and tirofiban; in fact, abciximab production was discontinued by the manufacturer a few years ago. However, the administration of aspirin is prevalently oral, and intravenous formulation is not marketed in many countries including the US (Table 18.1).

The use of complementary antiplatelet drugs administered with aspirin has undergone constant evolution in the last three decades [4–7]. Initially, GPIs were used along with aspirin during PCI before clopidogrel administration [4, 8, 9]. In the era of the newer $P2Y_{12}$ agents (i.e., prasugrel and ticagrelor) which provide more potent and stable platelet inhibition within 2 h compared to clopidogrel, GPIs play a marginal role during PCI and their use is limited to patients with thrombotic complications or no reflow [10, 11]. Nevertheless, some studies showed insufficient platelet inhibition with prasugrel and ticagrelor in the first hours after acute coronary syndrome (ACS) [12–14]. The weak point of oral antiplatelet agents is the dependence on enteric absorption [13, 15]. I.V. antiplatelet agents, mainly cangrelor, with fast onset and offset are mostly used during PCI and can address many drawbacks of oral antiplatelet drugs.

B. Cortese, S. Rigattieri (eds.), *High Bleeding Risk Patients in Interventional Cardiology*,
https://doi.org/10.1007/978-3-031-87302-7_18

Table 18.1 Key pharmacological characteristics of glycoprotein IIb/IIIa inhibitors and cangrelor

	Abciximab Fab fragment, chimeric	Eptifibatide Synthetic peptide	Tirofiban Nonpeptide mimetic	Cangrelor Analogue adenosine triphosphate
Molecule	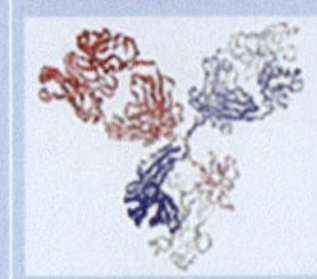	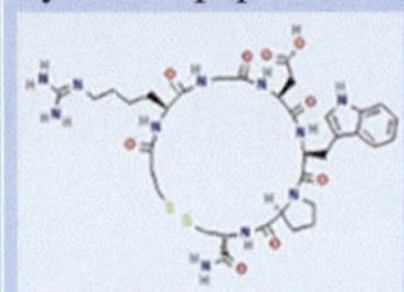	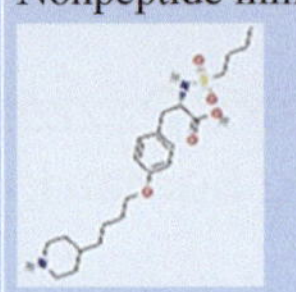	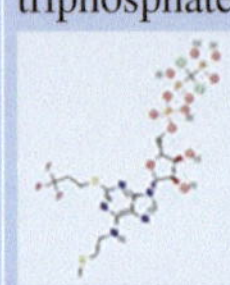
Binding	Non-competitive	Competitive	Competitive	Competitive
Half life	10–15 h	2–2.5 h	2 h	3–6 min
Dosage	Bolus: 0.25 mg/kg (10–60 min)	Bolus: 180 mcg/kg (10 min) + 180 mcg/kg	Bolus: 25 mcg/kg (over 3 min)	Bolus: 30 mg/kg
	Infusion: 0.125 mcg/kg/min (12 h)	Infusion: 2 mcg/kg/min (up to 18 h)	Infusion: 0.15 mcg/kg/min (up to 18 h)	Infusion: 4 mg/kg/min (at least 2 h and up to 4 h)
Renal adjustment	No	Yes	Yes	No
Commercially available	No	Yes	Yes	Yes

18.2 GP IIB/IIIA Inhibitors

18.2.1 Overview

The integrin GP IIB/IIIA is the most important membrane receptor for aggregation, acting as a mediator of bridging platelets. The idea in the pharmacological development of GPIs was to reach fast platelet inhibition, reducing the risk of thrombotic complications associated with PCI and/or ACS. In large-scale clinical trials, oral administration was associated with an increase in bleeding and thrombotic events and excess all-cause mortality [16]. Conversely, several clinical trials showed the benefits of I.V. administration in ACS patients. Nevertheless, GPI use is, nowadays, not recommended as part of routine upstream therapy in patients with ACS but represents a viable option for reducing thrombus burden in bail-out situations. The reasons for the marginal utilization of GPIs, in contemporary clinical practice, are related to the high bleeding risk associated with routine use and the availability of potent oral $P2Y_{12}$ inhibitors (prasugrel and ticagrelor) in the ACS setting.

18.2.2 Pharmacology

The currently available GPIs for clinical use are the small molecules tirofiban and eptifibatide, which act specifically on the α_{IIb}-chain of the GP IIb/IIIa. Tirofiban is a synthetic non-peptide tyrosine derivate inhibitor, while eptifibatide is a cyclic heptapeptide. They act as ligand-mimetic competitive platelet inhibitors, binding specifically to the arginine-glycine-aspartic acid (RGD) recognition site of GPIIb/IIIa, thereby impeding the binding of integrin with fibrinogen and the subsequent formation of platelet clot.

Due to their short plasma half-lives (2–2.5 h), continuous infusion is needed to obtain sustained platelet inhibition [16]. Accordingly, their antiplatelet effect is reduced within hours after beginning the infusion, because platelet function is reestablished as soon as the drug is excreted by the kidney in about 4–8 h [17].

The dosage of tirofiban in ACS is 25 mcg/kg I.V. over 3 min, followed by an infusion of 0.15 mcg/kg/min for up to 18 h. In case of chronic kidney disease (i.e. estimated glomerular filtration rate <30 ml/min/1.73 m^2), the loading dose is 25 mcg/kg I.V. over 5 min followed by a maintenance infusion of 0.075 mcg/kg/min continued for up to 18 h. The dosage of eptifibatide in ACS is 180 + 180 μg/kg (double bolus given at a 10-min interval) followed by infusion of 2 μg/kg/min for up to 18 h. In patients with renal impairment (defined as an estimated glomerular filtration rate <50 ml/min), only one bolus is given and the infusion dose is halved. Their use is contraindicated in patients with prior ICH, ischemic stroke within 30 days, fibrinolysis, or platelet count <100,000/mm^3. Additionally, in consideration of the class-related risk of thrombocytopenia, it is recommended to measure platelet counts before initiation of GPI treatment and within 24 h of their administration.

18.2.3 GPI Studies Across the Spectrum of Coronary Artery Disease

In the past decades, numerous studies of GPIs have been conducted, using a wide range of dosages and concomitant antithrombotic drugs [16]. An exhaustive description of each clinical trial goes beyond the scope of this chapter, which will discuss selected studies that have played a central role in the comprehension of benefits and risks associated with GPI use.

18.2.3.1 Chronic Coronary Syndromes

The relevance of many studies in low-risk patients undergoing elective PCI has scarce clinical relevance because conducted before the era of dual antiplatelet therapy (i.e. clopidogrel). The only clinical trials in patients with elective PCI and concomitant clopidogrel assumption (600 mg loading dose at least 2 h before the PCI) are ISAR-REACT (Intracoronary Stenting and Antithrombotic Regimen: Rapid Early Action for Coronary Treatment) and ISAR SWEET (Intracoronary Stenting and Antithrombotic Regimen: Is Abciximab a Superior Way to Eliminate Elevated Thrombotic Risk in Diabetics) trials, although the GPI investigated was abciximab which is no longer commercially available worldwide [18, 19]. Of note, abciximab demonstrated no benefit on the primary composite endpoint of death, MI, or urgent target vessel revascularization at 30 days and 1 year. Conversely, abciximab was associated with more frequent thrombocytopenia while not increasing major bleeding events.

In a meta-analysis of 22 trials and 10,123 patients on $P2Y_{12}$ inhibitors undergoing elective, the use of GPIs did not reduce the mortality and increased bleeding events [20].

18.2.3.2 Non-ST-segment Acute Myocardial Infarction

Before the advent of clopidogrel in clinical practice, numerous studies were conducted in patients with ACS undergoing PCI using GPIs. These trials and those involving abciximab alone will be not examined because no longer significant to current practice.

Some collateral data on the role of GPIs in patients with ACS undergoing PCI and treated with clopidogrel derive from some trials involving the use of bivalirudin.

The ACUITY (Acute Catheterization and Urgent Intervention Triage Strategy) trial ($n = 13{,}819$, three arms) reported no difference in terms of 30-day rates of death, MI, or unplanned revascularization between bivalirudin monotherapy and bivalirudin plus GPIs compared with heparin plus GPIs. To note, only bivalirudin monotherapy significantly reduced major bleeding reduction compared with heparin plus GPIs [21].

In the MATRIX (Minimizing Adverse Hemorrhagic Events by Transradial Access Site and Systemic Implementation of Angiox) trial ($n = 7213$), bleeding events were increased with heparin (2.5% versus 1.4%, $p < 0.001$) compared to bivalirudin, likely related to the higher rate of GPI usage [22]. Conversely, in the VALIDATE-SWEDEHEART (Bivalirudin versus Heparin in ST Segment and Non-ST-Segment Elevation Myocardial Infarction in Patients on Modern Antiplatelet Therapy in the Swedish Web System for Enhancement and Development of Evidence-based Care in Heart Disease Evaluated according to Recommended Therapies Registry), where the GPIs administration was 2% for both groups, no difference in bleeding events was reported between bivalirudin and heparin [23]. Therefore, GPIs probably acted as an adverse factor that increased bleeding events in the comparison between bivalirudin and heparin.

In contemporary clinical practice, the central role of prasugrel and ticagrelor, in place of clopidogrel, in the treatment of ACS was first established in the TRITON (Trial to Assess Improvement in Therapeutic Outcomes by Optimizing Platelet Inhibition with Prasugrel) and PLATO (Platelet inhibition and patient Outcomes) trials, respectively [6, 7]. In both trials, the benefit of the newer $P2Y_{12}$ thienopyridines was independent of the concomitant use of the GPIs use. Consequently, no evidence suggests the routinary use of GPIs in patients with non-ST-segment elevation ACS undergoing PCI.

18.2.3.3 ST-Segment Elevation Myocardial Infarction

Ideally, patients with acute ST-segment elevation MI (STEMI) and presence of high-burden thrombus may be the best candidates for the administration of GPIs. Two large meta-analyses, published in 2005 and 2007, described decreasing mortality and MI rates at 30 days in patients GPIs treated [24, 25].

Conversely, in the On-TIME 2 trial ($n = 984$), upstream tirofiban improved ST-segment resolution with tirofiban 1 h after PCI [26]. Nevertheless, the study was unable to demonstrate a survival benefit or a reduced risk of reinfarction [26]. A post hoc analysis of the trial revealed a reduction in the incidence of early stent thrombosis and urgent revascularization in the tirofiban group [27]. Additionally, early stent thrombosis and prehospital tirofiban were reported as independent predictors of 30-day mortality [27].

Similarly to non-ST-segment elevation ACS, GPIs were studied in STEMI in bivalirudin trials. The HORIZONS-AMI (Harmonizing Outcomes with Revascularization and Stents in Acute Myocardial Infarction) ($n = 3602$) trial evaluated patients undergoing primary PCI and randomized to heparin plus a GPI and bivalirudin. Bivalirudin reduced the net adverse clinical events (9.2% versus 12.1%) and major bleeding (4.9% versus 8.3%) at 30 days but led to an increased risk of acute stent thrombosis [28].

Finally, a meta-analysis of 14 studies ($n = 3754$) focused on intracoronary versus intravenous GPI administration did not show differences in major adverse cardiac events [29].

18.2.4 Studies with Different Administration Strategies to Improve Bleeding Outcomes

Numerous clinical trials have been conducted to compare different administration strategies (upstream *or* downstream use, shorter *or* longer infusions) have been conducted to improve bleeding outcomes. Early or delayed administration of GPIs in ACS was analyzed in the EARLY-ACS (Early Glycoprotein IIb/IIIa Inhibition in Non-ST-Segment Elevation Acute Coronary Syndrome) ($n = 9492$) trial. No difference was reported in early ischemic outcomes at 96 h and 30 days, along with a significantly higher transfusions and bleeding rate with early eptifibatide administration [30]. The ACUITY Timing (Acute Catheterization and Urgent Intervention Triage Strategy Timing) trial ($n = 9207$) reported no difference between upstream and downstream GPI use in terms of ischemic events at 30 days, but the deferred use was associated with a significant reduction of major bleeding [31]. The advent of $P2Y_{12}$ inhibitors and their use as a pretreatment strategy led to dismiss the upstream administration of GPIs. The BRIEF PCI (Brief Infusion of Eptifibatide Following Percutaneous Coronary Intervention) trial investigated shorter GPI use in attempting to reduce the risk of bleeding complications associated with their routinary administration. Patients with ACS were randomized to an 18-h or maximum 2-h eptifibatide infusion. The shorter regimen met non-inferiority for ischemic outcomes and paralleled decreased bleeding events (1.0% versus 4.2%, $p = 0.02$) [32].

18.2.5 GPIs in Clinical Practice Guidelines

The most recent guidelines for Coronary Artery Revascularization by the American College of Cardiology (ACC), American Heart Association (AHA) and Society for Cardiovascular Angiography and Interventions (SCAI) were published in 2021 [10].

GPIs are recommended in patients with ACS undergoing PCI with large thrombus burden, no-reflow, or slow flow, to improve procedural success (Class of Recommendation IIA, Level of Evidence C-LD) [10].

The 2023 European Society of Cardiology guidelines for the Management of Acute Coronary Syndrome state that GPIs should be considered if there is evidence of no-reflow or a thrombotic complication during PCI (Class of Recommendation IIA, Level of Evidence C) [11]. Additionally, it is suggested that another potential use for GPIs is in the setting of high-risk PCI in patients who have not been pretreated with P2Y12 receptor inhibitors [11].

In both clinical practice guidelines, routine pretreatment with GPIs is not recommended in any clinical condition (Class of Recommendation III, Level of Evidence A).

18.3 Cangrelor

18.3.1 Rationale

The platelet $P2Y_{12}$ receptor for adenosine 5′diphosphate (ADP) plays a central role in platelet function, hemostasis, and thrombosis [33]. In the past two decades, paramount clinical trials supported the relevant benefit of P2Y12 receptor inhibitors in adjunct to aspirin, in high-risk patients with coronary artery disease, such as those undergoing PCI or presenting with an ACS, reducing short- and long-term ischemic events [5–7]. Nevertheless, significant concerns remain about their onset of action. Most investigations have been conducted with oral formulations of $P2Y_{12}$ inhibitors. Their administration does not suppress the high residual platelet reactivity up to 4–6 h after the loading dose [13]. The availability of oral $P2Y_{12}$ inhibitors is closely related and limited by enteric absorption, leading to a delay between administration and the time to reach therapeutical platelet inhibition. The most important determinants involved in their absorption are stomach emptying, gastrointestinal motility, and perfusion of the gastrointestinal mucosa [34]. Furthermore, the time required to reach effective platelet inhibition after oral intake is different in distinct presentations of coronary artery disease impact. The platelet inhibition is faster for patients with chronic coronary syndromes undergoing PCI, slower for NSTE-ACS, and the slowest for STEMI patients [35, 36]. In patients with ACS, nausea and vomiting concur to reduce drug absorption as well. Lastly, the concomitant administration of morphine in ACS for the treatment of chest pain may induce nausea and vomiting, slowing gastric emptying and intestinal peristalsis. Another important concern about the effectiveness of oral $P2Y_{12}$ inhibitors is in intubated or unconscious patients related to the unpredictable timeframe of inadequate platelet inhibition after their administration and, potentially, increased risk of stent thrombosis and periprocedural MI. These observations underscore the need to define strategies that can bridge the gap in platelet inhibitory effects following the intake of oral $P2Y_{12}$ inhibitors. Finally, the rapid onset/offset pharmacological profile makes it suitable as bridging therapy after $P2Y_{12}$ inhibitor discontinuation in surgical candidates.

18.3.2 Pharmacology of Cangrelor

Cangrelor is a non-thienopyridine analog of adenosine triphosphate and a reversible antagonist of the platelet P2Y12 receptor. It binds to the P2Y12 receptor directly and hence does not require any bioactivation [37]. Therapeutic plasma concentrations are immediately achieved after I.V. bolus administration and its plasma half-life is short (3–5 min) [38, 39].

Cangrelor has an extremely fast onset and offset of action. The complete platelet inhibition is achieved in 2 min when administered as an I.V.

bolus (30 μg/kg) followed by a continuous infusion (2–4 μg/kg/min). Platelet function recovers within 60–90 min after the discontinuation of the infusion. Notably, unlike GPIs, cangrelor overdose is not associated with increased bleeding, owing to its short half-life, and rapid offset of action [40].

Body weight was associated with a higher clearance and a higher volume of distribution. However, this is accounted for by body weight-adjusted I.V. dosing.

Genetic polymorphisms of CYP enzymes do not impact the metabolism of cangrelor, because it is CYP enzyme independent. Also, its metabolism is liver independent and can be administered irrespective of hepatic function according to the label.

No dose adjustment in patients with mild, moderate, or severe renal impairment is required, at a variance of GPIs.

18.3.3 Safety and Efficacy of Cangrelor

18.3.3.1 The CHAMPION Program

Three large, double-blind, randomized clinical trials have allowed cangrelor to be recommended in European and American clinical practice guidelines (Table 18.2). The CHAMPION-PLATFORM (n = 5362) trial randomized clopidogrel-naïve patients to cangrelor or placebo at the time of PCI, followed by a clopidogrel loading dose of 600 mg. No difference was found for the primary composite endpoint (death, MI, or ischemia-guided revascularization at 48 h) between groups [41]. Conversely, the rate of major bleeding was highest in the cangrelor group (5.5% versus 3.5%), mainly driven by the increased rate of access-site hematoma [41]. The CHAMPION-PCI trial (n = 8877) randomized patients to receive cangrelor or clopidogrel 600 mg administered before PCI. At 48 h and 30 days, cangrelor was not superior to clopidogrel for the primary composite endpoint (death from any cause, myocardial infarction, or ischemia-driven revascularization). The rate of major bleeding was higher with cangrelor, but this difference did not reach a statistically significant difference. To note, the enrollment in both studies was terminated early due to futility. Finally, the CHAMPION PHOENIX trial (n = 11,145) randomized patients who were undergoing either urgent or elective PCI to receive cangrelor or a 300–600 mg loading dose of clopidogrel. In this

Table 18.2 CHAMPION Program

	CHAMPION PCI	CHAMPION PLATFORM	CHAMPION PHOENIX
Years	2007–2009	2007–2009	2010–2012
Patients	8.877	5.362	11.145
Presentation	STEMI (11.2%) NSTE-ACS (73.8%) Stable angina (1.5%)	NSTE-ACS (96.8%) Stable angina (5.2%)	STEMI (18%) NSTE-ACS (25.7%) Stable angina (62.3%)
Antiplatelet therapy	Clopidogrel	Clopidogrel naive	Clopidogrel naïve
Treatment arm	Cangrelor 30 mcg/kg bolus 4 mcg/kg/min infusion	Cangrelor 30 mcg/kg bolus 4 mcg/kg/min infusion	Cangrelor 30 mcg/kg bolus 4 mcg/kg/min infusion
Transition to clopidogrel	Clopidogrel 600 mg at the end of cangrelor infusion	Clopidogrel 600 mg at the end of cangrelor infusion	Clopidogrel 600 mg at the end of cangrelor infusion
Control arm	Clopidogrel 600 mg	Placebo	Clopidogrel 600 or 300 mg
Definition of myocardial infarction	Clinical	Clinical	Universal definition
Primary endpoint	Death, MI, IDR after 48 h	Death, MI, IDR after 48 h	Death, MI, IDR after 48 h
Results	OR 1.05 (95% CI 0.88–1.24; $p = 0.59$)	OR 0.87 (95% CI 0.71–1.07; $p = 0.17$)	OR 0.78 (95% CI 0.66–0.83; $p = 0.005$)

STEMI ST-segment acute myocardial infarction, *NSTEMI-ACS* non-ST-segment acute myocardial infarction-acute coronary syndrome, *MI* myocardial infarction, *IDR* ischemia-driven revascularization trial, unlike the previous CHAMPION trials, was used the universal MI definition. The primary composite endpoint (death, MI, ischemia-driven revascularization, or stent thrombosis at 48 h) was reduced by cangrelor (4.7% versus 5.9%, $p = 0.005$), without differences in terms of major bleeding [42]. Additionally, stent thrombosis and clinical outcomes at 30 days were reduced with the use of cangrelor [43].

A patient-level meta-analysis of the three CHAMPION studies confirmed the efficacy and safety of cangrelor in terms of death, MI, or stent thrombosis. No significant increase in major bleeding was documented. Specifically, cangrelor reduced the odds of the primary outcome by 19% and stent thrombosis by 41% [44]. Numerous post hoc sensitivity analyses confirmed the effectiveness of cangrelor with different endpoint definitions and subgroups and with respect to ACS [45, 46].

18.3.4 Role of Cangrelor and Recent $P2Y_{12}$ Inhibitors

The first trials of cangrelor mainly involved patients with stable or unstable CAD and a limited proportion of patients with STEMI.

The CANTIC Study (Platelet Inhibition with Cangrelor and Crushed TICagrelor in STEMI Patients Undergoing Primary Percutaneous Coronary Intervention) was the first prospective randomized study in patients undergoing primary PCI to explore the drug–drug interaction when cangrelor or placebo are concomitantly administered with ticagrelor [47]. The patients were randomized to receive either cangrelor or matching placebo (bolus followed by 2-h infusion). Additionally, crushed ticagrelor (180 mg) was administered in both groups. Following PCI, all patients were discharged on ticagrelor 90 mg and life-long aspirin. Cangrelor showed lower levels of platelet reactivity (measured with VerifyNow P2Y12 point-of-care testing as P2Y12 reaction units) compared to placebo at 5 min after bolus, 30 min, and until the termination of the 2-h infusion. Rates of high platelet reactivity were significantly higher with placebo than with cangrelor at any study time point. Therefore, this study ruled out a drug–drug interaction during concomitant administration of cangrelor and ticagrelor, since the levels of platelet reactivity were comparable between the two groups after drug infusion was stopped.

The findings of the CANTIC study were confirmed by the results of the prospective, randomized, double-blind, placebo-controlled, crossover, pharmacokinetic, and pharmacodynamic SWAP-5 (Pharmacodynamic and Pharmacokinetic Profiles of Switching Between Cangrelor and Ticagrelor Following Ticagrelor Pre-treatment: The Switching Antiplatelet-5 Study) trial, which ruled out drug–drug interaction also in the subset of patients with stable coronary artery disease treated with cangrelor who had been pretreated with ticagrelor [48].

The ARCANGELO (Italian Prospective Study on Cangrelor) was a multicenter, observational, prospective study that assessed the safety of cangrelor in daily clinical practice. The study included patients with ACS undergoing PCI who were oral P2Y12-naïve before the PCI procedure and in whom oral therapy with $P2Y_{12}$ inhibitors was not feasible [49]. Among 995 ACS patients undergoing PCI, 597 (60.0%) had ST-segment elevation myocardial infarction. Bolus and cangrelor infusion, between 2 and 4, were administered in 95% of the patients. Among them, 73.4% received ticagrelor, 12.8% prasugrel, and 13.9% clopidogrel as transition therapy. Bleeding, assessed until 30 days post-PCI, occurred in 5.2% of patients, of whom moderate and mild in 0.5% and 4.7% of the cases. Major adverse cardiac events occurred in 1.4% of the patients. Therefore, this study underscored the safety and effectiveness of cangrelor in ACS patients undergoing PCI and the transition strategy to $P2Y_{12}$ inhibitors.

18.3.5 Transition to $P2Y_{12}$ Inhibitors After Cangrelor

Patients undergoing PCI should receive a loading dose of an oral $P2Y_{12}$ inhibitor on top of aspirin. The precise timing for the administration of the loading dose of the $P2Y_{12}$ inhibitor depends on

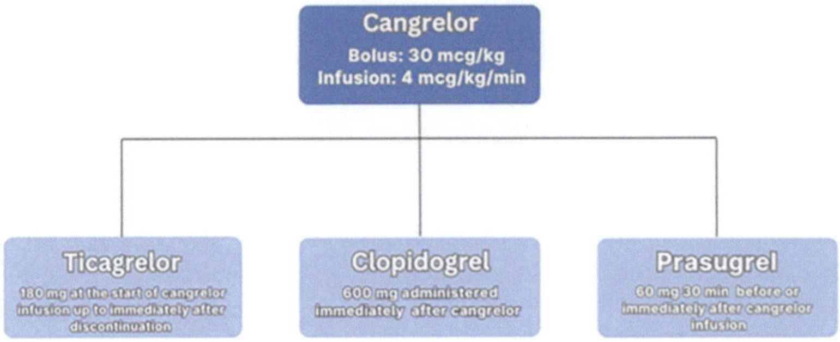

Fig. 18.1 Transitioning from cangrelor to oral $P2Y_{12}$ inhibitors

the pharmacology of the specific drug. The active metabolite of clopidogrel, less potent than cangrelor, is subjected to degradation if it does not bind its receptor. Thus, if cangrelor occupies and binds $P2Y_{12}$ receptor, the clopidogrel active metabolite is degraded, resulting in no platelet inhibition following the termination of cangrelor infusion. Given that, a loading dose of 600 mg clopidogrel must be administered only after cangrelor infusion cessation [50].

Pharmacodynamics of prasugrel is similar to clopidogrel. Therefore, the loading dose administration of prasugrel should be administered at the end of cangrelor infusion. A study found that the optimal administration time of prasugrel, to limit the recovery of platelet function, is 30 min before cangrelor cessation [51]. Therefore, the european medicines agency (EMA) recommends the administration of a prasugrel loading dose (60 mg) either 30 min before the cangrelor cessation or immediately after; the FDA recommends it only immediately after cangrelor cessation.

Ticagrelor is a reversible $P2Y_{12}$ inhibitor, and its binding site at the $P2Y_{12}$ receptor is different compared to cangrelor. Numerous studies showed that there are no drug–drug interactions between ticagrelor and cangrelor [52]. Thus, the FDA and EMA recommend the administration of a ticagrelor loading dose (180 mg) at any time during cangrelor infusions or at the end of it (Fig. 18.1).

18.3.6 Cangrelor in Emergency

Patients with cardiogenic shock and comatose survivors of out-of-hospital cardiac arrest undergoing PCI are at increased risk for stent thrombosis [53]. This may be explained by a delayed onset of P2Y12 inhibitors [54]. The role of cangrelor, with its immediate platelet inhibition, may be pivotal in this setting. The Cangrelor OHCA (Out-of-Hospital Cardiac Arrest), single-center, non-placebo controlled, randomized study enrolled 30 comatose survivors of out-of-hospital cardiac arrest undergoing PCI and target temperature management. The use of cangrelor was safe, inducing immediate and adequate platelet inhibition without drug–drug interaction with ticagrelor [55]. The design not powered for clinical endpoint and the small sample size are important limits of this pivotal study. Nevertheless, DAPT-SHOCK-AMI (Dual Antiplatelet Therapy for Shock Patients with Acute Myocardial Infarction; ClinicalTrials.gov Identifier: NCT03551964) multicenter, randomized, double-blind, ongoing trial will shed light on the use of cangrelor in this population. It will compare a combination of cangrelor and crushed ticagrelor versus ticagrelor alone in patients with MI complicated by initial cardiogenic shock and treated with primary PCI.

18.3.7 Bridge to Surgery with Cangrelor

Treatment with a $P2Y_{12}$ inhibitor increases the risk for peri- and post-operative bleedings. The recommendation for patients after PCI with DES implantation who require non-emergent surgery is to delay the operation until the termination of the prescribed DAPT regimen or minimum after 1 month of DAPT [56]. In patients who need earlier surgery, the recommended timing to stop

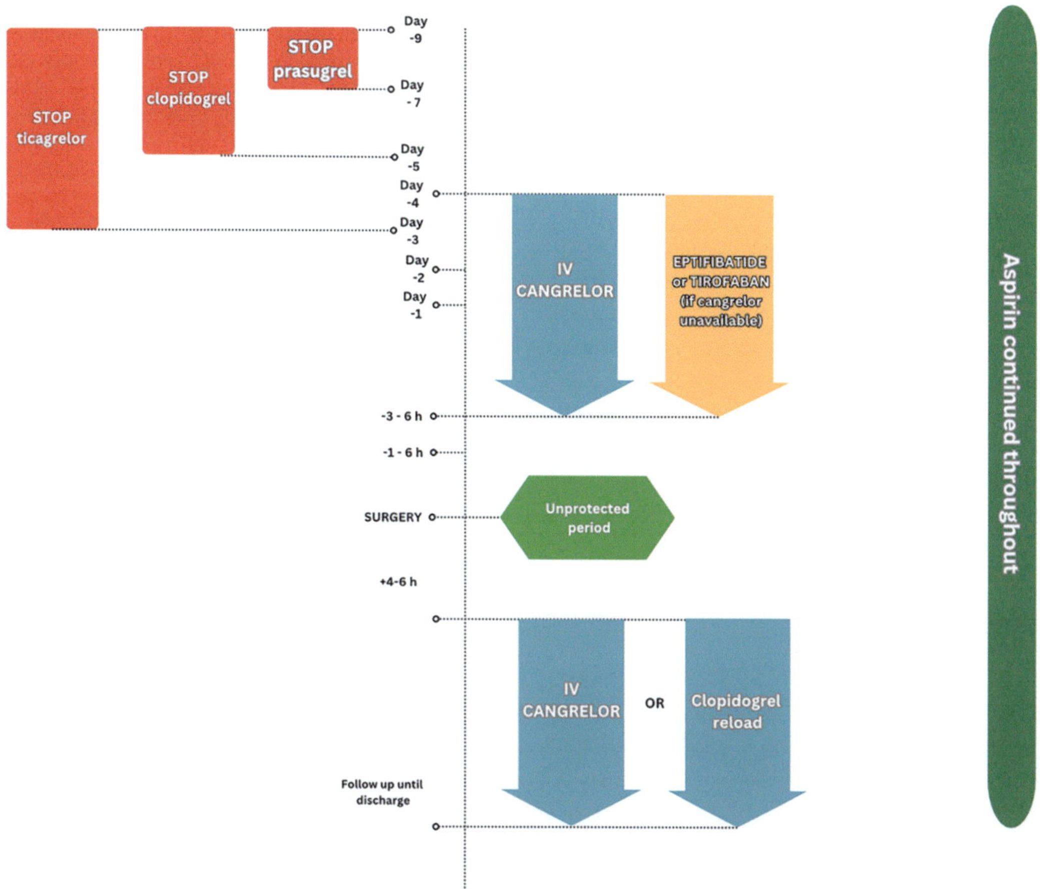

Fig. 18.2 Perioperative bridging protocol with cangrelor. I.V. = intravenous

$P2Y_{12}$ inhibitors before an operation is 7 days for prasugrel, 5 days for clopidogrel, and 3 days for ticagrelor before surgery. However, ACS patients with early stent implantation have a high ischemic risk profile, and the early cessation of DAPT is related to worse outcomes. In this population, the use of intravenous agents may be considered. Cangrelor, with its rapid onset/offset pharmacological profile, may be the ideal $P2Y_{12}$ "bridging" after DAPT discontinuation before surgery.

The BRIDGE trial (n = 210) randomized patients planned to undergo non-emergent CABG, after the discontinuation of the second oral antiplatelet, to cangrelor or placebo for at least 48 h, maintaining aspirin [57]. After an initial open-label phase to identify the correct bridging dose of cangrelor to achieve an antiplatelet effect after oral P2Y12 inhibitor discontinuation, the dose of 0.75 μg/kg/min showed a higher reduction in platelet activity compared to placebo. Additionally, cangrelor did not increase significantly CABG-related bleeding.

Based on the BRIDGE trial protocol, a consensus document advises starting cangrelor as a bridge regimen after the discontinuation of the oral P2Y12 inhibitors and its suspension 1 h before surgery [58]. After that, clopidogrel should be started, with a loading dose of 300 or 600 mg, as soon as possible after surgery. In case of intubation, cangrelor should be restarted. The use of ticagrelor and prasugrel is discouraged (Fig. 18.2).

The more recent MONET BRIDGE study assessed the infusion of cangrelor as I.V. antiplatelet bridge therapy in patients undergoing surgery within 1 year from stent implantation [59], showing that cangrelor as I.V. bridging antiplatelet therapy is safe and feasible in patients at high thrombotic risk. At the 30-day follow-up, no ischemic events were reported and the mean hemoglobin drop was <2 g/dL, with nine patients receiving blood transfusions consistent with the type of surgery. Notably, no life-threatening or fatal bleeding occurred.

The ongoing, multicenter, US national MARS registry (Management of Antiplatelet Regimen During Surgical Procedures; ClinicalTrials.gov Identifier: NCT03981835) will provide further data on perioperative antiplatelet therapy. It will collect preoperative, intraoperative, and postoperative clinical strategies, therapeutic interventions, and 30-day outcomes data of 1500 patients post-PCI scheduled to undergo cardiac or noncardiac surgery.

18.3.8 Cangrelor in Clinical Practice Guidelines

The 2021 American guidelines for Coronary Arteries Revascularization and the 2023 European Society of Cardiology guidelines for the Management of Acute Coronary Syndrome suggest to consider cangrelor in P2Y12 receptor inhibitor-naïve patients undergoing PCI (Class of Recommendation IIB, Level of Evidence B-R and A, respectively).

References

1. Angiolillo DJ, Ueno M, Goto S. Basic principles of platelet biology and clinical implications. Circ J. 2010;74:597–607. https://doi.org/10.1253/circj.cj-09-0982.
2. Capodanno D, Mehran R, Krucoff MW, et al. Defining strategies of modulation of antiplatelet therapy in patients with coronary artery disease: a consensus document from the Academic Research Consortium. Circulation. 2023;147:1933–44. https://doi.org/10.1161/CIRCULATIONAHA.123.064473.
3. Holmes DR, Kereiakes DJ, Garg S, et al. Stent thrombosis. J Am Coll Cardiol. 2010;56:1357–65. https://doi.org/10.1016/j.jacc.2010.07.016.
4. EPILOG Investigators. Platelet glycoprotein IIb/IIIa receptor blockade and low-dose heparin during percutaneous coronary revascularization. N Engl J Med. 1997;336:1689–96. https://doi.org/10.1056/NEJM199706123362401.
5. Mehta SR, Yusuf S, Peters RJ, et al. Effects of pretreatment with clopidogrel and aspirin followed by long-term therapy in patients undergoing percutaneous coronary intervention: the PCI-CURE study. Lancet. 2001;358:527–33. https://doi.org/10.1016/s0140-6736(01)05701-4.
6. Wallentin L, Becker RC, Budaj A, et al. Ticagrelor versus clopidogrel in patients with acute coronary syndromes. N Engl J Med. 2009;361:1045–57. https://doi.org/10.1056/NEJMoa0904327.
7. Wiviott SD, Braunwald E, McCabe CH, et al. Prasugrel versus clopidogrel in patients with acute coronary syndromes. N Engl J Med. 2007;357:2001–15. https://doi.org/10.1056/NEJMoa0706482.
8. Platelet Receptor Inhibition in Ischemic Syndrome Management in Patients Limited by Unstable Signs and Symptoms (PRISM-PLUS) Study Investigators. Inhibition of the platelet glycoprotein IIb/IIIa receptor with tirofiban in unstable angina and non-Q-wave myocardial infarction. N Engl J Med. 1998;338:1488–97. https://doi.org/10.1056/NEJM199805213382102.
9. Platelet Receptor Inhibition in Ischemic Syndrome Management (PRISM) Study Investigators. A comparison of aspirin plus tirofiban with aspirin plus heparin for unstable angina. N Engl J Med. 1998;338:1498–505. https://doi.org/10.1056/NEJM199805213382103.
10. Lawton JS, Tamis-Holland JE, Bangalore S, et al. 2021 ACC/AHA/SCAI Guideline for coronary artery revascularization: executive summary: a report of the American College of Cardiology/American Heart Association Joint Committee on clinical practice guidelines. Circulation. 2022;145:e4–e17. https://doi.org/10.1161/CIR.0000000000001039.
11. Byrne RA, Rossello X, Coughlan JJ, et al. 2023 ESC Guidelines for the management of acute coronary syndromes. Eur Heart J. 2023;44:3720–826. https://doi.org/10.1093/eurheartj/ehad191.
12. Michelson AD, Frelinger AL, Braunwald E, et al. Pharmacodynamic assessment of platelet inhibition by prasugrel vs. clopidogrel in the TRITON-TIMI 38 trial. Eur Heart J. 2009;30:1753–63. https://doi.org/10.1093/eurheartj/ehp159.
13. Parodi G, Valenti R, Bellandi B, et al. Comparison of prasugrel and ticagrelor loading doses in ST-segment elevation myocardial infarction patients: RAPID (Rapid Activity of Platelet Inhibitor Drugs) primary PCI study. J Am Coll Cardiol. 2013;61:1601–6. https://doi.org/10.1016/j.jacc.2013.01.024.
14. Kubica J, Adamski P, Ostrowska M, et al. Morphine delays and attenuates ticagrelor exposure and action in patients with myocardial infarction: the randomized, double-blind, placebo-controlled IMPRESSION trial. Eur Heart J. 2016;37:245–52. https://doi.org/10.1093/eurheartj/ehv547.
15. Hobl E-L, Stimpfl T, Ebner J, et al. Morphine decreases clopidogrel concentrations and effects: a randomized, double-blind, placebo-controlled trial. J Am Coll Cardiol. 2014;63:630–5. https://doi.org/10.1016/j.jacc.2013.10.068.

16. Kristensen SD, Würtz M, Grove EL, et al. Contemporary use of glycoprotein IIb/IIIa inhibitors. Thromb Haemost. 2012;107:215–24. https://doi.org/10.1160/TH11-07-0468.
17. Capodanno D, Milluzzo RP, Angiolillo DJ. Intravenous antiplatelet therapies (glycoprotein IIb/IIIa receptor inhibitors and cangrelor) in percutaneous coronary intervention: from pharmacology to indications for clinical use. Ther Adv Cardiovasc Dis. 2019;13:1753944719893274. https://doi.org/10.1177/1753944719893274.
18. Kastrati A, Mehilli J, Schühlen H, et al. A clinical trial of abciximab in elective percutaneous coronary intervention after pretreatment with clopidogrel. N Engl J Med. 2004;350:232–8. https://doi.org/10.1056/NEJMoa031859.
19. Mehilli J, Kastrati A, Schühlen H, et al. Randomized clinical trial of abciximab in diabetic patients undergoing elective percutaneous coronary interventions after treatment with a high loading dose of clopidogrel. Circulation. 2004;110:3627–35. https://doi.org/10.1161/01.CIR.0000148956.93631.4D.
20. Winchester DE, Wen X, Brearley WD, et al. Efficacy and safety of glycoprotein IIb/IIIa inhibitors during elective coronary revascularization: a meta-analysis of randomized trials performed in the era of stents and thienopyridines. J Am Coll Cardiol. 2011;57:1190–9. https://doi.org/10.1016/j.jacc.2010.10.030.
21. Stone GW, McLaurin BT, Cox DA, et al. Bivalirudin for patients with acute coronary syndromes. N Engl J Med. 2006;355:2203–16. https://doi.org/10.1056/NEJMoa062437.
22. Valgimigli M, Frigoli E, Leonardi S, et al. Radial versus femoral access and bivalirudin versus unfractionated heparin in invasively managed patients with acute coronary syndrome (MATRIX): final 1-year results of a multicentre, randomised controlled trial. Lancet. 2018;392:835–48. https://doi.org/10.1016/S0140-6736(18)31714-8.
23. Erlinge D, Omerovic E, Fröbert O, et al. Bivalirudin versus heparin monotherapy in myocardial infarction. N Engl J Med. 2017;377:1132–42. https://doi.org/10.1056/NEJMoa1706443.
24. De Luca G, Suryapranata H, Stone GW, et al. Abciximab as adjunctive therapy to reperfusion in acute ST-segment elevation myocardial infarction: a meta-analysis of randomized trials. JAMA. 2005;293:1759–65. https://doi.org/10.1001/jama.293.14.1759.
25. Montalescot G, Antoniucci D, Kastrati A, et al. Abciximab in primary coronary stenting of ST-elevation myocardial infarction: a European meta-analysis on individual patients' data with long-term follow-up. Eur Heart J. 2007;28:443–9. https://doi.org/10.1093/eurheartj/ehl472.
26. Van't Hof AWJ, Ten Berg J, Heestermans T, et al. Prehospital initiation of tirofiban in patients with ST-elevation myocardial infarction undergoing primary angioplasty (On-TIME 2): a multicentre, double-blind, randomised controlled trial. Lancet. 2008;372:537–46. https://doi.org/10.1016/S0140-6736(08)61235-0.
27. Heestermans AACM, Van Werkum JW, Hamm C, et al. Marked reduction of early stent thrombosis with pre-hospital initiation of high-dose Tirofiban in ST-segment elevation myocardial infarction. J Thromb Haemost. 2009;7:1612–8. https://doi.org/10.1111/j.1538-7836.2009.03573.x.
28. Stone GW, Witzenbichler B, Guagliumi G, et al. Bivalirudin during primary PCI in acute myocardial infarction. N Engl J Med. 2008;358:2218–30. https://doi.org/10.1056/NEJMoa0708191.
29. Elbadawi A, Elgendy IY, Megaly M, et al. Meta-analysis of randomized trials of intracoronary versus intravenous glycoprotein IIb/IIIa inhibitors in patients with ST-elevation myocardial infarction undergoing primary percutaneous coronary intervention. Am J Cardiol. 2017;120:1055–61. https://doi.org/10.1016/j.amjcard.2017.06.040.
30. Giugliano RP, White JA, Bode C, et al. Early versus delayed, provisional eptifibatide in acute coronary syndromes. N Engl J Med. 2009;360:2176–90. https://doi.org/10.1056/NEJMoa0901316.
31. Stone GW, Bertrand ME, Moses JW, et al. Routine upstream initiation vs deferred selective use of glycoprotein IIb/IIIa inhibitors in acute coronary syndromes: the ACUITY Timing trial. JAMA. 2007;297:591–602. https://doi.org/10.1001/jama.297.6.591.
32. Fung AY, Saw J, Starovoytov A, et al. Abbreviated infusion of eptifibatide after successful coronary intervention The BRIEF-PCI (Brief Infusion of Eptifibatide Following Percutaneous Coronary Intervention) randomized trial. J Am Coll Cardiol. 2009;53:837–45. https://doi.org/10.1016/j.jacc.2008.09.060.
33. Cattaneo M. P2Y12 receptors: structure and function. J Thromb Haemost. 2015;13(Suppl 1):S10–6. https://doi.org/10.1111/jth.12952.
34. Serenelli M, Pavasini R, Vitali F, et al. Efficacy and safety of alternative oral administrations of P2Y12-receptor inhibitors: systematic review and meta-analysis. J Thromb Haemost. 2019;17:944–50. https://doi.org/10.1111/jth.14434.
35. Alexopoulos D, Xanthopoulou I, Gkizas V, et al. Randomized assessment of ticagrelor versus prasugrel antiplatelet effects in patients with ST-segment-elevation myocardial infarction. Circ Cardiovasc Interv. 2012;5:797–804. https://doi.org/10.1161/CIRCINTERVENTIONS.112.972323.
36. Capranzano P, Angiolillo DJ. Tackling the gap in platelet inhibition with oral antiplatelet agents in high-risk patients undergoing percutaneous coronary intervention. Expert Rev Cardiovasc Ther. 2021;19:519–35. https://doi.org/10.1080/14779072.2021.1920925.
37. Akers WS, Oh JJ, Oestreich JH, et al. Pharmacokinetics and pharmacodynamics of a bolus and infusion of cangrelor: a direct, parenteral P2Y12 receptor antagonist. J Clin Pharmacol. 2010;50:27–35. https://doi.org/10.1177/0091270009344986.

38. Waite LH, Phan YL, Spinler SA. Cangrelor: a novel intravenous antiplatelet agent with a questionable future. Pharmacotherapy. 2014;34:1061–76. https://doi.org/10.1002/phar.1471.
39. Franchi F, Rollini F, Muñiz-Lozano A, et al. Cangrelor: a review on pharmacology and clinical trial development. Expert Rev Cardiovasc Ther. 2013;11:1279–91. https://doi.org/10.1586/14779072.2013.837701.
40. Angiolillo DJ, Bhatt DL, Steg PG, et al. Impact of cangrelor overdosing on bleeding complications in patients undergoing percutaneous coronary intervention: insights from the CHAMPION trials. J Thromb Thrombolysis. 2015;40:317–22. https://doi.org/10.1007/s11239-015-1233-3.
41. Bhatt DL, Lincoff AM, Gibson CM, et al. Intravenous platelet blockade with cangrelor during PCI. N Engl J Med. 2009;361:2330–41. https://doi.org/10.1056/NEJMoa0908629.
42. Bhatt DL, Stone GW, Mahaffey KW, et al. Effect of platelet inhibition with cangrelor during PCI on ischemic events. N Engl J Med. 2013;368:1303–13. https://doi.org/10.1056/NEJMoa1300815.
43. Généreux P, Stone GW, Harrington RA, et al. Impact of intraprocedural stent thrombosis during percutaneous coronary intervention: insights from the CHAMPION PHOENIX Trial (Clinical Trial Comparing Cangrelor to Clopidogrel Standard of Care Therapy in Subjects Who Require Percutaneous Coronary Intervention). J Am Coll Cardiol. 2014;63:619–29. https://doi.org/10.1016/j.jacc.2013.10.022.
44. Steg PG, Bhatt DL, Hamm CW, et al. Effect of cangrelor on periprocedural outcomes in percutaneous coronary interventions: a pooled analysis of patient-level data. Lancet. 2013;382:1981–92. https://doi.org/10.1016/S0140-6736(13)61615-3.
45. Gutierrez JA, Harrington RA, Blankenship JC, et al. The effect of cangrelor and access site on ischaemic and bleeding events: insights from CHAMPION PHOENIX. Eur Heart J. 2016;37:1122–30. https://doi.org/10.1093/eurheartj/ehv498.
46. Abtan J, Steg PG, Stone GW, et al. Efficacy and safety of cangrelor in preventing periprocedural complications in patients with stable angina and acute coronary syndromes undergoing percutaneous coronary intervention: the CHAMPION PHOENIX trial. JACC Cardiovasc Interv. 2016;9:1905–13. https://doi.org/10.1016/j.jcin.2016.06.046.
47. Franchi F, Rollini F, Rivas A, et al. Platelet inhibition with cangrelor and crushed ticagrelor in patients with ST-segment-elevation myocardial infarction undergoing primary percutaneous coronary intervention. Circulation. 2019;139:1661–70. https://doi.org/10.1161/CIRCULATIONAHA.118.038317.
48. Franchi F, Ortega-Paz L, Rollini F, et al. Cangrelor in patients with coronary artery disease pretreated with ticagrelor: the switching antiplatelet (SWAP)-5 study. JACC Cardiovasc Interv. 2023;16:36–46. https://doi.org/10.1016/j.jcin.2022.10.034.
49. De Luca L, Calabrò P, Capranzano P, et al. Safety of cangrelor and transition to oral P2Y12 inhibitors in patients undergoing percutaneous coronary intervention: the ARCANGELO study. Eur Heart J Open. 2023;3:oead076. https://doi.org/10.1093/ehjopen/oead076.
50. Angiolillo DJ, Schneider DJ, Bhatt DL, et al. Pharmacodynamic effects of cangrelor and clopidogrel: the platelet function substudy from the cangrelor versus standard therapy to achieve optimal management of platelet inhibition (CHAMPION) trials. J Thromb Thrombolysis. 2012;34:44–55. https://doi.org/10.1007/s11239-012-0737-3.
51. Schneider DJ, Seecheran N, Raza SS, et al. Pharmacodynamic effects during the transition between cangrelor and prasugrel. Coron Artery Dis. 2015;26:42–8. https://doi.org/10.1097/MCA.0000000000000158.
52. Schneider DJ, Agarwal Z, Seecheran N, et al. Pharmacodynamic effects during the transition between cangrelor and ticagrelor. JACC Cardiovasc Interv. 2014;7:435–42. https://doi.org/10.1016/j.jcin.2013.08.017.
53. Rauber M, Nicol P, Sabic E, et al. Timing and predictors of definite stent thrombosis in comatose survivors of out-of-hospital cardiac arrest undergoing percutaneous coronary intervention and therapeutic hypothermia (ST-OHCA study). EuroIntervention. 2022;18:740–8. https://doi.org/10.4244/EIJ-D-22-00336.
54. Steblovnik K, Blinc A, Mijovski MB, et al. Ticagrelor versus clopidogrel in comatose survivors of out-of-hospital cardiac arrest undergoing percutaneous coronary intervention and hypothermia: a randomized study. Circulation. 2016;134:2128–30. https://doi.org/10.1161/CIRCULATIONAHA.116.024872.
55. Kordis P, Bozic Mijovski M, Berden J, et al. Cangrelor for comatose survivors of out-of-hospital cardiac arrest undergoing percutaneous coronary intervention: the CANGRELOR-OHCA study. EuroIntervention. 2023;18:1269–71. https://doi.org/10.4244/EIJ-D-22-00675.
56. Valgimigli M, Bueno H, Byrne RA, et al. 2017 ESC focused update on dual antiplatelet therapy in coronary artery disease developed in collaboration with EACTS: the Task Force for dual antiplatelet therapy in coronary artery disease of the European Society of Cardiology (ESC) and of the European Association for Cardio-Thoracic Surgery (EACTS). Eur Heart J. 2018;39:213–60. https://doi.org/10.1093/eurheartj/ehx419.
57. Angiolillo DJ, Firstenberg MS, Price MJ, et al. Bridging antiplatelet therapy with cangrelor in

patients undergoing cardiac surgery: a randomized controlled trial. JAMA. 2012;307:265–74. https://doi.org/10.1001/jama.2011.2002.
58. Rossini R, Tarantini G, Musumeci G, et al. A multidisciplinary approach on the perioperative antithrombotic management of patients with coronary stents undergoing surgery: surgery after stenting 2. JACC Cardiovasc Interv. 2018;11:417–34. https://doi.org/10.1016/j.jcin.2017.10.051.
59. Rossini R, Masiero G, Fruttero C, et al. Antiplatelet therapy with cangrelor in patients undergoing surgery after coronary stent implantation: a real-world bridging protocol experience. TH Open. 2020;4:e437–45. https://doi.org/10.1055/s-0040-1721504.

Parenteral Anticoagulant Therapy 19

Francesco Franchi and Fabiana Rollini

Adjunctive pharmacotherapy, in particular antithrombotic therapy, has a pivotal role in optimizing outcomes in patients undergoing percutaneous coronary intervention (PCI). Plaque rupture or erosion leading to thrombosis in the coronary arteries represents the primary cause of acute coronary syndrome (ACS) [1]. This process is mediated by many activating factors, mainly thromboxane A_2, adenosine diphosphate, and thrombin, which activate intraplatelet signaling pathways leading to enhanced interactions among adherent platelets and further recruitment and activation of circulating platelets. In addition, vascular injury also exposes subendothelial tissue factor, which activates the coagulation cascade leading to thrombin generation [2]. Thrombin converts fibrinogen to fibrin, an essential component of arterial thrombus, and represents one of the most potent platelet activators by binding to protease-activated receptors (PARs) on the platelet membrane [1, 2]. Indeed, thrombin levels are known to be particularly high in the initial phase of an ACS [3]. Therefore, antithrombotic therapy in the early phase of an ACS plays a fundamental role in the reduction of thrombus burden and flow obstruction at the site of the culprit lesion [1, 4]. In addition, side branch occlusion, slow coronary flow, distal embolization, and iatrogenic plaque disruption are potential mechanisms of atherothrombotic complications during PCI for chronic coronary disease (CCD). The use of foreign surfaces, such as stent platforms and devices during PCI, can also trigger platelet activation and the coagulation cascade [1, 4, 5]. Therefore, the use of parenteral anticoagulation plays a fundamental role in the reduction of thrombus burden and flow obstruction at the site of the culprit lesion in ACS and of atherothrombotic complications associated to PCI, representing a key antithrombotic strategy to be used during PCI for both ACS and CCD patients [6–8].

Over the past four decades, there has been an evolution in the approach to antithrombotic treatment regimens used in patients undergoing PCI. This may be attributed to significant improvement in stent technologies, leading to safer (i.e., less thrombogenic) stent platforms, the development of new antithrombotic drugs, as well as an understanding of the prognostic implications associated with bleeding. This underscores the need to define antithrombotic strategies that mitigate bleeding without any trade-off in thrombotic events [9, 10]. This chapter is aimed to review currently available parenteral anticoagulant therapies for patients undergoing PCI, with a particular focus on patients with high bleeding risk (HBR).

F. Franchi (✉) · F. Rollini
Division of Cardiology, University of Florida College of Medicine-Jacksonville, Jacksonville, FL, USA
e-mail: francesco.franchi@jax.ufl.edu

B. Cortese, S. Rigattieri (eds.), *High Bleeding Risk Patients in Interventional Cardiology*,
https://doi.org/10.1007/978-3-031-87302-7_19

19.1 Pharmacology and Clinical Trial Development of Parenteral Anticoagulants in PCI

Anticoagulant therapy is mandatory during PCI [6–8]. Anticoagulant drugs available for parenteral use are (1) factor II inhibitors (antithrombin), which include indirect thrombin inhibitors (unfractionated heparin [UFH] and low-molecular-weight heparin [LMWH]), and the direct thrombin inhibitors bivalirudin and argatroban, and (2) the factor X inhibitor fondaparinux. These agents have different mechanisms of action, binding specificity, pharmacokinetic and pharmacodynamic consistency, risks of heparin-induced thrombocytopenia (HIT), effects on platelet function, and half-lives (Table 19.1) [4]. Because of the high rate of catheter thrombosis recorded in the OASIS-6 trial, fondaparinux is not recommended as background anticoagulant for PCI, and therefore it will not be discussed.

19.2 Unfractionated Heparin

UFH is a sulfated polysaccharide with a molecular weight range of 3000–30,000 kDa (mean, 15,000 kDa). Its major anticoagulant effect is based on inactivation of thrombin and activated factor X (factor Xa) by forming a complex with antithrombin (AT). The heparin/AT complex inactivates not only thrombin but also factors Xa, IXa, XIa, and XIIa (Fig. 19.1) [4, 11]. Besides hemorrhagic complications, the major side effect of UFH is the risk of HIT, which is a serious, potentially lethal, immunologically mediated adverse drug reaction to UFH or, less commonly, to LMWH. It occurs in 0.1–5.0% of patients receiving heparin when the heparin molecule binds to platelet factor 4. The treatment of HIT includes termination of heparin therapy (both UFH and LMWH), use of alternative anticoagulants which do not bind to platelet factor 4 (i.e. the direct thrombin inhibitors argatroban or bivalirudin), and platelet transfusion in severely thrombocytopenic patients with bleeding [12].

Table 19.1 Pharmacological properties of parenteral anticoagulants

	UFH	Enoxaparin	Bivalirudin
Administration route	IV	IV, SC	IV
Factor Xa:IIa inhibition	1:1	3–4:1	Only IIa
Action independent of AT	No	No	Yes
Nonspecific binding	Yes	Partial	No
Variable PK/PD measures	Yes	Yes (<UFH)	No
Inhibits fibrin-bound thrombin	No	No	Yes
Effect on platelets	Activation	Activation	Inhibition
Half-life	~60 min	90–120 min[a]	25 min
Risk of HIT	Yes	Yes (<UFH)	No
Dose in PCI	70–100 U/kg bolus with GPIs[b] 50–70 U/kg bolus without GPIs[b]	0.5 mg/kg IV bolus	0.75 mg/kg IV bolus 1.75 mg/kg/h infusion
Reversal agent	Protamine sulfate	No	No

Modified with permission from Franchi et al. [4]

AT antithrombin, *GPIs* glycoprotein IIb/IIIa inhibitors, *HIT* heparin-induced thrombocytopenia, *IV* intravenous, *PD* pharmacodynamic, *PK* pharmacokinetic, *PCI* percutaneous coronary intervention, *SC* subcutaneous, *UFH* unfractionated heparin

[a]After IV administration of 0.5 mg/kg

[b]Further boluses needed to maintain therapeutic activated clotting time

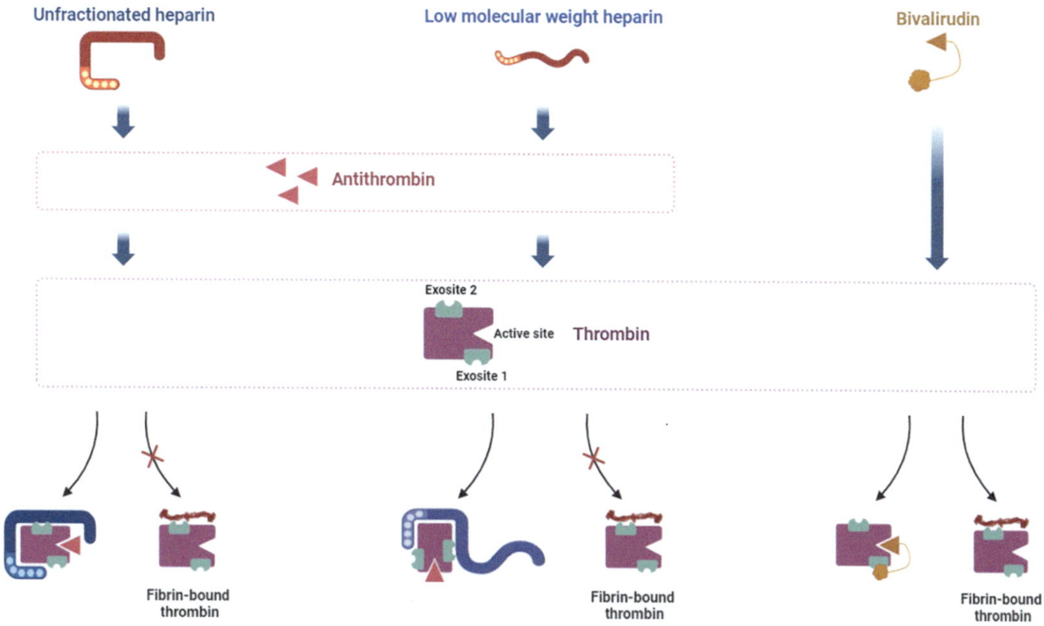

Fig. 19.1 Mechanism of action of unfractionated heparin, low-molecular-weight heparin and bivalirudin. The anticoagulant activity of UFH and LMWH is dependent on the presence of antithrombin and the ability to generate a ternary heparin–thrombin–antithrombin complex that binds exosite 2 (heparin-binding site) and the active site. Bivalirudin, a direct thrombin inhibitor, simultaneously binds the exosite 1 (fibrin binding site) and the active site. Because bivalirudin, but not the heparin–antithrombin complex, can bind exosite 1, only bivalirudin is able to inhibit the activity of both soluble thrombin and thrombin bound to fibrin, as is the case of an already formed blood clot. UFH: unfractionated heparin; LMWH: low-molecular-weight heparin. (Reproduced with permission from Galli et al. [18])

As the only parenteral anticoagulant available for many years, UFH has been the standard of care for PCI and the primary comparator for trials with newer anticoagulants. No placebo-controlled trials have evaluated UFH in PCI, but intravenous UFH titrated to an optimal activated clotting time (ACT) represents a familiar and extensively experienced strategy during PCI for both ACS and CCD [6–8]. Dosage should follow standard recommendations for PCI, taking into account the use of GPIs (70- to 100-U/kg bolus with no GPIs use planned and 50- to 70-U/kg bolus with GPIs), to achieve therapeutic ACT (250–300 s without GPIs use and 200–250 s with GPIs use). In patients who had received previous anticoagulant therapy before PCI, additional UFH should be administered as needed (e.g., 2000–5000 U) to achieve the target ACT [6–8].

19.3 Low-Molecular-Weight Heparin

LMWHs are derived from UFH by chemical or enzymatic depolymerization to yield fragments approximately one-third the molecular weight of UFH (mean molecular weight of 4000–5000 kDa) [4, 11]. The lower molecular weight translates into reduced binding to protein and cells compared with UFH, a longer plasma half-life and a more predictable dose–response profile. This allows LMWHs to be administered in weight-adjusted fixed doses, without the need for laboratory monitoring, and leads to lower risk of osteopenia and HIT [4, 11]. Similar to UFH, LMWHs produce their major anticoagulant effect by enhancing AT activity (Fig. 19.1) [4, 11]. Different LMWHs are approved for use in the

USA, Europe, and Canada. However, the most extensively tested in the setting of PCI is enoxaparin. The major limitation of this class of agents is that clearance is predominantly renal and use is generally not recommended in patients with creatinine clearance of less than 30 mL/min, due to increased risk of bleeding [13].

Enoxaparin has been tested in trials both in ACS and CCD and is overall considered a safe alternative to UFH. The STEEPLE trial, conducted in patients ($n = 3528$) undergoing elective PCI, showed that enoxaparin was associated with a reduction in major bleeding events as compared to UFH, with more predictable anticoagulation levels [14]. In patients with non-ST-segment elevation (NSTE)-ACS, the SYNERGY [15] and A–Z [16] trials showed enoxaparin to be non-inferior to UFH, with no difference in rates of death, myocardial infarction (MI), or major bleeding. Enoxaparin was compared with UFH in primary PCI patients in the ATOLL trial [17]. In this trial, patients (n = 910) with ST-segment elevation MI (STEMI) were randomly assigned to receive an intravenous bolus of 0.5 mg/kg of enoxaparin or UFH before primary PCI. Enoxaparin did not significantly reduce the incidence of the primary endpoint of the trial (a composite of death, complication of MI, procedure failure, or major bleeding at 30 days) as compared with UFH. However, enoxaparin led to a significant 41% relative reduction of the composite main secondary endpoint of death, recurrent ACS, or urgent revascularization (7% vs. 11%; p = 0.015), without increasing the risk of major bleeding (5% vs. 5%; p = 0.79). Of note, crossover between anticoagulants or simultaneous administration of both was associated with the worst outcomes.

19.4 Bivalirudin

The direct thrombin inhibitor bivalirudin is a synthetic derivative of hirudin. It's a polypeptide of 20 amino acids that binds to thrombin at both the active site and the fibrinogen-binding site (exosite 1) without the need for a cofactor [4, 11, 18]. Given its mechanism of action, bivalirudin can bind to and inhibit the activity of not only soluble thrombin but also thrombin bound to fibrin, as is the case of an already formed blood clot (Fig. 19.1). Administered with intravenous infusion, bivalirudin has a linear dose–response profile which translates into an immediate (2–15 min) and predictable anticoagulant effect, with no need for routine coagulation monitoring and rapid offset after stopping the infusion [4, 11, 18]. Only 20% of bivalirudin clearance is dependent on kidneys and its half-life increases from 25 min to 1 h in patients with severe kidney disease and 3.5 h in patients undergoing hemodialysis. Additionally, bivalirudin does not bind extensively to blood proteins and is associated with a notably lower incidence of HIT compared with UFH. Bivalirudin is used as bolus (0.75 mg/kg i.v.) followed by a low (0.25 mg/kg/h)- or high-dose (1.75 mg/kg/h) infusion lasting 2–6 h [4, 11, 18].

Several clinical trials have been conducted in the last two decades comparing bivalirudin vs. heparin in patients with NSTE-ACS and STEMI.

19.4.1 NSTE-ACS

ACUITY was the first trial testing bivalirudin in patients (n = 13,819) with NSTE-ACS undergoing PCI. Patients were randomized to either: (1) UFH or enoxaparin plus glycoprotein IIb/IIIa inhibitor (GPI), (2) bivalirudin plus GPI, and (3) bivalirudin alone [19]. A GPI was used during PCI in 9.1% of patients treated with bivalirudin alone. The primary outcomes of the trial were the 30-day rates of composite ischemic endpoints (including death, MI, or unplanned revascularization for ischemia), major bleeding, and the net clinical outcome (net adverse clinical event [NACE], a combination of composite ischemic or major bleeding). Bivalirudin plus GPI was non-inferior to UFH plus GPI for all the three outcomes. Importantly, bivalirudin alone resulted in non-inferiority for the composite ischemic endpoint compared with UFH plus GPI but showed significantly lower rates of major bleeding and NACE [19]. Limitations of this study lie in the fact that it did not compare bivalirudin versus

UFH regardless of GPI use (i.e., bivalirudin alone versus UFH alone) and that bivalirudin infusion was not continued after PCI. Moreover, the use of radial access and potent $P2Y_{12}$ inhibitors was far lower than in current practice.

The ISAR-REACT trial randomized NSTE-ACS patients ($n = 1721$) to either abciximab plus UFH (70 UI/kg) or bivalirudin (bolus of 0.75 mg/kg, followed by high-dose infusion of 1.75 mg/kg/h for the duration of PCI) [20]. The primary endpoint was a composite of death, large recurrent MI, urgent target-vessel revascularization, or major bleeding within 30 days. No statistically significant differences were observed between the two treatment groups in terms of the primary endpoints at 30 days. However, bivalirudin significantly reduced rates of 30-day major bleeding events. Limitations of the study include that a GPI was routinely used in the UFH group, bivalirudin infusion was not continued after PCI, and clopidogrel was the only $P2Y_{12}$ inhibitor used [20].

19.4.2 STEMI

Major trials comparing bivalirudin vs. heparin in STEMI are summarized in Table 19.2. HORIZONS-AMI was the first trial comparing UFH plus GPI versus bivalirudin alone in STEMI patient ($n = 3602$) undergoing PCI [21]. The primary endpoints were major bleeding and NACE (major bleeding plus major adverse cardiovascular events [MACE]). At 30 days, bivalirudin alone showed a significant 40% reduction of NACE, mainly due to a reduction in major bleeding, compared with UFH plus GPI. Notably, bivalirudin significantly reduced cardiac death by 38% and death from all causes by 34% compared with UFH plus GPI. Although MACE were similar between the two treatments, bivalirudin use led to a fourfold increase in the rate of acute (≤24 h) stent thrombosis (ST, 1.3% vs. 0.3%; $p < 0.001$) with no differences in subacute (>24 h to 30 days) [21]. The high incidence of acute ST in the bivalirudin group might have been related to the use of clopidogrel (300 mg in one-third of patients) and the termination of bivalirudin infusion at the end of PCI in most of the patients. Interestingly, a post hoc analysis of this trial suggested that a UFH bolus administered before bivalirudin administration could lead to an attenuated risk of acute ST without increasing major bleeding [22].

The EUROMAX trial aimed to investigate whether the benefit of bivalirudin over heparin in primary PCI persisted in the setting of a more contemporary approach characterized by the optional use of GPI and use of radial access and of the more potent $P2Y_{12}$ receptor inhibitors prasugrel and ticagrelor [23]. In the trial, patients ($n = 2218$) with STEMI transported for primary PCI were randomly assigned to receive either bivalirudin or heparin plus optional GPI, initiated in the ambulance or in a non-PCI-capable hospital. Bivalirudin was administered as a bolus of 0.75 mg/kg, and differently from HORIZON-AMI, it was followed by an infusion lasting at least 4 h after PCI (1.75 mg/kg/h during PCI and 0.25 mg/kg/h after PCI). The use of GPI was allowed in both treatment arms: in the bivalirudin group only as a bailout strategy and in the UFH arm either as a routine or bailout strategy according to physician preferences. This design led to a very high use of GPI in the UFH group (69%). The primary endpoint of death or major bleeding not associated with coronary artery bypass grafting at 30 days was reduced with bivalirudin compared to heparin (5.1% vs. 8.5%, $p = 0.001$), mainly driven by a 57% reduction in major bleeding. Although no differences in mortality were observed, bivalirudin use was associated with a sixfold increase in the rate of acute ST (1.1% vs. 0.2%; $p = 0.007$). This occurred despite prolonged bivalirudin infusion post-PCI (in 93% of patients, of whom 22.5% received the PCI dose) and the use of prasugrel or ticagrelor in half the patients [23]. However, the risk of ST seemed to be mitigated by prolonging the bivalirudin infusion at the PCI dose [24]. A meta-analysis combining the results from HORIZONS-AMI and EUROMAX trials confirmed that patients receiving bivalirudin had a higher rate of ST compared to UFH plus GPI, mainly in the first 4 h after PCI. However, bivalirudin was associated with a 26% reduction in 30-day NACE and a significant reduction in bleeding, thrombocytopenia, and transfusion rates compared to UFH plus GPI [25].

Table 19.2 Major randomized clinical trials of bivalirudin vs. heparin in STEMI

	HORIZONS-AMI	EUROMAX	HEAT-PPCI	BRIGHT	BRIGHT-4
Trial design					
Patient population	3602 STEMI undergoing PPCI	2218 STEMI transported for PPCI	1812 STEMI undergoing PPCI	2194 acute MI undergoing emergency PCI (87.7% STEMI)	6016 STEMI undergoing primary PCI
Type of heparin	UFH	UFH or enoxaparin	UFH	UFH	UFH
Heparin dose[a]	60 U/kg with subsequent boluses targeted to ACT of 200–250 s	UFH: 100 U/kg without GPI or 60 U/kg with GPI Enoxaparin: 0.5 mg/kg	70 U/kg	100 U/kg in heparin only group 60 U/kg in heparin plus tirofiban group	70 U/kg
GPI use in heparin arm	Routine (97.7% of patients)	Routine or bailout (69% of patients)	Bailout (14% of patients)	Bailout (5.6% of patients) in heparin only group; Routine (100%) in heparin plus tirofiban group	Bailout (13.7% of patients)
GPI use in bivalirudin arm	Bailout (7.5% of patients)	Bailout (11.5% of patients)	Bailout (14% of patients)	Bailout (4.4% of patients)	Bailout (11.5% of patients)
Post-PCI bivalirudin infusion	None (but could be continued at low doses if clinically indicated)	4 h after PCI at 0.25 mg/kg/h. Continuation of PCI dose was also permitted (22.5%)	None	30 min to 4 h after PCI (mean 180 min) at PCI dose	2–4 h after PCI (median 3 h) at PCI dose
$P2Y_{12}$ receptor inhibitor	Clopidogrel 300–600 mg	Clopidogrel (50%), prasugrel (30%), or ticagrelor (20%)	Clopidogrel (11%), prasugrel (27%), or ticagrelor (62%)	Clopidogrel 300–600 mg	Clopidogrel (34%) or ticagrelor (66%)
Radial access	No	47% of patients	81% of patients	78% of patients	93% of patients
Primary endpoint	NACE [major bleeding or MACE (death, reinfarction, target-vessel revascularization for ischemia, and stroke)] at 30 days Non-CABG major bleeding at 30 days	Death or non-CABG-related major bleeding at 30 days	Efficacy: MACE (all-cause death, CVA, reinfarction, or additional unplanned TLR) at 28 days Safety: Major bleeding at 28 days	NACE (MACE [all-cause death, reinfarction, ischemia-driven TVR, or stroke] or any bleeding) at 30 days	All-cause death or BARC types 3–5 bleeding at 30 days
Bleeding definition	Protocol-defined[b]	Protocol-defined[c]	BARC type 3–5	BARC	BARC
Study results					

(continued)

Table 19.2 (continued)

	HORIZONS-AMI	EUROMAX	HEAT-PPCI	BRIGHT	BRIGHT-4
Primary endpoint(s)	NACE: Bivalirudin 9.2% Heparin 12.1% $p = 0.005$ Non-CABG major bleeding: Bivalirudin 4.9% Heparin 8.3% $p < 0.001$	Bivalirudin 5.1% Heparin 8.5% $p = 0.001$	NACE: Bivalirudin 8.7% Heparin 5.7% $p = 0.02$ Major bleeding: Bivalirudin 3.5% Heparin 3.1% $p = 0.59$	Bivalirudin 8.8% Heparin 13.2% Heparin plus tirofiban 17.0% $p < 0.001$	Bivalirudin 3.06% Heparin 4.39% $p = 0.007$
MACE	Bivalirudin 5.4% Heparin 5.5% $p = 0.95$	Bivalirudin 6.0% Heparin 5.5% $p = 0.64$	See primary endpoint	Bivalirudin 5.0% Heparin 5.8% Heparin plus tirofiban 4.9% $p = 0.83$	Bivalirudin 4.09% Heparin 5.15% $p = 0.051$ All-cause death: Bivalirudin 2.96% Heparin 3.92% $p = 0.042$
Major bleeding	See primary endpoint	Bivalirudin 2.6% Heparin 6.0% $p < 0.001$	See primary endpoint	BARC type 3–5: Bivalirudin 0.5% Heparin 1.5% Heparin plus tirofiban 2.1% p = n/a	Bivalirudin 0.17% Heparin 0.80% $p = 0.001$
Acute stent thrombosis (≤24 h)	Bivalirudin 1.3% Heparin 0.3% $p < 0.001$	Bivalirudin 1.1% Heparin 0.2% $p = 0.007$	Bivalirudin 2.9% Heparin 0.9% $p = 0.007$	Bivalirudin 0.3% Heparin 0.3% Heparin plus tirofiban 0.3% p = n/a	Bivalirudin 0.13% Heparin 0.47% $p = 0.027$

Modified with permission from Franchi et al. [4]

Bivalirudin dose was 0.75 mg/kg bolus followed by 1.75 mg/kg/h for the duration of PCI in all studies

ACS acute coronary syndrome, *BARC* Bleeding Academic Research Consortium, *CABG* coronary artery bypass graft, *CVA* cardiovascular accident, *GPI* glycoprotein IIb/IIIa inhibitors, *MACE* major adverse cardiovascular events, *NACE* net adverse clinical events, *STEMI* ST-segment elevation myocardial infarction, *PPCI* primary percutaneous coronary intervention, *TLR* target lesion revascularization, *TVR* target vessel revascularization, *UFH* unfractionated heparin

[a]Initial bolus dose. Subsequent UFH boluses were to be administered to maintain target ACT

[b]Major bleeding: intracranial or intraocular hemorrhage; bleeding at the access site, with a hematoma that was 5 cm or larger or that required intervention; a decrease in the hemoglobin level of 4 g/dL or more without an overt bleeding source or 3 g/dL or more with an overt bleeding source; reoperation for bleeding; or blood transfusion

[c]Major bleeding: intracranial, retroperitoneal, or intraocular bleeding; access-site hemorrhage requiring radiologic or surgical intervention; a reduction in the hemoglobin level of more than 4 g/dL without an overt source of bleeding; a reduction in the hemoglobin level of more than 3 g/dL with an overt source of bleeding; reintervention for bleeding; or use of any blood-product transfusion

The single-center open-label HEAT-PPCI trial was designed to overcome potential biases in previous studies, such as the unbalanced use of GPI among arms observed in EUROMAX. In the trial, STEMI patients ($n = 1812$) were randomly allocated to bivalirudin (bolus of 0.75 mg/kg, followed by infusion of 1.75 mg/kg/h until the end of PCI) or UFH, and only provisional use of GPI was allowed in both groups [26]. The study showed that UFH led to a lower incidence of 28-day MACE compared to bivalirudin, without any difference in major bleeding events. Remarkably, the study highlighted that the use of UFH could substantially reduce drug costs. Bivalirudin use was associated with a more than threefold increase in the rate of acute ST (2.9%

vs. 0.9%; $p = 0.007$). Of note, the acute ST rate with bivalirudin was two to three times higher than in any prior study, likely related to the very short duration of infusion, which was not continued post-PCI.

In the BRAVE-4 trial, STEMI patients with planned primary PCI were randomly assigned to a strategy based on prasugrel plus bivalirudin or a strategy based on clopidogrel plus UFH. The trial was terminated early due to slow recruitment after 548 patients (of the 1240 planned) were randomized. No difference in the primary outcome (a composite of 30-day MACE or major bleeding) was shown between the two strategies, although the results should be interpreted with caution because the trial was underpowered [27].

In the BRIGHT trial, a total of 2194 patients with acute MI undergoing emergency PCI were randomized to three treatment arms: (1) bivalirudin with post-PCI high-dose 1.75 mg/kg/h infusion (median duration 3 h), (2) UFH alone, and (3) UFH plus tirofiban with a post-PCI infusion. Although the trial was designed to include both NSTEMI and STEMI patients, nearly 90% of enrolled patients were STEMI. Bivalirudin with a post-PCI infusion decreased NACE compared with the other two arms, driven by a reduction in bleeding events, without any increase in MACE or ST, likely due to the routine use of a prolonged post-procedural bivalirudin infusion at PCI dose [28].

The recent BRIGHT-4 trial is a large, open-label, multicenter trial conducted in China and involving 6016 STEMI patients undergoing PCI by radial artery access [29]. Patients were randomly assigned to receive bivalirudin with a high-dose post-PCI infusion (mean duration 3 h) vs. UFH alone. Moreover, GPIs were allowed solely as bailout strategy in both arms, minimizing potential confounding effects. Bivalirudin significantly reduced the primary endpoint (composite of all-cause death or Bleeding Academic Research Consortium [BARC] 3–5 bleeding) at 30 days, compared to UFH. Moreover, bivalirudin significantly reduced BARC 3–5 bleeding, acute ST, and cardiovascular death, compared with UFH. However, it is important to acknowledge that this trial, similarly to BRIGHT, was conducted exclusively in China, and these findings might not be generalizable to non-east Asian populations [29].

19.4.3 NSTE-ACS and STEMI

In the MATRIX trial, patients ($n = 7213$) with ACS for whom PCI was anticipated were randomized to receive either bivalirudin or UFH [30]. The co-primary outcomes were the incidence of MACE (a composite of death, MI, or stroke) and NACE (a composite of non-CABG BARC 3 or 5 bleeding or MACE) at 30 days. The trial showed that the rates of MACE and NACE were not significantly lower with bivalirudin than with UFH, despite a significant reduction in major bleeding, all-cause death, and cardiac death. Acute ST rates were similar between treatment groups. Of note, the effects were consistent in both the NSTE-ACS and STEMI cohorts. However, bivalirudin seemed to be more effective and safer than heparin in the subgroup of STEMI patients with chronic kidney disease and in those with prior use of UFH [31]. Additionally, in the trial, patients in the bivalirudin group were further randomized to receive or not a post-PCI bivalirudin infusion (full or reduced dose at operator discretion). Bivalirudin infusion following PCI was not associated with a decreased rate of urgent target-vessel revascularization, definite ST, or NACE at 30 days, compared with UFH. However, the full dose compared with the reduced-dose infusion regimen was associated with a significant reduction in urgent target-vessel revascularization, definite ST, or NACE, that was consistent across ACS types [32].

VALIDATE-SWEDEHEART was a multicenter, randomized, registry-based, open-label clinical trial, enrolling NSTE-ACS ($n = 3001$) and STEMI ($n = 3005$) patients undergoing PCI using radial access and receiving treatment with a potent $P2Y_{12}$ inhibitor (ticagrelor, prasugrel, or cangrelor), without the planned use of a GPI [33]. Patients were randomized to bivalirudin alone (bolus of 0.75 mg/kg, followed by high-dose infusion of 1.75 mg/kg/h) or UFH. The primary endpoint (death, MI, or major bleeding at 180 days), as well as the individual outcome of ST and major bleeding, did not differ between the two treatment arms. The results were consistent in patients with STEMI and in those with NSTEMI and across other major subgroups. Limitations of this study are being registry-based, the open-label design, and the fact that post-PCI bivalirudin infusion was not used in all patients (65%) and was relatively short (mean 57 min).

Recently, an individual patient data meta-analysis of patients (n = 12,155) with NSTEMI in all five large trials that randomized patients with any MI undergoing PCI to bivalirudin versus heparin showed that procedural anticoagulation with bivalirudin or heparin did not result in significantly different rates of mortality or ischemic events, including ST and reinfarction. However, bivalirudin reduced serious bleeding compared with heparin arising both from the access site and nonaccess sites [34]. Another recent meta-analysis of trials comparing bivalirudin followed by a post-PCI high-dose infusion versus heparin without routine GPI in ACS, accounting for a total of 16,920 patients, showed bivalirudin to be associated with a nonsignificant reduction in 30-day all-cause death compared with UFH. In addition, bivalirudin followed by a high-dose infusion seemed to be associated with reduced ST and NACE [35].

19.5 Guideline Recommendations

The latest guideline recommendations for the use of intravenous anticoagulant agents in patients undergoing PCI are summarized in Table 19.3.

UFH currently has a class of recommendations (COR) 1 for anticoagulation during PCI for both ACS and CCD patients in both American College of Cardiology (ACC)/American Heart

Table 19.3 Current guideline recommendations for parenteral anticoagulants

	Recommendations	COR/LOE
CCD		
ACC/AHA/SCAI	In patients undergoing PCI, administration of intravenous UFH is useful to reduce ischemic events.	1 C-EO
	In patients with HIT undergoing PCI, bivalirudin or argatroban should be used to replace UFH to avoid thrombotic complications	1 C-LD
ESC	Unfractionated heparin is indicated as the standard anticoagulant (70–100 U/kg)	1 B
	Bivalirudin (0.75 mg/kg bolus, 1.75 mg/kg/h for up to 4 h after the procedure) is indicated in the case of HIT.	1 C
	Enoxaparin (IV 0.5 mg/kg) should be considered as an alternative agent	2a B
ACS		
ACC/AHA/SCAI	In patients undergoing PCI, administration of intravenous UFH is useful to reduce ischemic events	1 C-EO
	In patients with ACS, intravenous enoxaparin may be considered as an alternative to UFH at the time of PCI to reduce ischemic events	2b B-R
	In patients with STEMI undergoing PCI, bivalirudin is useful as an alternative to UFH to reduce mortality and bleeding	1 B-R
ESC	Routine use of a UFH bolus (70–100 U/kg) is recommended in patients undergoing PCI.	1 C
	IV enoxaparin at the time of PCI should be considered in patients pretreated with subcutaneous enoxaparin.	2a B
	Enoxaparin should be considered as an alternative to UFH in patients with STEMI undergoing primary PCI.	2a A
	For patients with NSTE-ACS in whom early invasive angiography (i.e. within 24 h) is anticipated, enoxaparin should be considered as an alternative to UFH.	2a B
	Bivalirudin with a full-dose post-PCI infusion should be considered as an alternative to UFH in patients with STEMI undergoing primary PCI.	2a A

ACC American College of Cardiology, *ACS* acute coronary syndrome, *AHA* American Heart Association, *CCD* chronic coronary disease, *COR* class of recommendation, *ESC* European Society of Cardiology, *EO* expert opinion, *HIT* heparin-induced thrombocytopenia, *IV* intravenous, *LD* limited data, *LOE* level of evidence, *NSTE-ACS* non-ST-segment elevation acute coronary syndrome, *PCI* percutaneous coronary intervention, *R* randomized, *SCAI* Society for Cardiovascular Angiography and Interventions, *STEMI* ST-segment elevation myocardial infarction, *UFH* unfractionated heparin

Association (AHA) and European Society of Cardiology (ESC) guidelines [6–8].

The ACC/AHA guidelines suggest in patients with ACS, intravenous enoxaparin may be considered as an alternative to UFH at the time of PCI to reduce ischemic events (COR 2b). ESC guidelines recommend that i.v. enoxaparin (0.5 mg/kg) should be considered as an alternative agent to standard UFH for patients with CCD, NSTE-ACS undergoing early invasive angiography, and STEMI undergoing primary PCI, as well as in patients pretreated with subcutaneous enoxaparin (COR IIa) [6–8].

Despite the favorable pharmacodynamic and pharmacokinetic characteristics resulting into improved safety compared to UFH, both North American and European guidelines had previosuly downgraded the recommendation in the use of bivalirudin in the last years, from a COR 1 to 2a and 2b in the setting of STEMI and NSTE-ACS, respectively [6–8]. This downgrade was mainly attributable to an excess of acute ST associated with the use of bivalirudin not followed by post-PCI infusion. Interestingly, bivalirudin has been for years recommended as an alternative to UFH and GPI, particularly in HBR patients. Recently, likely due to the results of BRIGHT-4 trial, ACC/AHA guidelines have upgraded the recommendations for the use of bivalirudin, which has now a COR 1 in patients with STEMI undergoing PCI, as an alternative to UFH to reduce mortality and bleeding. Notably, when bivalirudin is used to support primary PCI for STEMI, a postprocedure 2- to 4-hour infusion at full dose is recommended.

19.6 Clinical Perspective and Practical Recommendations

The ultimate goal of antithrombotic therapy is to provide a rapid onset of potent pharmacodynamic effect to prevent ST and periprocedural MI, without increasing serious bleeding. The use of intravenous anticoagulant agents is mandatory during PCI, and the choice among agents should be based on the patient's hemorrhagic risk and, for some centers, financial resources, given the higher costs of bivalirudin. While UFH titrated to an optimal ACT has represented for many years the standard approach, enoxaparin has been shown to have a safety and efficacy profile similar to UFH but with a more predictable effect and should therefore be considered as a valuable alternative irrespective of ischemic and bleeding risk. In addition, it is preferable to avoid the administration of UFH in patients that have received enoxaparin in the previous 12 h to reduce risk of bleeding, particularly in HBR patients.

Randomized trials on bivalirudin have been characterized by many confounding factors and limitations, complicating the interpretation of its safety and efficacy compared with UFH among the spectrum of ACS patients. These include the concomitant use of GPI in the treatment and/or comparison arms, the use of different dosing regimens of bivalirudin, and the selective inclusion in some of the trials of East Asian patients, known to be characterized by peculiar thrombotic and bleeding risks compared with other ethnicities. Further limitations include the low use of radial access and of potent $P2Y_{12}$ inhibitors in early compared to more recent trials, limiting their applicability in the modern setting of ACS. Despite a clear reduction in bleeding risk, regardless of clinical presentation and HBR status, the main concern in the use of bivalirudin is represented by the increased rates of acute ST as compared with UFH. However, more recent data have now demonstrated that the risk of acute ST could be effectively mitigated by using a full-dose post-PCI infusion for a duration of 3–4 h, without any trade-off in bleeding risk. The rationale of such post-PCI infusion is counterbalancing the short half-life of bivalirudin potentially leading to an early hypercoagulable state after the stop of infusion in the peri-PCI phase, in which the thrombotic milieu and the risk of ST are the highest.

Residual limitations on the use of bivalirudin in clinical practice include its high costs compared with UFH. However, advantages of bivalirudin use, including a trivial incidence of HIT, the consistent pharmacological effect without the need for monitoring, the reduction in major bleeding, and the reduction in mortality shown in some trials, should prompt detailed cost-effectiveness analysis to better define the level of recommendations for the anticoagulant of choice. In addition, the increased understanding of the prognostic relevance of bleeding events and the excellent safety profile of bivalirudin make bivalirudin an attractive strategy, particularly in HBR patients.

In clinical practice, for patients at low bleeding risk, the use of heparin, in particular UFH, as an anticoagulant during PCI appears to be the most cost-effective option. In many systems, in STEMI patients, a fixed bolus of UFH (generally 4000–5000 IU) is routinely administered upstream, at the time of clinical presentation, as this strategy has been associated with better clinical outcomes, particularly for those patients who then are treated with bivalirudin in the catheterization lab. For patients who remain on UFH during PCI, additional bolus should be administered based on ACT levels. Enoxaparin can be considered a safe and effective alternative to UFH, especially for those patients already pretreated with subcutaneous enoxaparin. On the other hand, bivalirudin should be considered in case of HBR, such as elderly patients or those with anemia, thrombocytopenia, or chronic kidney disease, particularly in STEMI. If bivalirudin is used, strategies to reduce the risk of acute stent thrombosis should be employed, such as an initial bolus of UFH or prolonging the infusion at PCI-dose for up to 4 h after reperfusion.

Disclosures Dr. Franchi declares that he has received payment as an individual for consulting fee or honoraria from AstraZeneca and institutional payments for grants from PLx Pharma and The Scott R. MacKenzie Foundation.

Dr. Rollini has no conflict of interest to report.

References

1. Franchi F, Angiolillo DJ. Novel antiplatelet agents in acute coronary syndrome. Nat Rev Cardiol. 2015;12:30–47.
2. Davì G, Patrono C. Platelet activation and atherothrombosis. N Engl J Med. 2007;357:2482–94.
3. Brummel-Ziedins K, Undas A, Orfeo T, et al. Thrombin generation in acute coronary syndrome and stable coronary artery disease: dependence on plasma factor composition. J Thromb Haemost. 2008;6:104–10.
4. Franchi F, Rollini F, Angiolillo DJ. Antithrombotic therapy for patients with STEMI undergoing primary PCI. Nat Rev Cardiol. 2017;14:361–79.
5. Angiolillo DJ, Galli M, Collet JP, et al. Antiplatelet therapy after percutaneous coronary intervention. EuroIntervention. 2022;17:e1371–96.
6. Rao SV, O'Donoghue ML, Ruel M, et al. ACC/AHA/ACEP/NAEMSP/SCAI Guideline for the Management of Patients With Acute Coronary Syndromes: A Report of the American College of Cardiology/American Heart Association Joint Committee on Clinical Practice Guidelines. J Am Coll Cardiol. 2025; Published online February 27, 2025. https://doi.org/10.1016/j.jacc.2024.11.009.
7. Neumann FJ, Sousa-Uva M, Ahlsson A, et al. 2018 ESC/EACTS Guidelines on myocardial revascularization. Eur Heart J. 2019;40:87–165.
8. Byrne RA, Rossello X, Coughlan JJ, et al. ESC Scientific Document Group. 2023 ESC Guidelines for the management of acute coronary syndromes. Eur Heart J. 2023;44:3720–826.
9. Urban P, Mehran R, Colleran R, et al. Defining high bleeding risk in patients undergoing percutaneous coronary intervention. Circulation. 2019;140:240–61.
10. Capodanno D, Morice MC, Angiolillo DJ, et al. Trial design principles for patients at high bleeding risk undergoing PCI: JACC scientific expert panel. J Am Coll Cardiol. 2020;76:1468–83.
11. Garcia DA, Baglin TP, Weitz JI, Samama MM. Parenteral anticoagulants: Antithrombotic Therapy and Prevention of Thrombosis, 9th ed: American College of Chest Physicians Evidence-Based Clinical Practice Guidelines. Chest. 2012;141(2 Suppl):e24S–43S.
12. Salter BS, Weiner MM, Trinh MA, et al. Heparin-induced thrombocytopenia: a comprehensive clinical review. J Am Coll Cardiol. 2016;67:2519–32.
13. Palm M, Mattsson C. Pharmacokinetics of heparin and low molecular weight heparin fragment (Fragmin) in rabbits with impaired renal or metabolic clearance. Thromb Haemost. 1987;58:932–5.
14. Montalescot G, White HD, Gallo R, et al. Enoxaparin versus unfractionated heparin in elective percutaneous coronary intervention. N Engl J Med. 2006;355:1006–17.
15. Ferguson JJ, Califf RM, Antman EM, et al. Enoxaparin vs unfractionated heparin in high-risk patients with non-ST-segment elevation acute coronary syndromes managed with an intended early invasive strategy: primary results of the SYNERGY randomized trial. JAMA. 2004;292:45–54.
16. Blazing MA, de Lemos JA, White HD, et al. Safety and efficacy of enoxaparin vs unfractionated heparin in patients with non-ST-segment elevation acute coronary syndromes who receive tirofiban and aspirin: a randomized controlled trial. JAMA. 2004;292:55–64.
17. Montalescot G, Zeymer U, Silvain J, et al. Intravenous enoxaparin or unfractionated heparin in primary percutaneous coronary intervention for ST-elevation

myocardial infarction: the international randomised open-label ATOLL trial. Lancet. 2011;378:693–703.
18. Galli M, Bernardi M, Ortega-Paz L, et al. Bivalirudin in acute coronary syndromes. Expert Rev Cardiovasc Ther. 2023;21:901–11.
19. Stone GW, McLaurin BT, Cox DA, et al. Bivalirudin for patients with acute coronary syndromes. N Engl J Med. 2006;355:2203–16.
20. Kastrati A, Neumann FJ, Schulz S, et al. Abciximab and heparin versus bivalirudin for non-ST-elevation myocardial infarction. N Engl J Med. 2011;365:1980–9.
21. Stone GW, Witzenbichler B, Guagliumi G, et al. Bivalirudin during primary PCI in acute myocardial infarction. N Engl J Med. 2008;358:2218–30.
22. Dangas GD, Mehran R, Nikolsky E, et al. Effect of switching antithrombin agents for primary angioplasty in acute myocardial infarction: the HORIZONS-SWITCH analysis. J Am Coll Cardiol. 2011;57:2309–16.
23. Steg PG, Van't Hof A, Hamm CW, et al. Bivalirudin started during emergency transport for primary PCI. N Engl J Med. 2013;369:2207–17.
24. Clemmensen P, Wiberg S, Van't Hof A, et al. Acute stent thrombosis after primary percutaneous coronary intervention: insights from the EUROMAX trial (European Ambulance Acute Coronary Syndrome Angiography). JACC Cardiovasc Interv. 2015;8:214–20.
25. Stone GW, Mehran R, Goldstein P, et al. Bivalirudin versus heparin with or without glycoprotein IIb/IIIa inhibitors in patients with STEMI undergoing primary percutaneous coronary intervention: pooled patient-level analysis from the HORIZONS-AMI and EUROMAX trials. J Am Coll Cardiol. 2015;65:27–38.
26. Shahzad A, Kemp I, Mars C, et al. Unfractionated heparin versus bivalirudin in primary percutaneous coronary intervention (HEAT-PPCI): an open-label, single centre, randomised controlled trial. Lancet. 2014;384:1849–58.
27. Schulz S, Richardt G, Laugwitz KL, et al. Prasugrel plus bivalirudin vs. clopidogrel plus heparin in patients with ST-segment elevation myocardial infarction. Eur Heart J. 2014;35:2285–94.
28. Han Y, Guo J, Zheng Y, et al. Bivalirudin vs heparin with or without tirofiban during primary percutaneous coronary intervention in acute myocardial infarction: the BRIGHT randomized clinical trial. JAMA. 2015;313:1336–46.
29. Li Y, Liang Z, Qin L, et al. Bivalirudin plus a high-dose infusion versus heparin monotherapy in patients with ST-segment elevation myocardial infarction undergoing primary percutaneous coronary intervention: a randomised trial. Lancet. 2022;400:1847–57.
30. Valgimigli M, Frigoli E, Leonardi S, Rothenbühler M, Gagnor A, Calabrò P, et al. Bivalirudin or unfractionated heparin in acute coronary syndromes. N Engl J Med. 2015;373:997–1009.
31. Leonardi S, Frigoli E, Rothenbühler M, et al. Bivalirudin or unfractionated heparin in patients with acute coronary syndromes managed invasively with and without ST elevation (MATRIX): randomised controlled trial. BMJ. 2016;354:i4935.
32. Gargiulo G, Carrara G, Frigoli E, et al. Post-procedural bivalirudin infusion at full or low regimen in patients with acute coronary syndrome. J Am Coll Cardiol. 2019;73:758–74.
33. Erlinge D, Omerovic E, Frobert O, Linder R, Danielewicz M, Hamid M, et al. Bivalirudin versus heparin monotherapy in myocardial infarction. N Engl J Med. 2017;377:1132–42.
34. Bikdeli B, Erlinge D, Valgimigli M, et al. Bivalirudin versus heparin during PCI in NSTEMI: individual patient data meta-analysis of large randomized trials. Circulation. 2023;148:1207–19.
35. Galli M, Gargiulo G, Benenati S, et al. Bivalirudin plus a high-dose infusion versus heparin in patients with acute coronary syndrome. Eur Heart J Cardiovasc Pharmacother. 2023;9:666–8.

DAPT After Coronary Stenting: For How Long and Which Drug

20

Simone Fezzi, Sara Sgreva, Domenico Tavella, and Flavio Ribichini

20.1 Introduction

Dual antiplatelet therapy (DAPT) with aspirin and a P2Y12 receptor blocker is the standard antithrombotic regimen following percutaneous coronary intervention (PCI), irrespectively of the clinical presentation, either acute coronary syndrome (ACS) or chronic coronary syndrome (CCS) [1, 2]. The need for DAPT emerged subsequently to the development of drug-eluting stents (DES) that, while allowing to mitigate the risk of stent restenosis, led to an increased risk of late and very late stent thrombosis. DAPT decreases the risk of ischemic events by preventing stent thrombosis and by reducing the risk of thrombosis in non-stented coronary segments (plaque rupture at sites remote from the stented location). Therefore, DAPT provides with a pivotal measure to reduce ischemic events that is counterbalanced by an increased risk of bleeding events, associated with increased mortality [3–5]. Over the past four decades, an evolution in antiplatelet regimens has occurred, mostly thanks to the advancements in stent technologies, the development of new drugs, and the understanding of the prognostic implications associated with bleeding events.

S. Fezzi (✉) · S. Sgreva · D. Tavella · F. Ribichini
Division of Cardiology, Department of Medicine, University of Verona, Verona, Italy

20.2 Rationale for DAPT Use After PCI

Intraluminal arterial thrombus formation, responsible for acute coronary syndromes (ACS) onset, is an intricate and dynamic pathological process initiated within an injured blood vessel wall, mostly due to plaque rupture, plaque erosion, or eruptive calcified nodules [6]. Nonetheless, plaque instability seldom leads to clinical events, as it is well established that plaques with mild obstruction and vulnerable characteristics can undergo subclinical rupture and healing cycles, with subsequent plaque progression [7]. An acute coronary event could potentially arise due to an unfortunate combination (i.e., "perfect storm") of prothrombotic factors within the context of a rupture or erosion of a coronary atherosclerotic plaque that deviates from the usual outcome of asymptomatic plaque healing [8]. Platelets and their activation play a pivotal role in this process, as the hemostatic system, and inflammatory pathways are crucial in atherosclerotic development and thrombotic complications following plaque destabilization, with plaque rupture and erosion that activate the coagulation cascade and platelets, leading to sub-occlusive or occlusive thrombosis and symptomatic events [9]. The rationale for employing antiplatelet agents in CAD patients extends beyond treating the acute thrombotic clinical event to include the modulation of atherosclerotic disease progression, by acting on the subclinical healing process (Fig. 20.1).

B. Cortese, S. Rigattieri (eds.), *High Bleeding Risk Patients in Interventional Cardiology*,
https://doi.org/10.1007/978-3-031-87302-7_20

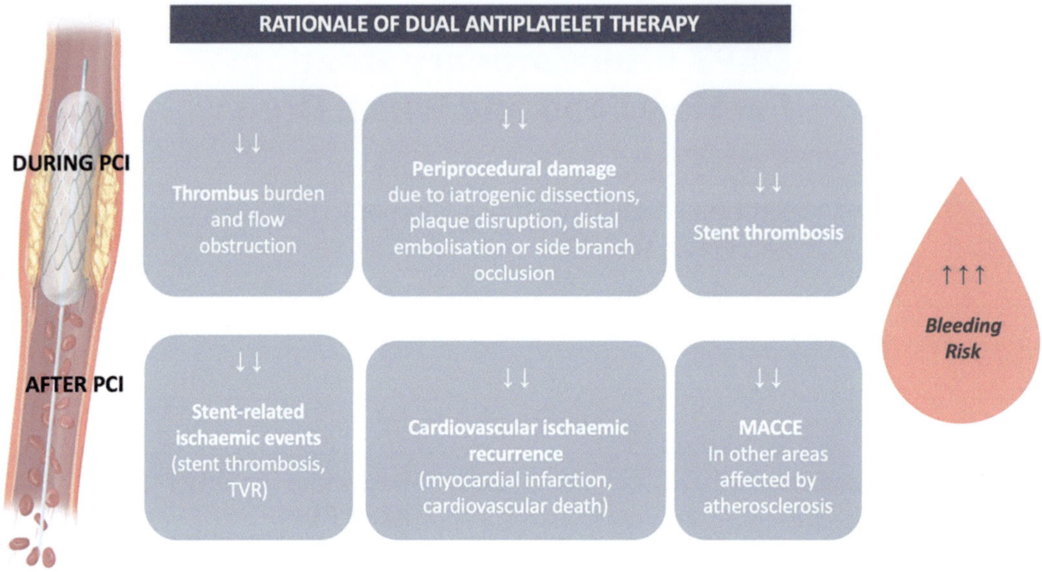

Fig. 20.1 Rationale for the use of dual antiplatelet therapy during and after PCI. The rationale for employing antiplatelet agents during and after PCI extends beyond treating the acute thrombotic clinical event to include the modulation of atherosclerotic disease progression, by acting on the subclinical healing process, but it is inevitably associated with increased risk of bleeding. MACCE: major adverse cardiac and cerebrovascular events; PCI: percutaneous coronary intervention; TVR: target vessel revascularization

20.3 P2Y12 Molecules and Therapy

P2Y12 inhibitors block the P2Y12 ADP receptor expressed on platelet surface. P2Y12 is a G-protein-coupled receptor that binds ADP and thereby enhances sustained platelet aggregation through intracellular signal activation and conformational changes of the GPIIB/IIIA receptor augmenting the affinity for its major ligand, soluble fibrinogen [10]. Drugs that inhibit the P2Y12 receptor include several thienopyridine and non-thienopyridine agents: clopidogrel, ticlopidine, prasugrel, ticagrelor, and cangrelor. Clopidogrel, ticlopidine, and prasugrel are irreversible platelet function inhibitors. These are thienopyridine prodrugs that require a metabolic process by cytochrome P450 enzymes to be activated. Platelet inhibition occurs within 24–48 h of the first dose, becomes maximal after 4–6 days, and may last for 4–10 days after drug discontinuation, due to their extended pharmacokinetic and pharmacodynamic half-life. Ticlopidine is usually not used in clinical practice anymore due to its multiple side effects and is not recommended in the current guidelines. Ticagrelor and cangrelor are not thienopyridines (ticagrelor is a modified pyrimidine; cangrelor is an ATP analog). They do not require metabolic conversion to an active form, so they have the advantage of a more rapid onset of action. Being reversible inhibitors, these are associated with a more rapid recovery of platelet function after their discontinuation [11] (Table 20.1).

Table 20.1 Pharmacokinetic and pharmacodynamic characteristics of P2Y12 inhibitors

	Clopidogrel	Prasugrel	Ticagrelor	Cangrelor
Target	P2Y12 irreversible	P2Y12 irreversible	P2Y12 reversible	P2Y12 reversible
Application	Oral	Oral	Oral	i.v.
Time to Cmax	2 h (after loading dose 600 mg)	0.5 h (after loading dose 60 mg)	0.5 h (after loading dose 180 mg)	2 min
Prodrug	Yes	Yes	No	No
Bioavailability (%)	50%	80%	36%	100%
Drug interactions	CYP3A4, CYP3A5 or CYP2C19 inhibitors or inducers	CYP3A4/A5 and CYP2B6 inhibitor	CYP3A4 inducers or inhibitors	None
Plasma half-life	0.5–1 h (active metabolite)	0.5–1 h (active metabolite)	6–12 h	3–6 min
Duration of action after last dose	3–10 days	7–10 days	3–5 days	1–2 h
Renal clearance of the active metabolite (%)	NR	NR	NR	58%
Dose regimen	o.d.	o.d.	b.i.d.	Bolus, infusion

Cmax maximum serum concentration, *i.v.* intravenous, *NR* non relevant, *o.d.* once a day, *b.i.d.* twice a day

20.4 Clopidogrel

Clopidogrel is recommended in patients undergoing elective PCI and should be initiated preferably more than 6 h before the planned intervention with a loading dose of 300 (to 600) mg and followed by 75 mg daily. Such pretreatment is no longer routinely recommended in all CCS patients before diagnostic coronary angiogram as no evidence of benefit is available, while it should be offered to those patients with a high probability of PCI [12]. In ACS setting, clopidogrel has been replaced by more potent agents (i.e., ticagrelor or prasugrel) [1]. These should be preferred as up to 25% of individuals are nonresponders or low responders to clopidogrel. This is partially based on genetic polymorphisms and other nongenetic reasons when a consistent optimal inhibition of platelet function cannot be guaranteed. Homozygote carriers of the most important loss-of-function polymorphism (CYP2C19*2; 2–3% of all patients) are nonresponders to therapy, while heterozygotes might react to increasing doses of clopidogrel [13] (Table 20.1).

20.5 Prasugrel

Prasugrel (oral intake, 60 mg LD followed by 10 mg/day MD, dose reduction to 5 mg/day in patients >75 years and low-weight patients) is an irreversible, but fast-acting blocker of the $P2Y_{12}$ receptor. In TRITON-TIMI 38 trial, prasugrel was superior to clopidogrel with respect to the combined primary endpoint (cardiovascular [CV] mortality, reinfarction, and stroke) [14]. Prasugrel seems to be especially effective in diabetic patients and high-risk patients with recurrent thromboembolic events, but should be avoided in patients with prior stroke or transient ischemic attack (TIA). The main side effect is an increase in spontaneous major bleeding events (an absolute increase of 0.6%) compared to clopidogrel. Such an increased risk of bleeding offsets the benefits of prasugrel in certain patient cohorts, resulting in neutral effects in the elderly (aged ≥75 years) and low body weight (<60 kg) patients. The ischemic benefits of prasugrel in ACS patients undergoing PCI have been confirmed in meta-analyses showing reduced risk of myocardial infarction (MI) and ST but yielding a 25–30% increase in major bleeding compared to clopidogrel [15]. Prasugrel activation is not adversely affected by the common CYP polymorphisms that can reduce the effectiveness of clopidogrel (Table 20.1).

20.6 Ticagrelor

Ticagrelor (oral intake, 180 mg LD followed by 2x90 mg/day MD) is a reversible and fast-acting (>80% platelet inhibition in 60–90 min) ADP-receptor blocker. Ticagrelor has been investigated in the PLATO trial and has been shown to be superior to clopidogrel with respect to a combined primary endpoint (cardiovascular mortality, reinfarction, and stroke) in primarily conservative, as well as primarily invasive, NSTE-ACS patients [16]. Ticagrelor has demonstrated a significant reduction of all-cause and cardiovascular mortality, which was also shown in a prespecified subgroup analysis for patients with diabetes and those referred for coronary bypass surgery. Potential side effects, besides an increase in spontaneous major bleeding events (an absolute increase of 0.6%), include dyspnea and bradycardia, both of which have been associated with the adenosine-like properties of the agent. Although in the PLATO in any subgroups, bleeding risk offset the efficacy of ticagrelor, absolute bleeding rates increased among the elderly patients. Subsequent meta-analyses in ACS showed ticagrelor to be the only P2Y12 inhibitor associated with a reduction in all-cause and CV death, but yielding a 20–30% increase of major bleeding compared to clopidogrel. This finding can potentially be attributed to the pleiotropic mechanisms of ticagrelor, including increased plasma levels of adenosine, and supports the concept that there may be a mortality benefit independent from a reduction of ischemic events. However, such observations have not been further confirmed in other studies. Ultimately, in patients with CCS undergoing high-risk elective PCI, ticagrelor was not superior to clopidogrel in reducing periprocedural myocardial damage [17] (Table 20.2).

Table 20.2 Randomized controlled trials testing antiplatelet strategies aiming at reducing bleeding events among patients undergoing PCI

Study, year	*N*	Clinical		Treatment arms and population	Primary endpoint definition	Primary endpoint results	Follow-up	Inclusion criteria	Major exclusion criteria
		ACS	CCS						
EXCELLENT, 2012	1443	51	49	6 versus 12 months DAPT	CV death, MI and ischemia- driven target vessel revascularisation	HR 1.14 (0.70–1.86) *P* 0.60	12	1 lesion stenosis of >50% and myocardial ischemia such as stable angina, UA, recent MI, silent ischemia, a positive functional study, or reversible changes on ECG	MI within 72 h; cardiogenic shock; LVEF <25%; prior stent in target vessel; true bifurcation lesions requiring 2 stents strategy; left main stenosis >50%; CTO
RESET, 2012	2148	54	46	3 versus 12 months DAPT	CV death, MI, ST, target vessel revascularization and bleeding	Difference: 0.0%; 95% confidence interval [CI]: −2.5–2.5; p 0.84; $p = 0.001$ for noninferiority	12	Angina or acute myocardial infarction with more than 50% diameter stenosis in a coronary artery by visual estimation	STEMI within 48 h; cardiogenic shock; LVEF <40%; cerebral/ peripheral atherosclerotic disease; thromboembolic disease; prior ST; left main disease; CTO; re-stenotic lesion
OPTIMIZE, 2013	3211	32	68	3 versus 12 months DAPT	All death, MI, stroke, and major bleeding	Risk difference, 0.17 [95% CI, −1.52–1.86]; $p = 0.002$ for noninferiority	12	Stable coronary artery disease or history of low-risk acute coronary syndrome (ACS) undergoing PCI with zotarolimus-eluting stents	Primary or rescue PCI for STEMI; BMS in nontarget vessel in the last 6 months; previous DES; saphenous vein graft lesion
SECURITY, 2014	1404	39	61	6 versus 12 months DAPT	CV death, MI, stroke, definite or probable ST and BARC bleeding 3–5	Risk difference 0.8%; 95% confidence interval [CI]: −2.4–1.7%; $p = 0.469$	12	Patients with a stable or unstable angina diagnosis or documented silent ischemia undergoing revascularization with at least 1 s-generation DES	Saphenous vein graft, in-stent restenosis, unprotected left main coronary artery, ST-segment elevation MI in the 48 h before the procedure, or non–ST-segment elevation MI in the previous 6 months; LVFE<30%

(continued)

Table 20.2 (continued)

Study, year	N	Clinical ACS	Clinical CCS	Treatment arms and population	Primary endpoint definition	Primary endpoint results	Follow-up	Inclusion criteria	Major exclusion criteria
ISAR-SAFE, 2015	4005	39	61	6 versus 12 months DAPT	All death, MI, ST, stroke, and TIMI major bleeding	Difference 20.1%, 95% CI 0.5%; 97.5% CI 0.6%; p for noninferiority, 0.001, HR 0.91, 95% CI: 0.55–1.50	9	DES implantation due to symptoms or signs of coronary artery disease, i.e. even patients with ACS	Previous stent thrombosis, DES implantation in the left main coronary artery, myocardial infarction during the 6 months after DES implantation, malignancies
I-LOVE-IT 2, 2016	1829	85	15	3 versus 12 months DAPT	CV death, target vessel MI or clinically indicated target lesion revascularization	6.8% versus 5.9%; difference and 95% confidence interval, 0.87% [−1.37–3.11%], p for noninferiority = 0.0065	18	With stable coronary artery disease or acute coronary syndromes (ACSs) undergoing PCI	Life expectancy <1 year; re-stenosed lesions; stent implantation within 1 year; LVFE<40%; severe renal or hepatic dysfunction
NIPPON, 2017	3773	32	68	6 versus 12 months DAPT	All death, MI, stroke, and major bleeding	Difference 0.6%, 95% CI: 1.5–0.3	36	Stable or acute coronary syndromes undergoing Nobori stent implantation	In-stent restenosis (bare-metal stent or DES) and index PCI for saphenous vein graft disease or unprotected left main trunk disease
DAPT-STEMI, 2018	1100	100	0	6 versus 12 months DAPT	All death, MI, any revascularization, stroke, and TIMI major bleeding	HR 0.73, (95% confidence interval 0.41–1.27, $P = 0.26$). $p = 0.004$ for noninferiority	18	STEMI that underwent primary percutaneous coronary intervention (PCI) with second generation DES	History of stent thrombosis Drug eluting stent in main left coronary artery
SMART-DATE, 2018	2712	100	0	6 versus 12 months DAPT	All death, MI, or stroke	Cumulative event rate 4.7% vs 4.2%; absolute risk difference 0.5%; upper limit of one-sided 95% CI 1.8%; p for noninferiority = 0.03 with a predefined noninferiority margin of 2.0%	18	Patients with ACS	Active pathological bleeding, major bleeding within the previous 3 months, or major surgery within the previous 2 months;

OPTIMA-C, 2018	1368	51	49	6 versus 12 months DAPT	All death, MI or ischemia-driven target lesion revascularization	Risk difference 0.6%; 95% confidence interval [CI]: −0.4–1.6%; $p = 0.24$ p for noninferiority <0.05	12	Indication of percutaneous coronary intervention (PCI)	ST-elevation MI and treatment of the left main artery, true bifurcation lesions requiring two stents, and target lesions with CTO
ONE MONTH DAPT, 2021	3020	39	61	1 versus 6–12 months DAPT in noncomplex PCI	CV death, MI, target vessel revascularization, stroke and major bleeding	Difference 0.7%; 97.5% CI: 1.33%; $p < 0.001$ for noninferiority	12	Nonemergent percutaneous coronary intervention (PCI)	Acute MI and complex morphologies, CTO, graft, thrombosis
MASTER DAPT, 2021	4434	49	51	1 versus 5 months DAPT among HBR patients	All death, MI, stroke, or major bleeding All death, MI, stroke, major or clinically relevant nonmajor bleeding	HR 0.83 [95% CI, 0.60–1.15] *p* 0.35; HR, 0.88 [95% CI, 0.60–1.30] *p* 0.45	11	Patients at high risk for bleeding who underwent treatment of all planned coronary artery stenoses	Implantation of a nonstudy stent within the previous 6 months or a bioresorbable scaffold at any time before the index procedure, or in-stent restenosis or stent thrombosis.
GLOBAL-LEADERS, 2018	15,968	47	53	Ticagrelor monotherapy for 23 months versus DAPT with ticagrelor for 12 months	All death or MI	Rate ratio 0·87 [95% CI 0·75–1·01]; $p = 0.073$	24	Patients undergoing PCI for stable angina or ACS	Ongoing long-term treatment with oral anticoagulants
TWILIGHT, 2019	7119	64	36	Ticagrelor monotherapy after 3 months of DAPT versus standard DAPT in uneventful patients with high-risk PCI	BARC bleeding type 2, 3, or 5 and all-cause death or MI and stroke	Hazard ratio, 0.56; 95% confidence interval [CI], 0.45–0.68; $p < 0.001$	15	Patients undergoing PCI with at least one locally approved DES and one additional clinical feature and one angiographic feature associated with a high risk of ischemic or bleeding events	ST-segment elevation MI, cardiogenic shock, ongoing long-term treatment with oral anticoagulants
SMART-CHOICE, 2019	2993	58	42	P2Y12 inhibitor monotherapy after 3 months of DAPT versus standard DAPT	All death, MI, or stroke	Difference, 0.4% [1-sided 95% CI, $-\infty$% to 1.3%]; $p = 0.007$ for noninferiority	12	Patients undergoing PCI	Hemodynamic instability or cardiogenic shock; active pathologic bleeding

(continued)

Table 20.2 (continued)

Study, year	*N*	Clinical		Treatment arms and population	Primary endpoint definition	Primary endpoint results	Follow-up	Inclusion criteria	Major exclusion criteria
		ACS	CCS						
STOPDAPT-2, 2019	3045	38	62	Clopidogrel monotherapy after 1 month of DAPT versus standard DAPT	CV death, MI, stroke, ST, and TIMI major or minor bleeding	Absolute difference, −1.34% [95% CI, −2.57% to −0.11%]; hazard ratio [HR], 0.64 [95% CI, 0.42–0.98], noninferiority $p < 0.001$	12	Patients undergoing PCI with CoCr-EES without concomitant use of other types of DES or in-hospital major complications other than periprocedural MI	Oral anticoagulation or antiplatelet therapy other than aspirin and P2Y12 receptor blockers, history of intracranial bleeding
TICO, 2020	3056	100	0	Ticagrelor monotherapy after 3 months of DAPT versus standard DAPT	TIMI major bleeding, all-cause death, MI, ST, stroke, and target vessel revascularization	Difference, −1.98% [95% CI, −3.50% to −0.45%]; hazard ratio [HR], 0.66 [95% CI, 0.48 to 0.92]; $p = 0.01$	12	Patients with ACS treated with DES	Increased risk of bleeding due to prior hemorrhagic stroke, traumatic brain injury or brain surgery, internal bleeding, need of oral anticoagulation therapy, and anemia
STOPDAPT-2-ACS, 2021	4169	100	0	Clopidogrel monotherapy after 1 month of DAPT versus standard DAPT among ACS	CV death, MI, stroke, ST, and TIMI major or minor bleeding	Difference, 0.37% [95% CI, −0.68–1.42%]; HR, 1.14 [95% CI, 0.80–1.62]; *p* for noninferiority = 0.06	12	Patients with ACS who underwent successful PCI using cobalt-chromium everolimus-eluting stents	Oral anticoagulants and previous history of hemorrhagic stroke
ANTARCTIC, 2016	877	100	0	PFT-guided de-escalation versus standard DAPT	CV death, MI, stroke, ST, urgent revascularization, and BARC 2–5 bleeding	HR 1.003, 95% CI 0.78–1.29; $p = 0.98$	12	Patients aged 75 years or older undergoing PCI for ACS	Previous history of stroke or TIA, fibrinolytic therapy in the past 48 h, chronic oral anticoagulation, concomitant medical illness
TROPICAL-ACS, 2017	2610	100	0	PFT-guided de-escalation versus standard DAPT	CV death, MI, stroke, ST, urgent revascularization and BARC 2–5 bleeding	HR 0.99 (0.58–1.70), $p = 0.97$	12	Biomarker-positive ACS patients between 18 and 80 years under- going successful PCI	Patients requiring chronic oral anticoagulation
POPular, 2019	2488	100	0	Genotype-guided de-escalation versus standard DAPT	All death, MI, definite ST, stroke, or PLATO major bleeding and PLATO major or minor bleeding	OR 0.87 [95% CI, 0.49–1.55]; $p = 0.64$	12	Patients undergoing CABG with ≥1 SVG	Oral anticoagulation, indication for use of a P2Y12 inhibitor or other antithrombotic agents after CABG

TOPIC, 2017	646	100	0	Clopidogrel-based DAPT versus standard DAPT	CV death, urgent revascularization, stroke and BARC 2–5 bleeding	HR 0.78; 95% CI: 0.40–1.49; $p = 0.45$	12	Patients with ACS undergoing primary PCI	History of intracranial bleeding
HOST-REDUCE-POLYTHEC-ACS, 2020	3429	100	0	Prasugrel 5-mg-based DAPT versus prasugrel 10 mg-based DAPT	All death, MI, ST, repeat revascularization, stroke and BARC 2–5 bleeding	Absolute risk difference, −1.2%; 97.5% CI, 0.4%; p for noninferiority <0.001	12	Clinical diagnosis of ACS and with at least 1 culprit coronary lesion	History of TIA or stroke, active bleeding
TALOS-MI, 2021	2697	100	0	Clopidogrel-based DAPT versus ticagrelor-based DAPT	CV death, MI, stroke and BARC 2–5 bleeding	–	12	Patients with bio-marker-positive AMI (non-ST-segment elevation or ST-segment elevation MI) undergoing PCI with DES	Cardiogenic shock, bleeding, history of intracranial bleeding, anemia, oral anticoagulant agent, malignancy

ACS acute coronary syndrome, *CCS* chronic coronary syndrome, *DAPT* dual antiplatelet therapy, *CV* cardiovascular, *MI* myocardial infarction, *HR* hazard ratio, *UA* unstable angina, *ECG* electrocardiogram, *LVFE* left ventricular ejection fraction, *CTO* chronic total occlusion, *ST* stent thrombosis, *CI* confidence interval, *PCI* percutaneous coronary intervention, *STEMI* ST elevation myocardial infarction, *BMS* bare metal stent, *DES* drug eluting stent, *HBR* high bleeding risk, *PFT* platelet function testing, *TIA* transient ischemic attack, *CABG* coronary artery bypass graft, *NSTEMI* non-ST elevation myocardial infarction

20.7 Cangrelor

Cangrelor is an intravenous (non-thienopyridine) adenosine triphosphate analog that blocks the adenosine diphosphate $P2Y_{12}$ receptor. The advantages of cangrelor, which might improve clinical outcomes over other antiplatelet agents, are its rapid onset of action and rapid return of platelet function after cessation. Two early trials evaluated cangrelor in patients undergoing PCI, either for CCS or ACS, and both failed to show clinical superiority to clopidogrel, either with administration before (CHAMPION PCI) and following (CHAMPION PLATFORM and CHAMPION PHOENIX) PCI. A meta-analysis of these trials showed that the benefit of cangrelor with respect to major ischemic endpoints was counterbalanced by an increase in minor bleeding complications. It is also important to note that the benefit of cangrelor with respect to ischemic endpoints was attenuated in CHAMPION PCI with upfront administration of clopidogrel, and data for its use in conjunction with ticagrelor or prasugrel treatment are limited. Due to its proven efficacy in preventing intra-procedural and post-procedural stent thrombosis in P2Y12 receptor inhibitor-naïve patients, cangrelor may be considered on a case-by-case basis in P2Y12 receptor inhibitor-naïve ACS patients undergoing PCI, including in patients for whom it may not be feasible to give oral drugs in the setting of emergent PCI (e.g., cardiogenic shock patients and/or patients on mechanical ventilation) [18–20] (Table 20.1).

20.8 Guidelines and Recommendations on DAPT After PCI

In individuals diagnosed with CCS, the commencement of oral P2Y12 inhibitors is usually postponed until the coronary anatomy is clearly identified and the decision to proceed with PCI is achieved. Clopidogrel, given as a 600 mg loading dose followed by a 75 mg maintenance dose, is the preferred P2Y12 inhibitor. The default DAPT duration is set at 6 months, followed by a lifelong regimen of aspirin monotherapy. Premature discontinuation of a P2Y12 inhibitor is associated with an increased risk of stent thrombosis and is discouraged. For patients at higher bleeding risk, especially in case of lower ischemic risk, a shorter course of DAPT followed by antiplatelet monotherapy may be appropriate (i.e., 1 month in case of extremely high bleeding risk).

For patients at higher ischemic risk, especially in case of low bleeding risk, a longer course of DAPT may be reasonable. Potent P2Y12 inhibitors may be considered after PCI in CCS patients in specific high ischemic risk situations [2].

In patients with ACS, post-interventional antiplatelet treatment is mandatory. The default DAPT regimen, recommended by the American and European guidelines, consists of a potent P2Y12 receptor inhibitor (prasugrel or ticagrelor) and aspirin for 12 months [1]. According to the latest STE-ACS guidelines [1], prasugrel should be considered as the preferred option over ticagrelor for patients with ACS undergoing PCI. This recommendation is based on the findings of the Intracoronary Stenting and Antithrombotic Regimen Rapid Early Action for Coronary Treatment (ISAR-REACT) 5 trial, where a treatment approach involving prasugrel (loading dose administered as soon as possible after randomization for patients undergoing primary PCI and after clarification of coronary anatomy for patients with NSTE-ACS) demonstrated a significant reduction in the composite endpoint of death, myocardial infarction, or stroke (6.9% vs. 9.3%, $p = 0.006$) without an associated increase in bleeding complications (4.8% vs. 5.4%, $p = 0.46$) (Fig. 20.2).

Oral P2Y12 inhibitor loading time is still a matter of debate: the rationale for preloading lies in providing enhanced antiplatelet protection by the time of PCI, theoretically reducing the risk of acute thrombosis. Nevertheless, this may also increase the risk of periprocedural bleeding in patients treated with PCI or coronary artery bypass grafting (CABG), thus increasing the length of stay and hospital costs [21–23]. Notably, in randomized clinical trials providing insights on DAPT loading time, the rate of ACS patients referred to CABG was

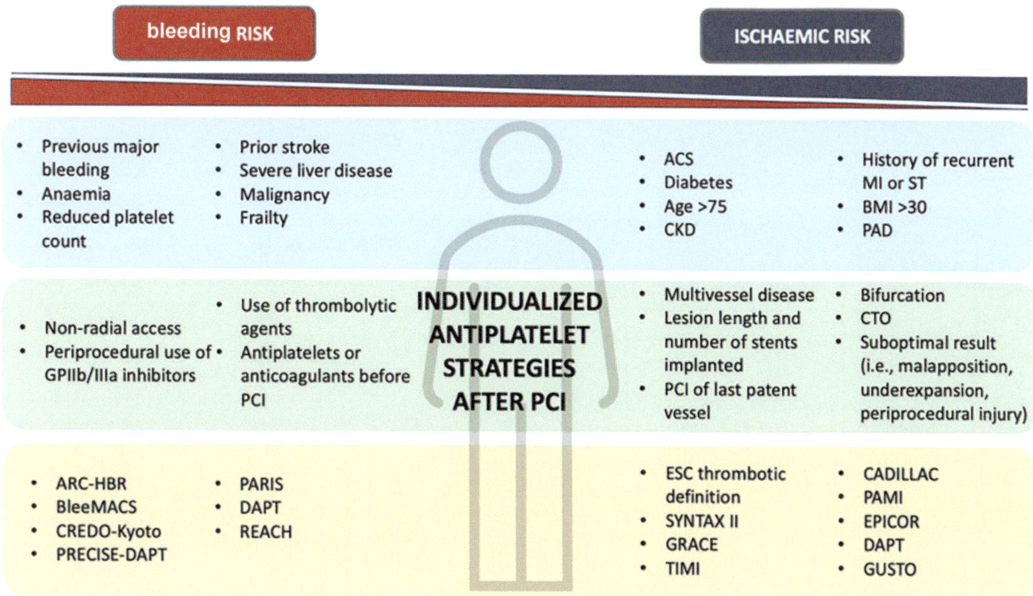

Fig. 20.2 Individualized risk assessment to guide dual antiplatelet therapy strategy. The default DAPT duration can be shortened or extended according to the ischemic/bleeding risk balance. Bleeding and ischemic risk assessments are based on clinical variables, procedural features, and the use of scores/definitions. ACS: acute coronary syndrome; BMI: body mass index; CKD: chronic kidney disease; CTO: chronic total occlusion; MI myocardial infarction; PAD polyvascular atherosclerotic disease; PCI percutaneous coronary intervention; ST stent thrombosis

around 3–6% and to medical management 14–25% [24, 25]. The Administration of Ticagrelor in the Cath Lab or in the Ambulance for New ST Elevation Myocardial Infarction to Open the Coronary Artery (ATLANTIC) trial is the only randomized study examining the safety and effectiveness of different initiation timings for P2Y12 receptor inhibitors in STEMI patients undergoing primary PCI. During the trial, participants were randomly assigned to receive a ticagrelor loading dose either during transfer to a PPCI center or immediately before angiography, with a median time difference of 31 min between the two strategies. Pretreatment approach did not meet the predefined primary endpoint of improved ST-segment elevation resolution or TIMI flow before intervention [26]. Notably, rates of major and minor bleeding events were comparable in both treatment groups. Such findings were further supported by real-world data from the SWEDEHEART registry [27]. While prasugrel pretreatment did not yield favorable results, investigations into ticagrelor-based strategies, such as the ISAR-REACT 5 trial, indicated inferiority to a prasugrel-based strategy with a deferred loading dose in NSTE-ACS patients. Additionally, the DUBIUS trial, focusing on upstream vs. downstream oral P2Y12 administration in NSTE-ACS patients scheduled for early coronary angiography, was stopped early due to futility, revealing no difference between the two approaches [24] (Fig. 20.3).

In summary, for patients diagnosed with STEMI undergoing PPCI, pretreatment with a P2Y12 receptor inhibitor may be considered. Conversely, routine pretreatment in NSTE-ACS patients before knowing the coronary anatomy for those undergoing an early invasive strategy (<24 h) is not recommended. In cases where there is an anticipated delay to invasive angiography (>24 h) for NSTE-ACS patients, pretreatment with a P2Y12 receptor inhibitor may be considered based on patient's bleeding risk. For all ACS patients proceeding to PCI without prior P2Y12 receptor inhibitor pretreatment, a loading dose is recommended at the time of PCI [1].

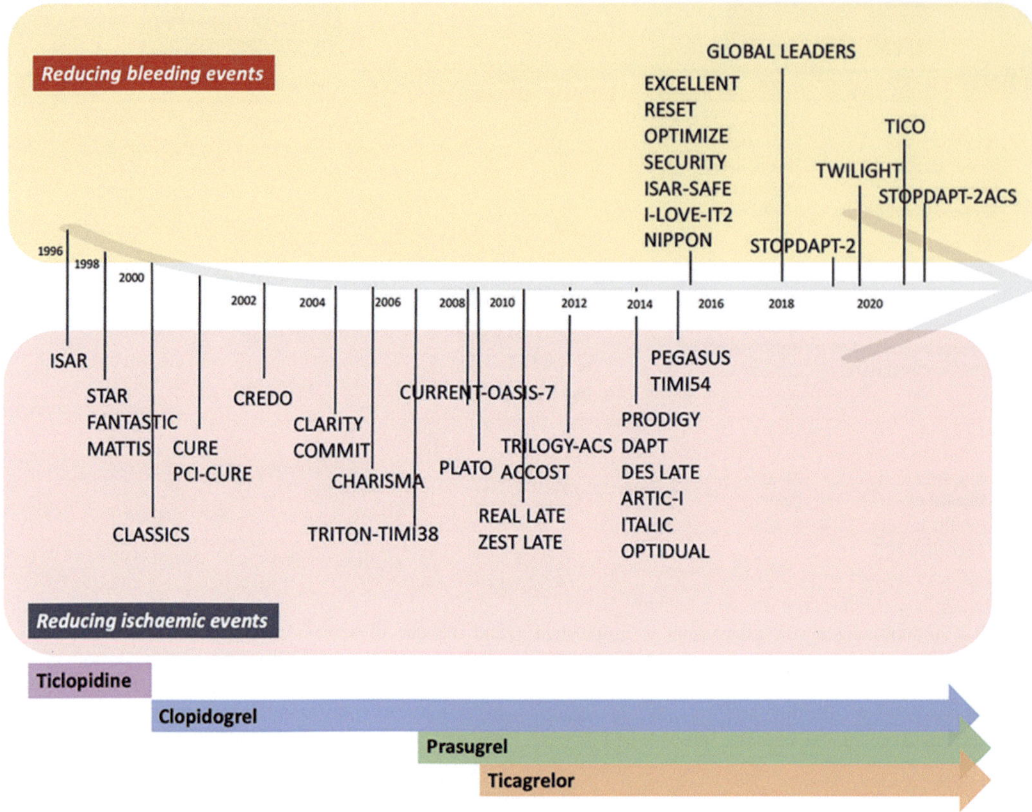

Fig. 20.3 Timeline of randomized controlled trials on dual antiplatelet therapy focusing on strategies aiming at reducing ischemic or bleeding events

20.9 Ischemic Risk Assessment and DAPT Prolongation

The default DAPT duration in ACS can be shortened (<12 months) or extended (>12 months) according to the ischemic/bleeding risk balance (Fig. 20.2). A patient is deemed at high ischemic risk when several angiographic/procedural or clinical factors are present (bifurcation lesion, left main coronary artery, total stent length, saphenous vein grafts, ≥3 stents implanted or ≥3 lesions treated, implantation of older-generation DES, bioresorbable scaffolds, prior stent thrombosis, diabetes mellitus, chronic kidney disease (CKD), ischemic events after PCI, vascular disease including myocardial infarction or peripheral vascular disease). Patient with ACS/CCS and high ischemic risk may benefit from longer DAPT duration [28].

The DAPT trial [29] is the largest randomized clinical trial to compare longer (than 12 months) with 12 months DAPT duration after DES implantation. The study randomized a total number of 9961 patients. Prolonged DAPT, conducted either with clopidogrel (75 mg/od) or prasugrel (10 mg/od), significantly reduced MACE rate by 29%. However, this advantage came with a notable rise in moderate and severe bleeding. Notably, prolonged DAPT was associated with a decrease in MACE especially in patients with previous history of MI. Moreover, in this trial an apparent increased risk for ischemic events during the 3 months after P2Y12 inhibition withdrawal was described.

The PEGASUS-TIMI 54 trial [30] investigated the efficacy of a prolonged P2Y12 inhibiting therapy, either ticagrelor 90 mg/bid or 60 mg/bid in addition to aspirin, compared to a placebo, involving 21,162 patients. Patients experienced a MI 1–3 years earlier and were at least 50 years old, with additional high-risk factors such as age ≥65, diabetes mellitus requiring medication, a second prior MI, multivessel CAD, or CKD. Over a 33-month period, both ticagrelor doses significantly reduced MACE rate by 15%. However, this reduction came at the cost of increased major bleeding with both ticagrelor regimens (2.60% with 90 mg and 2.30% with 60 mg) as compared to placebo (1.06%; $p = 0.001$), while with no difference in terms of intracranial hemorrhage (ICH). However, the 60 mg/bid dose showed a more favorable safety profile, in terms of non-bleeding side effects like dyspnea, leading to its recommendation for long-term secondary prevention beyond 1 year in practice guidelines.

The THEMIS study [31] further focused on patients with type 2 diabetes mellitus and stable CAD (with 58% of the total population having undergone prior PCI), randomly allocating 19,220 patients either to ticagrelor 60 mg/bid or to placebo, added to aspirin 75–150 mg/od. At 39 months, DAPT reduced MACE rate by 10% (7.7% vs. 8.5%; hazard ratio, 0.90; 95% CI 0.81–0.99; $p = 0.04$), whereas the incidence of TIMI major bleeding was higher (2.2% vs. 1.0%; hazard ratio, 2.32; 95% CI, 1.82–2.94; $p < 0.001$), as was the incidence of intracranial hemorrhage (0.7% vs. 0.5%; hazard ratio, 1.71; 95% CI, 1.18–2.48; $p = 0.005$). The net clinical benefit was more favorable among patients with a history of PCI compared to those without. An important aspect observed in both the PEGASUS-TIMI 54 and THEMIS studies was the consistent efficacy of low-dose ticagrelor over time, irrespective of the time from the most recent MI and PCI.

Lastly, the combination of a low dose of the new-oral anticoagulant rivaroxaban (2.5 mg/od) and aspirin represents a further prolonged therapeutic strategy for ischemic risk reduction, namely, the dual pathway inhibition (DPI). In the COMPASS trial, the vascular dose regimen of rivaroxaban (2.5 mg/bid) added to low-dose aspirin was assessed in patients with stable CAD at risk for recurrences. In this trial, 27,395 patients were randomized to receive either rivaroxaban (2.5 mg twice daily) plus aspirin (100 mg once daily), rivaroxaban (5 mg twice daily), or aspirin (100 mg once daily). Rivaroxaban 2.5 mg plus aspirin, but not rivaroxaban 5 mg twice daily, led to a 24% reduction in MACE compared to aspirin alone (4.1% vs. 5.4%; HR 0.76; 95% CI 0.66–0.86; $p < 0.001$), but major bleeding events occurred more frequently in the rivaroxaban-plus-aspirin group (3.1% vs. 1.9%; HR 1.70; 95% CI 1.40–2.05; $p < 0.001$), while no significant difference in intracranial or fatal bleeding between these two groups was noted.

Accordingly, long-term DAPT therapy should be considered in patients deemed at high thrombotic risk and without an increased risk of major or life-threatening bleeding [15, 26–28]. According to the DAPT score, which includes clinical and procedural variables, DAPT extension up to 30 months may be considered with a score ≥2.

20.10 Hemorrhagic Risk Assessment

Several scores have been developed and validated to assess hemorrhagic risk in patients undergoing PCI. To evaluate the combination of ischemic and bleeding risks at patient's discharge, the PRECISE-DAPT score was validated (Table 20.3). This score may be helpful to guide and inform decision-making on DAPT duration. Among HBR patients based on PRECISE-DAPT (score ≥25), standard DAPT (12 months) was associated with no ischemic benefit but an increase in the risk of bleeding events. Conversely, longer treatment in patients without HBR (PRECISE-DAPT score <25) was not associated with an increase in bleeding but was associated with a significant reduction in the composite ischemic endpoint of myocardial infarction, definite stent thrombosis, stroke, and TVR. The findings remained valid in analyses restricted to ACS patients [1, 32, 33]. It is worth mentioning that both DAPT and PRECISE-DAPT scores were validated excluding patients on oral anticoagulation, although there is only limited evidence available in this scenario.

Table 20.3 Risk scores: several scores have been developed and validated to assess hemorrhagic/ischemic risk in patients undergoing PCI

RISK-SCORES

Score	Criteria	Cut off
HBR ARC Bleeding risk	**MAJOR CRITERIA** Severe CKD (eGFR<30), thrombocytopenia, liver cirrhosis, severe anaemia (Hb<11), past haemorrhagic stroke, anticoagulation **MINOR CRITERIA** Age ≥75 years, moderate CKD, mild anaemia, past ischemic stroke	**Cut off:** ≥ 1 major or ≥ 2 minor
HASBLED Bleeding risk	Hypertension, abnormal renal/liver function, stroke, bleeding tendency, labile INR, age>65	**Cut off:** - Low 0-2 - Intermediate 2 - High >2
PRECISE-DAPT At the time of PCI: Short DAPT (3-6 months) vs. standard/long DAPT	HB, WBC, Age, Creatinine clearance, prior bleeding	**Cut off:** ≥25 short DAPT <25 standard/long DAPT
CRUSADE Bleeding risk	0-96 points: Baseline haematocrit, creatinine clearance, heart rate, sex, sign of CHF at presentation, prior vascular disease, diabetes mellitus, systolic blood pressure	**Cut off:** - Moderate 31-40 - High 41-50 - Very high >50
ACUITY Bleeding risk in patients with ACS	Gender, age, serum creatinine, WBC, anaemia, presentation, antithrombotic medications	**Cut off:** - Low <10 - Intermediate 10-14 - High >14
PRAISE Risk assesment post ACS	*Clinical*: age, HB, LVFE, eGFR, sex, HT, hyperlipidaemia, PAD, prior AMI or CABG or stroke or bleeding, malignancy, NSTEMI, STEMI, diabetes *Therapeutic*: BB, ACEinhibitors/ARB, statin, PPI, OAC *Procedural*: multivessel, complete revascularization, vascular access, DES	**Cut off:** *probability* of all-cause death, recurrent MI and major bleeding at 1year
PARIS Risk assesment after PCI	**PARIS-ISCHEMIC** diabetes mellitus, ACS, current smoking, CrCl<60, prior PCI, prior CABG **PARIS-BLEEDING** age, BMI, current smoking, anaemia, CrCl<60, triple therapy on discharge	**Cut off:** - Ischemic 4 - Bleeding 9
CREDO-KYOTO Risk assesment after PCI	**CREDO-ISCHEMIC** severe chronic kidney disease, AF, peripheral vascular disease, anaemia, age ≥75, HF, diabetes, chronic total occlusion **CREDO-BLEEDING** platelet count<100/ml, severe chronic kidney disease, peripheral vascular disease, HF, prior MI, malignancy, AF	**Cut off:** - Ischemic 5 - Bleeding 2
DAPT score After 12 months of uneventful DAPT vs. long DAPT (30 months)	Age, cigarette smoking, diabetes, MI at presentation, prior PCI or MI paclitaxel-eluting stent, stent diameter <3 mm, CHF or LVEF <30%, vein graft stent	**Cut off:** ≥2 long DAPT <2 standard DAPT

CKD chronic kidney disease, *eGFR* estimated glomerular filtration rate, *INR* international normalized ratio, *HB* hemoglobin, *WBC* white blood cells, *DAPT* dual antiplatelet therapy, *CHF* chronic heart failure, *ACS* acute coronary syndrome, *LVFE* Left ventricular ejection fraction, *HT* hypertension, *PAD* polyvascular atherosclerotic disease, *AMI* acute myocardial infarction, *CABG* coronary artery bypass graft, *NSTEMI* non-ST elevation myocardial infarction, *STEMI* ST elevation myocardial infarction, *BB* beta blokers, *ACE* angiotensin-converting enzyme, *ARB* angiotensin receptor blockers, *PPI* proton pump inhibitors, *OAC* oral anticoagulant, *DES* drug eluting stent, *PCI* percutaneous coronary intervention, *CrCl* creatinine clearance, *BMI* body mass index, *HF* heart failure, *MI* myocardial infarction, *AF* atrial fibrillation

Moreover, increased ischemic and bleeding risk often concur in the same patient, and, when these risks align, observational data indicate that bleeding, rather than the ischemic risk, should primarily guide decisions regarding the duration of DAPT [34]. Bleeding risk should also play a pivotal role in defining DAPT duration following PCI. Major bleedings have relevant prognostic implications, with mortality rates similar to or exceeding those of major ischemic events. Minor bleedings can lead to an abrupt cessation of antiplatelet therapy, potentially resulting in elevated rates of subsequent ischemic events. According to the Academic Research Consortium for High Bleeding Risk (ARC-HBR), a patient is considered to be at high bleeding risk (HBR) if one major (oral anticoagulation, estimated glomerular filtration rate [eGFR] <30 ml/min, hemoglobin <11 g/dL, spontaneous bleeding requiring hospitalization or transfusion in the past 6 months, platelet count <100 × 109/L, chronic bleeding diathesis, liver cirrhosis with portal hypertension, active malignancy within the past 12 months, previous spontaneous intracranial hemorrhage, previous traumatic intracranial hemorrhage within the past 12 months, presence of a brain arteriovenous malformation, moderate or severe ischemic stroke within the past 6 months, nondeferrable major surgery on DAPT, recent major surgery, or major trauma within 30 days before PCI) or two minor criteria (age ≥75 years, eGFR 30–59 mL/min, hemoglobin 11–12.9 g/dL for men and 11–11.9 g/dL for women, spontaneous bleeding requiring hospitalization or transfusion within the past 12 months not meeting the major criterion, long-term use of oral NSAIDs or steroids, any ischemic stroke at any time not meeting the major criterion) for major bleeding are present. HBR is defined as bleeding risk of ≥4% at 1 year or a risk of an intracranial hemorrhage (ICH) of ≥1% at 1 year [35]. Strategies aiming at bleeding risk mitigation encompass DAPT shortening, P2Y12 monotherapy, and DAPT de-escalation.

20.10.1 DAPT Shortening

DAPT duration following ACS can be shortened to 1, 3, or 6 months, aiming at bleeding mitigation (Table 20.3). Current guidelines recommend DAPT duration should be minimized to 1 and up to 3 months in HBR patients [1]. Theoretically, lowering bleeding events by means of DAPT duration shortening may be associated with an increased risk of ischemic complications. Generally, the risk of stent thrombosis is highest soon after DES implantation, as the re-endothelialization is expected to be completed within 3–6 months. Several trials compared 1-, 3-, and 6-month therapy versus 12-month DAPT duration and despite the presence of high ischemic risk features, such as complex PCI or ACS, support that a shorter DAPT duration (3–6 months) was associated with superior net clinical benefit in HBR patients [34]. Therefore, DAPT duration should be adapted based on patients' characteristics and bleeding risk that should be prioritized as compared to ischemic risk in HBR patients [36]. Among others, the Management of High Bleeding Risk Patients Post Bioresorbable Polymer Coated Stent Implantation with an Abbreviated versus Standard DAPT Regimen (MASTER-DAPT) trial [37] was the first RCT specifically including HBR patients. In total 4434 HBR patients were randomly assigned to 1- vs. 3-month DAPT regimen. Abbreviated DAPT therapy was seen to be noninferior as compared to 3-month regimen, both in terms of 12-month net adverse clinical events (7.5% vs. 7.7%; 95% CI −1.80–1.33; $p < 0.001$ for noninferiority) and MACCE (6.1% vs 5.9%; 95% CI, −1.29–1.51; $p = 0.001$ for noninferiority). Interestingly, abbreviated DAPT was associated with a lower incidence of major or clinically relevant nonmajor bleedings (6.5% vs. 9.4%; 95% CI, −4.40 to −1.24; $p < 0.001$ for superiority).

In general, early discontinuation of P2Y12 inhibitor reduces bleeding, including major bleeding, without a significant increase in thrombotic events. However, it has been argued that dedicated clinical trials included patients at low ischemic risk or were not adequately powered to investigate hard ischemic endpoints. Therefore, whether such findings should be reliably extended to patients deemed at high-ischemic risk is still a matter of debate. Moreover, short DAPT should not be employed routinely in all-comers ACS population. The STOPDAPT-2 ACS study which randomized 4136 unselected ACS patients to 1- to 2-month or a 12-month DAPT regimen after PCI failed to demonstrate the noninferiority of the abbreviated DAPT regimen [38].

20.10.2 P2Y12 Monotherapy

Several investigations over time conducted in vitro and ex vivo have suggested that aspirin provides limited antithrombotic effects in addition to potent P2Y12 blockade. This, along with the recognized gastrointestinal risks associated with aspirin, has spurred investigations into assessing the safety and effectiveness of P2Y12 monotherapy regimens [39, 40] (Table 20.3). The GLOBAL-LEADERS [41] trial firstly investigated this strategy, comparing 1-month DAPT followed by 23 months of ticagrelor 90 mg/bid monotherapy against standard DAPT, based on 75–100 mg aspirin daily plus either 75 mg clopidogrel daily (for patients with stable coronary artery disease) or 90 mg ticagrelor twice daily (for patients with acute coronary syndromes) for 12 months followed by aspirin. The trial was designed as a superiority RCT, enrolling 15,968 all-comers patients undergoing PCI. At 2 years, P2Y12 monotherapy failed to meet the prespecified superiority margin both in terms of ischemic (rate ratio 0.87 [95% CI 0.75–1.01]; $p = 0.073$) and BARC 3–5 bleeding events (2.04% vs 2.12%; rate ratio 0.97 [95% CI 0.78–1.20]; $p = 0.77$).

The Ticagrelor With Aspirin or Alone in High-Risk Patients After Coronary Intervention (TWILIGHT) trial [42], utilizing a double-blind, placebo-controlled design, enrolled 7119 patients with high risk of ischemic or bleeding events. Following 3 months of uneventful DAPT with ticagrelor plus aspirin, patients were randomized to continue ticagrelor with aspirin or placebo for 1 year. Results showed a significant 44% reduction in the primary endpoint of BARC 2–5 bleeding with ticagrelor monotherapy, with no difference in MACE between groups. Notably, consistent MACE results were observed among high-risk subgroups, including those with diabetes mellitus and ACS and those undergoing complex PCI.

While the use of prasugrel monotherapy in P2Y12 monotherapy strategies is limited, preliminary studies show promising results. However, caution is warranted, particularly in high-risk patients like those with ACS, where the choice of P2Y12 inhibitor may influence outcomes. The ShorT and OPtimal Duration of Dual AntiPlatelet Therapy-2 ACS study (STOPDAPT-2 ACS), involving a total of 4169 patients, failed to demonstrate noninferiority for the primary endpoint of net adverse clinical events clopidogrel monotherapy after 1-month DAPT versus the standard 12-month DAPT, mainly due to an increase in myocardial infarction. These findings underscore the need for caution when considering early discontinuation of aspirin among high-risk patients, such as those with ACS, especially when using a less potent P2Y12 inhibitor as monotherapy [43].

The STOPDAPT-3 trial [44] enrolled 6002 patients diagnosed with ACS or deemed to be at HBR, randomized to receive either prasugrel monotherapy (3.75 mg/day) or DAPT with aspirin and prasugrel (3.75 mg/day) after a loading dose of 20 mg of prasugrel in both groups. At 1 month, the no-aspirin group did not demonstrate superiority over the DAPT group in terms of major bleeding (4.47% and 4.71%, HR 0.95 [95% CI 0.75–1.20]; p for superiority = 0.66). However, the no-aspirin group was found to be noninferior to the DAPT group regarding the composite cardiovascular endpoint (4.12% and 3.69%; HR 1.12 [95% CI, 0.87–1.45]; p for noninferiority = 0.01). Nevertheless, the aspirin-free strategy showed indications of increased ischemic coronary events, displaying higher rates of unplanned coronary revascularization (1.05% vs. 0.57%; HR 1.83 [95% CI, 1.01–3.30]) and subacute definite or probable stent thrombosis (0.58% vs. 0.17%; HR 3.40 [95% CI, 1.26–9.23]) compared to the DAPT group.

20.10.3 Antiplatelet Drug Reactivity and Guided DAPT De-escalation

The process of reducing the intensity of P2Y12 inhibiting therapy, known as de-escalation, involves transitioning from more potent agents (prasugrel or ticagrelor) to less potent ones such as clopidogrel (Table 20.3). Its aim is to minimize bleeding risks without compromising protection against ischemic events. De-escalation can be either guided or unguided. A guided approach involves utilizing platelet function or genetic tests to exclude individuals with clopidogrel resistance (clopidogrel-HPR) or those carrying CYP2C19 LoF alleles, which are associated with an elevated risk of thrombotic complications post-PCI. Conversely, an unguided approach entails de-escalation without such diagnostic assistance. Guided de-escalation permits early adjustment of therapy post-PCI, whereas unguided de-escalation at this stage has been linked to an increased incidence of thrombotic complications. Consequently, deferring de-escalation until the highest risk period for thrombotic complications post-PCI has passed, typically around 1 month, provides a safer window for considering unguided de-escalation [45].

A guided de-escalation approach has been investigated in three RCTs enrolling ACS patients, assessing platelet function testing or genetic testing. The Testing Responsiveness to Platelet Inhibition on Chronic Antiplatelet Treatment for Acute Coronary Syndromes Trial (TROPICAL-ACS) [46] represents the largest study utilizing platelet function testing to guide DAPT de-escalation. Based on a cohort of 2610 ACS patients, platelet function testing-guided de-escalation was found to be noninferior to the standard of care for the primary composite endpoint of net adverse cardiac events (7% vs. 9%; HR 0.81 [95% CI 0.62–1.06]; p noninferiority = 0.0004; p superiority = 0.12), with a trend toward reduced bleeding observed at 12 months compared to the standard group (5% vs 6%; HR 0.82 [95% CI 0.59–1.13]; $p = 0.23$).

In the Cost-effectiveness of Genotype Guided Treatment With Antiplatelet Drugs in ST-segment elevation MI (STEMI) Patients: Optimization of Treatment (POPular Genetics) trial, genetic testing was employed to guide de-escalation. This study involved 2488 STEMI patients undergoing primary PCI who were randomized to either a genotype-guided de-escalation or a standard-of-care approach (mostly using ticagrelor, 91%) for the selection of oral P2Y12 inhibitors [47]. The genotype-guided strategy was deemed noninferior for NACE and superior in terms of PLATO major or minor bleeding compared to the standard of care at the 12-month follow-up.

Genetic testing DAPT de-escalation needs to be followed by platelet function testing, as some patients who de-escalate to clopidogrel exhibit high platelet reactivity and thus require escalation to more potent P2Y12 inhibition, which increases the risk of bleeding. It's worth noting that a maintenance treatment period of 7–14 days with clopidogrel is necessary after de-escalation before assessing platelet responsiveness. During this time, patients with high platelet reactivity are at an elevated risk of thrombotic events [48].

20.11 Conclusions

Antiplatelet therapy is the cornerstone therapy following PCI with stent implantation, being crucial in preventing both local and systemic ischemic complications. Over time, various antiplatelet regimens involving aspirin and P2Y12 inhibitors have been developed and integrated into clinical practice. Understanding individual patient profiles regarding ischemic and bleeding risks, as well as responsiveness to antiplatelet agents, is essential in determining the most suitable regimen and tailor a targeted therapy to individual patients' characteristics. Recent evidence and guidelines recommend to carefully weigh ischemic and bleeding risk profiles of each patient, with bleeding risk being the most relevant factor, to guide the appropriate therapeutic choice.

Strategies to mitigate bleeding risk include shortening of DAPT duration, using P2Y12 inhibitor monotherapy, and P2Y12-guided de-escalation. On the other side, patients deemed at low bleeding risk presenting with high ischemic risk (e.g., ACS, DM) may consider prolonging DAPT therapy.

A comprehensive approach, which considers scores/definitions for assessing ischemic and bleeding risks, procedural characteristics, and tools for evaluating drug response, offers the most promising avenue for personalized antiplatelet agent selection among PCI patients.

References

1. Byrne RA, Rossello X, Coughlan JJ, et al. 2023 ESC Guidelines for the management of acute coronary syndromes. Eur Heart J. 2023. https://doi.org/10.1093/eurheartj/ehad191.
2. Neumann FJ, Sechtem U, Banning AP, et al. 2019 ESC Guidelines for the diagnosis and management of chronic coronary syndromes. Eur Heart J. 2020;41:407–77.
3. Généreux P, Giustino G, Witzenbichler B, et al. Incidence, predictors, and impact of post-discharge bleeding after percutaneous coronary intervention. J Am Coll Cardiol. 2015;66(9):1036–45.
4. Valgimigli M, Costa F, Lokhnygina Y, Clare RM, Wallentin L, Moliterno DJ, Armstrong PW, White HD, Held C, Aylward PE, Van de Werf F, Harrington RA, Mahaffey KW, Tricoci P. Trade-off of myocardial infarction vs. bleeding types on mortality after acute coronary syndrome: lessons from the Thrombin Receptor Antagonist for Clinical Event Reduction in Acute Coronary Syndrome (TRACER) randomized trial. Eur Heart J. 2017;38:804–10.
5. Bergmark BA, Scirica BM. First, do no (irreparable) harm: infarction, bleeding, and subsequent risk of death. The dangers of false equivalency. Eur Heart J. 2017;38:811–3.
6. Arbab-Zadeh A, Fuster V. From detecting the vulnerable plaque to managing the vulnerable patient. J Am Coll Cardiol. 2019;74:1582–93.
7. Ahmadi A, Leipsic J, Blankstein R, Taylor C, Hecht H, Stone GW, Narula J. Do plaques rapidly progress prior to myocardial infarction? Circ Res. 2015;117:99–104.
8. Arbab-Zadeh A, Nakano M, Virmani R, Fuster V. Acute coronary events. Circulation. 2012;125:1147–56.
9. Stark K, Massberg S. Interplay between inflammation and thrombosis in cardiovascular pathology. Nat Rev Cardiol. 2021;18:666–82.
10. Cunningham MR, Nisar SP, Mundell SJ. Molecular mechanisms of platelet P2Y(12) receptor regulation. Biochem Soc Trans. 2013;41:225–30.
11. Cattaneo M. New P2Y12 blockers. J Thromb Haemost. 2009;7(Suppl 1):262–5.
12. Knuuti J, Wijns W, Saraste A, et al. 2019 ESC Guidelines for the diagnosis and management of chronic coronary syndromes. Eur Heart J. 2020;41:407–77.
13. Bonello L, Tantry US, Marcucci R, et al. Consensus and future directions on the definition of high on-treatment platelet reactivity to adenosine diphosphate. J Am Coll Cardiol. 2010;56:919–33.
14. Wiviott SD, Braunwald E, McCabe CH, et al. Prasugrel versus clopidogrel in patients with acute coronary syndromes. N Engl J Med. 2007;357:2001–15.
15. Navarese EP, Khan SU, Kołodziejczak M, et al. Comparative efficacy and safety of oral $P2Y_{12}$ inhibitors in acute coronary syndrome. Circulation. 2020;142:150–60.
16. Wallentin L, Becker RC, Budaj A, et al. Ticagrelor versus clopidogrel in patients with acute coronary syndromes. N Engl J Med. 2009;361:1045–57.
17. Silvain J, Lattuca B, Beygui F, et al. Ticagrelor versus clopidogrel in elective percutaneous coronary intervention (ALPHEUS): a randomised, open-label, phase 3b trial. Lancet. 2020;396:1737–44.
18. Capodanno D, Milluzzo RP, Angiolillo DJ. Intravenous antiplatelet therapies (glycoprotein IIb/IIIa receptor inhibitors and cangrelor) in percutaneous coronary intervention: from pharmacology to indications for clinical use. Ther Adv Cardiovasc Dis. 2019;13:175394471989327.
19. Bhatt DL, Stone GW, Mahaffey KW, et al. Effect of platelet inhibition with cangrelor during PCI on ischemic events. N Engl J Med. 2013;368:1303–13.
20. Cavender MA, Bhatt DL, Stone GW, et al. Consistent reduction in periprocedural myocardial infarction with cangrelor as assessed by multiple definitions. Circulation. 2016;134:723–33.
21. Capodanno D, Angiolillo DJ. Pretreatment with antiplatelet drugs in invasively managed patients with coronary artery disease in the contemporary era. Circ Cardiovasc Interv. 2015. https://doi.org/10.1161/CIRCINTERVENTIONS.114.002301.
22. Capodanno D, Angiolillo DJ. Reviewing the controversy surrounding pre-treatment with $P2Y_{12}$ inhibitors in acute coronary syndrome patients. Expert Rev Cardiovasc Ther. 2016;14:811–20.
23. Montalescot G, Bolognese L, Dudek D, et al. Pretreatment with prasugrel in non–ST-segment elevation acute coronary syndromes. N Engl J Med. 2013;369:999–1010.
24. Tarantini G, Mojoli M, Varbella F, et al. Timing of oral P2Y12 inhibitor administration in patients with non-ST-segment elevation acute coronary syndrome. J Am Coll Cardiol. 2020;76:2450–9.
25. Schüpke S, Neumann F-J, Menichelli M, et al. Ticagrelor or prasugrel in patients with acute coronary syndromes. N Engl J Med. 2019;381:1524–34.
26. Montalescot G, van't Hof AW, Lapostolle F, et al. Prehospital ticagrelor in ST-segment elevation myocardial infarction. N Engl J Med. 2014;371:1016–27.
27. Koul S, Smith JG, Götberg M, et al. No benefit of ticagrelor pretreatment compared with treatment during percutaneous coronary intervention in patients with ST-segment–elevation myocardial infarction undergoing primary percutaneous coronary intervention. Circ Cardiovasc Interv. 2018. https://doi.org/10.1161/CIRCINTERVENTIONS.117.005528.
28. Xu J, Song Y, Gao Z, et al. Long-term outcomes of extending dual antiplatelet therapy after drug-eluting

stent implantation for acute coronary syndrome: a large single-center study. Platelets. 2020;31:869–76.
29. Garratt KN, Weaver WD, Jenkins RG, Pow TK, Mauri L, Kereiakes DJ, Winters KJ, Christen T, Allocco DJ, Lee DP. Prasugrel plus aspirin beyond 12 months is associated with improved outcomes after Taxus Liberté paclitaxel-eluting coronary stent placement. Circulation. 2015;131:62–73.
30. Bonaca MP, Bhatt DL, Steg PG, et al. Ischaemic risk and efficacy of ticagrelor in relation to time from $P2Y_{12}$ inhibitor withdrawal in patients with prior myocardial infarction: insights from PEGASUS-TIMI 54. Eur Heart J. 2016;37:1133–42.
31. Bhatt DL, Steg PG, Mehta SR, et al. Ticagrelor in patients with diabetes and stable coronary artery disease with a history of previous percutaneous coronary intervention (THEMIS-PCI): a phase 3, placebo-controlled, randomised trial. Lancet. 2019;394:1169–80.
32. Valgimigli M, Bueno H, Byrne RA, et al. 2017 ESC focused update on dual antiplatelet therapy in coronary artery disease developed in collaboration with EACTS. Eur Heart J. 2018;39:213–54.
33. Laudani C, Greco A, Occhipinti G, et al. Short duration of DAPT versus de-escalation after percutaneous coronary intervention for acute coronary syndromes. JACC Cardiovasc Interv. 2022;15:268–77.
34. Costa F, Van Klaveren D, Feres F, et al. Dual antiplatelet therapy duration based on ischemic and bleeding risks after coronary stenting. J Am Coll Cardiol. 2019;73:741–54.
35. Urban P, Mehran R, Colleran R, et al. Defining high bleeding risk in patients undergoing percutaneous coronary intervention. Circulation. 2019;140:240–61.
36. Costa F, Montalto C, Branca M, et al. Dual antiplatelet therapy duration after percutaneous coronary intervention in high bleeding risk: a meta-analysis of randomized trials. Eur Heart J. 2023;44:954–68.
37. Smits PC, Frigoli E, Tijssen J, et al. Abbreviated antiplatelet therapy in patients at high bleeding risk with or without oral anticoagulant therapy after coronary stenting: an open-label, randomized, controlled trial. Circulation. 2021;144:1196–211.
38. Watanabe H, Morimoto T, et al. Comparison of clopidogrel monotherapy after 1 to 2 months of dual antiplatelet therapy with 12 months of dual antiplatelet therapy in patients with acute coronary syndrome the STOPDAPT-2 ACS randomized clinical trial. JAMA Cardiol. 2022;7:407–17.
39. O'Donoghue ML, Murphy SA, Sabatine MS. The safety and efficacy of aspirin discontinuation on a background of a $P2Y_{12}$ inhibitor in patients after percutaneous coronary intervention. Circulation. 2020;142:538–45.
40. Capodanno D, Mehran R, Valgimigli M, et al. Aspirin-free strategies in cardiovascular disease and cardioembolic stroke prevention. Nat Rev Cardiol. 2018;15:480–96.
41. Vranckx P, Valgimigli M, Jüni P, et al. Ticagrelor plus aspirin for 1 month, followed by ticagrelor monotherapy for 23 months vs aspirin plus clopidogrel or ticagrelor for 12 months, followed by aspirin monotherapy for 12 months after implantation of a drug-eluting stent: a multicentre, open-label, randomised superiority trial. Lancet. 2018;392:940–9.
42. Mehran R, Baber U, Sharma SK, et al. Ticagrelor with or without aspirin in high-risk patients after PCI. N Engl J Med. 2019;381:2032–42.
43. Watanabe H, Morimoto T, Natsuaki M, et al. Comparison of clopidogrel monotherapy after 1 to 2 months of dual antiplatelet therapy with 12 months of dual antiplatelet therapy in patients with acute coronary syndrome. JAMA Cardiol. 2022;7:407.
44. Natsuaki M, Watanabe H, Morimoto T, et al. An aspirin-free versus dual antiplatelet strategy for coronary stenting: STOPDAPT-3 randomized trial. Circulation. 2024;149:585–600.
45. De Luca L, D'Ascenzo F, Musumeci G, Saia F, Parodi G, Varbella F, Marchese A, De Servi S, Berti S, Bolognese L. Incidence and outcome of switching of oral platelet P2Y12 receptor inhibitors in patients with acute coronary syndromes undergoing percutaneous coronary intervention: the SCOPE registry. EuroIntervention. 2017;13:459–66.
46. Sibbing D, Aradi D, Jacobshagen C, et al. A randomised trial on platelet function-guided de-escalation of antiplatelet treatment in ACS patients undergoing PCI. Thromb Haemost. 2017;117:188–95.
47. Willemsen LM, Janssen PWA, Peper J, et al. Effect of adding ticagrelor to standard aspirin on saphenous vein graft patency in patients undergoing coronary artery bypass grafting (POPular CABG). Circulation. 2020;142:1799–807.
48. Angiolillo DJ. Dual antiplatelet therapy guided by platelet function testing. Lancet. 2017;390:1718–20.

21 De-escalation of DAPT

Placido Maria Mazzone, Antonino Imbesi, and Davide Capodanno

21.1 Introduction

Dual antiplatelet therapy (DAPT) is the cornerstone of pharmacological therapy for patients with an acute coronary syndrome (ACS), with the ability to act on two distinct platelet activation pathways (i.e., the COX-1 pathway via aspirin and the ADP pathway via $P2Y_{12}$ inhibitors), thus reducing the risk of recurrent ischemic and thrombotic events [1]. Current European and American guidelines recommend the administration of DAPT with aspirin and a $P2Y_{12}$ inhibitor for 12 months after an acute coronary event, followed by long-term aspirin alone (class I). The oral $P2Y_{12}$ inhibitors prasugrel and ticagrelor, when available and in the absence of contraindications, are preferred to clopidogrel given their superiority in preventing major adverse cardiac events (MACE) (class I), although this benefit comes at the price of an increased risk of bleeding [2–5].

In the attempt to balance the risks and benefits that come from using of a more intense antiplatelet strategy, ischemic and hemorrhagic risk scores have been introduced to individualize decisions around DAPT [6]. One of such scores is the PRECISE-DAPT score, which considers age, creatinine clearance, hemoglobin, leukocyte count, and previous spontaneous bleeding to determine the risk of out-of-hospital bleeding in patients treated with DAPT. A PRECISE-DAPT score ≥25 identifies patients at high risk of bleeding. In this subset, it has been demonstrated that a standard DAPT duration of 12 months is associated with a high risk of bleeding without ischemic benefit, while in patients with a PRECISE-DAPT score <25, this strategy is associated with a significant reduction in ischemic events without increase in bleeding [7]. An alternative is the assessment of bleeding risk using the Academic Research Consortium for High Bleeding Risk criteria (i.e., 14 major and 6 minor criteria), where patients who meet at least one major or two minor criteria are considered to be at high risk of bleeding defined as a 1-year risk of BARC (Bleeding Academic Research Consortium) 3 or 5 bleeding ≥4% or a 1-year risk of intracranial hemorrhage ≥1% [8]. According to the 2023 guidelines for ACS from the European Society of Cardiology (ESC), in patients who are not at high ischemic risk, a short DAPT lasting 3–6 months followed by monotherapy preferably with a $P2Y_{12}$ should be considered (Class IIa); in patients at high risk of bleeding, a further shortening of DAPT to 1 month followed by monotherapy with aspirin or a $P2Y_{12}$ inhibitor may be considered (Class IIb) [5]. Importantly, bleeding and thrombosis share common risk factors, and patients at high risk for bleeding are often frequently also at high risk for thrombosis. Additionally, tools used to identify

P. M. Mazzone · A. Imbesi · D. Capodanno (✉)
Cardio-Thoracic-Vascular and Transplantation Department, Policlinico "G. Rodolico-San Marco", Catania, Italy

B. Cortese, S. Rigattieri (eds.), *High Bleeding Risk Patients in Interventional Cardiology*,
https://doi.org/10.1007/978-3-031-87302-7_21

patients at high risk for bleeding do not consider the broad interindividual variability of response to $P2Y_{12}$ inhibitors, especially clopidogrel [9].

After an acute coronary event, the risk of ischemic events is usually higher in the initial period (e.g., the first 30 days) while the risk of bleeding is uniformly distributed over time [1]. Consequently, the net benefit of antithrombotic therapy in some patients varies over time, with a higher relative risk of thrombosis than bleeding in the first few months and a higher relative risk of bleeding than thrombosis in the long term [1, 10, 11]. This evidence has led to the development of a therapeutic strategy that is able to ensure a high level of platelet inhibition and consequently a high level of ischemic protection during the initial stages of ACS, followed by a higher level of bleeding protection in the chronic phase. This strategy consists of switching the oral $P2Y_{12}$ inhibitors from a more potent to a less potent agent (e.g., prasugrel or ticagrelor to clopidogrel) or reducing the dose of the $P2Y_{12}$ inhibitor (e.g., prasugrel 5 mg) after an initial course of DAPT with potent $P2Y_{12}$ inhibitors (Fig. 21.1). This therapeutic approach, broadly known as de-escalation, is gaining attention as one of the most promising strategies to individualize antiplatelet therapy in patients with ACS and high risk of bleeding [9, 12–15]. The comparative efficacy and safety of short DAPT versus de-escalation was indirectly evaluated in a network meta-analysis of 29 randomized controlled trials, where there were no statistically significant differences between the two strategies for the primary endpoint of all-cause death (RR, 0.98; 95% CI, 0.68–1.43). However, de-escalation reduced the risk for net adverse clinical events (NACE) and increased major bleeding compared with short DAPT [16]. Another network meta-analysis included 37 trials with 103,497 patients and compared standard DAPT with several DAPT duration reduction strategies including short-term DAPT, unguided de-escalation, and guided selection of DAPT with genotype or platelet function testing (PFT). In this case, short DAPT emerged as the best strategy to reduce major bleeding and all-cause death, while unguided de-escalation was associated with the lowest risk of MACE and combined minor and major bleeds [17]. Given these mixed results and in the absence of a direct randomized comparison, the comparative efficacy and safety of short DAPT and de-escalation remain unclear. Semantically, the discontinuation of the $P2Y_{12}$ inhibitor or aspirin (i.e., short DAPT) can also be regarded as de-escalation [18]. This latter approach is discussed separately in another chapter, while this chapter will focus specifically on de-escalation by switch or dose reduction.

Based on the European guidelines, de-escalation by switch or dose reduction may be considered (class IIb) in selected ACS patients unsuitable for potent platelet inhibition based on clinical judgment (unguided) or guided by the results of PFT (e.g., with clopidogrel given only to patients without high on-treatment platelet reactivity) or CYP2C19 genotyping (e.g. clopidogrel given only to patients without loss-of-function [LoF] alleles indicating a genetic propensity to impaired clopidogrel-induced inhibition), depending on their individual risk profiles and assays availability [5]. The recent American guidelines for coronary revascularization did not provide specific recommendations in support of de-escalation by switch or dose reduction [2].

The European recommendations derive from several randomized trials that have demonstrated the ability of guided and unguided de-escalation to reduce bleeds without increasing the risk of ischemic events. A meta-analysis of 10,133 patients with ACS suggested that de-escalation, compared to standard DAPT, is effective in reducing not just bleeding events but also ischemic events, possibly as a consequence of reduced disruption of DAPT due to bleeding [19]. As such, this therapeutic approach could be valid not only for patients at high risk of bleeding and therefore ineligible for potent platelet inhibition but also for the broad spectrum of patients with ACS, the population actually included in the pivotal trials of de-escalation, as described in the following sections.

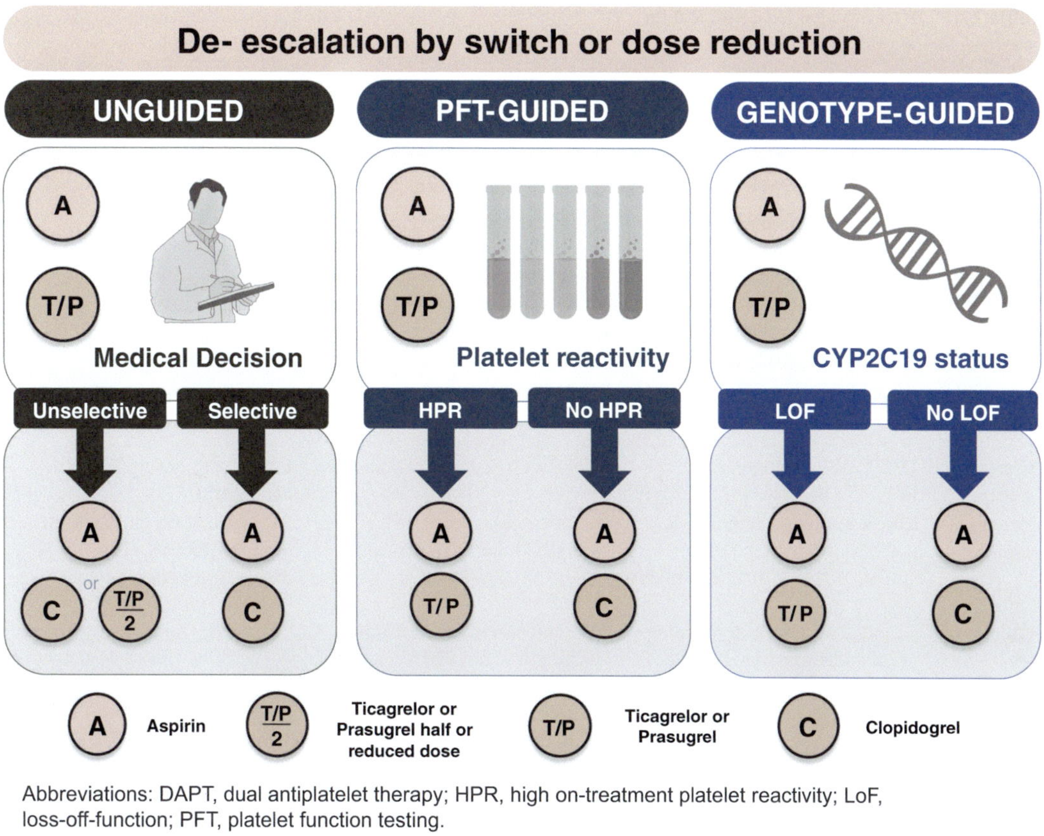

Fig. 21.1 Unguided and guided de-escalation strategies. Abbreviations: DAPT, dual antiplatelet therapy; HPR, high on-treatment platelet reactivity; LoF, loss-off-function; PFT, platelet function testing

21.2 Unguided De-escalation

Unguided de-escalation by switch or dose reduction is based on the above-mentioned principle that the risk of ischemic events after an acute event is higher during the first 30 days and subsequently tends to progressively decrease. In contrast, the risk of bleeding is uniformly distributed over time. Consequently, the high potency of prasugrel and ticagrelor compared to clopidogrel may be more necessary during the initial stages after an ACS. The rationale for de-escalation also stems from two additional consideration. Firstly, the advent of second- and third-generation drug-eluting stents has reduced the risk of myocardial infarction related to late stent thrombosis, one of the most feared complications of percutaneous coronary intervention (PCI) [20]. Secondly, the impact of some types of bleeding on mortality in patients with ACS undergoing PCI is widely recognized as being at least comparable to the risk of recurrent thrombotic events [21, 22].

In contrast to guided de-escalation, which may be readily accomplished post-PCI by utilizing genetic or platelet function tests, the implementation of unguided de-escalation poses a challenge in determining the optimal timing. Given the temporal variability of ischemic and bleeding risks, a reasonable compromise is to perform unguided de-escalation at the conclusion of the initial month after the acute event, as advocated by the landmark trials of unguided de-escalation and current ESC guidelines, which do not recommend its implementation in the first 30 days after the acute event [5, 23–25]. The strategy of delaying the de-escalation after the

Table 21.1 Trials of unguided de-escalation

	TOPIC	TALOS-AMI	HOST-REDUCE
Study design	Open-label, single center, superiority, randomized	Open-label, assessor-blinded, multicenter, non-inferiority, randomized	Open-label, assessor-blinded, multicenter, non-inferiority, randomized
No. of patients	646	2,697	2,338
Population	Stabilized AMI undergoing PCI on DAPT with prasugrel or ticagrelor and aspirin for 1 month without thrombotic/ischemic or bleeding events	Stabilized AMI undergoing PCI on DAPT with ticagrelor and aspirin for 1 month without thrombotic/ischemic or bleeding events	ACS undergoing PCI
Strategy	Unguided switch from prasugrel or ticagrelor and aspirin (100 mg) to clopidogrel and aspirin (75 mg)	Unguided switch from ticagrelor to clopidogrel	Unguided dose reduction from prasugrel 10 mg to 5 mg at 1 month after PCI
Control group	DAPT with prasugrel or ticagrelor and aspirin (100 mg)	DAPT with ticagrelor and aspirin	DAPT with prasugrel (10 mg) and aspirin
Primary endpoints	Cardiovascular death, urgent coronary revascularization, stroke, or BARC type 2 or higher	Cardiovascular death, MI, stroke, or BARC type 2, 3, or 5	All-cause death, nonfatal MI, stent thrombosis, clinically driven revascularization, stroke, or BARC type 2 or higher
Follow-up	11 months from randomization (12 months from AMI)	11 months from randomization (12 months from PCI)	12 months from randomization
Result	HR, 0.48; 95% CI, 0.34–0.68; *P* for superiority <0.01	HR, 0.55; 95% CI, 0.40–0.76; *P* for non-inferiority <0.001; *P* for superiority = 0.0001	HR, 0.70; 95% CI, 0.52–0.92; *P* for non-inferiority <0.0001; *P* for equivalence = 0.012

Abbreviations: *ACS* acute coronary syndrome, *AMI* acute myocardial infarction, *BARC* Bleeding Academic Research Consortium, *CI* confidence interval, *DAPT* dual antiplatelet therapy, *HR* hazard ratio, *MI* myocardial infarction, *PCI* percutaneous coronary intervention

initial vulnerable period is also supported by the SCOPE registry, a multicenter study that enrolled 1,363 patients with ACS undergoing PCI, which examined the safety of switching oral $P2Y_{12}$ inhibitors over a 3-month interval [26]. Earlier de-escalation, in the first month after PCI, resulted in a higher incidence of MACE, mainly driven by recurrent myocardial infarction [26].

Pharmacodynamic investigations have demonstrated that the transition from prasugrel to clopidogrel or from ticagrelor to clopidogrel results in a tenfold rise in platelet reactivity, which can be partly mitigated by administering a 600 mg loading dose at the time of switching [27, 28]. Moreover, this de-escalation approach raises the likelihood of pharmacological interactions between ticagrelor and clopidogrel, as their active metabolites have different sites of action and different affinities for the $P2Y_{12}$ platelet receptor. Specifically, the binding of ticagrelor to $P2Y_{12}$ receptors could impede the active metabolites of clopidogrel from attaching to the receptor, necessitating a waiting period of 12–24 h from the last maintenance dose of ticagrelor before administering the loading dose of clopidogrel [27]. In this scenario, early de-escalation would substantially decrease the level of antithrombotic protection during an extremely critical and highly vulnerable phase with respect to thrombotic or ischemic events.

Investigated strategies of unguided de-escalation include switching from ticagrelor or prasugrel to clopidogrel in the TOPIC and TALOS-AMI trial or reducing the prasugrel dose in the HOST-REDUCE-POLYTECH-ACS trial (Table 21.1) [23–25]. The TOPIC trial was the first study to investigate the efficacy and safety of unguided de-escalation in 646 ACS patients who underwent PCI [23]. The trial demonstrated the superiority of de-escalation over standard DAPT in terms of a composite outcome of ischemic and bleeding events (HR, 0.48; 95% CI, 0.34–0.68; $P < 0.01$), primarily due to a reduction in bleeding events, with no significant difference in the rate of ischemic or thrombotic occurrences. However, the primary composite endpoint did not include myocardial infarction, the trial was of modest size (which limits the interpretation of the observed differences in adverse events), and the patient population consisted mostly of individuals who underwent noncomplex PCI. Furthermore, the advantages of de-escalation were mainly due to BARC bleeding type 2, which are generally regarded as clinically significant but not major events.

In the TALOS-AMI trial, 2,697 individuals with acute myocardial infarction who underwent PCI were enrolled. De-escalation was not only non-inferior but also superior to standard DAPT in reducing NACE (HR, 0.55; 95% CI, 0.40–0.76; $P < 0.001$ for non-inferiority and 0.0001 for superiority), with the difference, like in TOPIC, primarily driven by a significant reduction in BARC type 2 bleeding. However, since the trial included East Asian patients who possess distinct thrombotic/ischemic and bleeding traits, the generalizability of the study to other ethnicities is uncertain. Moreover, since only ticagrelor was used before switching to clopidogrel, it remains unclear whether the findings are also relevant to de-escalation from prasugrel [24].

In the HOST-REDUCE-POLYTECH-ACS trial, a distinct de-escalation approach was investigated, wherein the 2,338 enrolled patients were randomized to standard DAPT or a reduction in prasugrel dosage from 10 mg to 5 mg [25]. Once again, de-escalation was found to be non-inferior to standard DAPT in terms of NACE (HR, 0.70; 95% CI, 0.52–0.92; $P < 0.0001$ for non-inferiority; $P = 0.012$ for equivalence) and was linked to a decrease in bleeding without an increase in thrombotic or ischemic events. Limitations of this study include the relatively large non-inferiority margin of 2.5% and the relatively low statistical power of 75% set by the investigators (although the study ended with more events than expected in the control arm). Again, the patient population studied was East Asian. Moreover, the trial employed a 2 × 2 multifactorial design (including another randomization of stent types), and although the two randomizations were independent, this type of design carries an inherent risk for lower potency due to multiple testing.

In comparison to the guided approach, de-escalation based on clinical judgment offers the benefit of greater practicality, as it does not necessitate multiple drug switches, such as transitioning from prasugrel to clopidogrel and potentially switching to prasugrel in the event of high platelet reactivity on a platelet function test. Additionally, it is important to acknowledge that the instruments required to conduct these tests have limited availability in routine clinical practice and are quite costly.

One area of the knowledge gap is the direct comparison of the two strategies in terms of efficacy and safety. Two meta-analyses have demonstrated that, compared with guided de-escalation, unguided de-escalation has the benefit of a significantly lower rate of bleeding complications, which in turn has a significant impact on the rate of ischemic events [19, 29]. In fact, a substantial proportion of patients undergoing guided de-escalation continue taking potent $P2Y_{12}$ inhibitors beyond the first month of ACS, regardless of changes over time in ischemic and bleeding risk. Additionally, numerous other factors, such as age, body mass index, chronic kidney disease, and diabetes mellitus, play a crucial role in determining the individual response to clopidogrel [30, 31]. Hence, these patients are potentially exposed to a heightened risk of bleeding, which, combined with other side effects of potent $P2Y_{12}$ inhibitors, such as epigastric pain or even dyspnea from ticagrelor, may lead to discontinuation of antithrombotic agents and an increased risk of ischemic events. Conversely, unguided de-escalation may reduce bleeding events uniformly and potentially improve medication adherence, resulting in fewer ischemic events.

21.3 Guided De-escalation

Clopidogrel is the most prescribed and studied $P2Y_{12}$ inhibitor. Although its efficacy has been widely demonstrated in the setting of coronary artery disease, the individual response to clopidogrel appears to be widely variable [32–34]. This results in an inadequate level of platelet inhibition in approximately 30% of treated patients, which can be explained mainly, but not necessarily, by genetic polymorphisms of the cytochrome CYP450 involved in the biotransformation of clopidogrel into its active metabolite in the liver, resulting in high platelet reactivity and an increased risk of thrombotic complications [35]. Carriers of CYP2C19*2 and CYP2C19*3 LoF alleles have diminished enzyme activity, while CYP2C19*17 gain-of-function (GoF) alleles have increased activity [36, 37]. As such, five phenotypes can be identified based on the distribution of CYP2C19 alleles: ultrarapid, rapid, normal, intermediate, and poor metabolizers. Poor metabolizers carry two CYP2C19 LoF alleles, while intermediate metabolizers carry only one allele. Several studies have shown intermediate metabolizers and particularly poor metabolizers phenotypes to be associated with reduced levels of the active metabolite of clopidogrel, diminished platelet inhibition, and a higher rate of MACE following PCI, including stent thrombosis, as compared to other phenotypes [38, 39].

On this background, the mechanism of the inadequate response to clopidogrel appears to be much more complex and multifactorial. For example, East Asian patients, despite having a higher prevalence of CYP2C19*2 and *3 LoF alleles, are more susceptible to bleeding rather than ischemic events than Caucasians during treatment with clopidogrel, a phenomenon known as the "East Asian paradox" [40]. Consequently, a different therapeutic window of platelet inhibition has been proposed to minimize ischemic and bleeding complications in East Asian versus Caucasian patients undergoing PCI, with higher cutoffs for high platelet reactivity, and multiple clinical trials are ongoing to find the best strategy for achieving the desirable clinical benefit in this population (NCT03465644, NCT04755387). This represents an important limitation of the current guided de-escalation studies as they have been conducted exclusively on the European population, which makes the applicability of these results to other ethnicities relatively unknown [40, 41].

The goal of guided de-escalation is to obtain an optimal level of platelet inhibition through the modulation of antiplatelet therapy after assessing the level of platelet reactivity through PFT or by assessing the patient's genotype [1]. This approach enables reducing the risk of bleeding linked to the administration of potent $P2Y_{12}$ inhibitors in patients without on-clopidogrel high platelet reactivity and in patients who do not have the CYP2C19 LoF alleles following genotyping, reserving the use of ticagrelor and prasugrel for patients with a suboptimal level of platelet inhibition to clopidogrel. Moreover, unlike unguided de-escalation, it can be theoretically implemented immediately or soon after PCI without waiting for the safety window of the first month post-PCI [9, 13]. This approach is currently not recommended by the guidelines (Class III); however it is important to underline that this is a generic recommendation for de-escalation, and there are currently no specific recommendations for guided de-escalation [5].

In recent years, new point-of-care tests have emerged that can be used at the patient's bedside, but their use is still limited by logistical problems and costs. PFT has the advantage of being able to identify two phenotypes, high platelet reactivity and low platelet reactivity, characterized by a high thrombotic and hemorrhagic risk, respectively. One major limitation of these tests is the requirement for patients to be treated with an antiplatelet therapy to determine their response to the drug and possibly modify it multiple times (e.g. firstly from prasugrel or ticagrelor to clopidogrel before PFT and secondly from clopidogrel to prasugrel or ticagrelor if they have high platelet reactivity [42]). This latter aspect is particularly problematic in the case of ACS, where prasugrel and ticagrelor are the first choice and one may need to switch to clopidogrel, maintain it for 7–14 days, and then perform the test, at the risk of providing inadequate antithrombotic protection in a critical phase where the ischemic risk is higher. Additionally, some of these tests require a blood sample and are therefore only viable in a laboratory setting, making them unavailable in nonspecialized centers. Common platelet aggregation tests include thromboelastography, the assessment of vasodilator-stimulated phosphoprotein (VASP), light transmission aggregometry, and the Multiplate, VerifyNow, PFA-100, and PL-12 analyzers. Among these, VerifyNow, PFA-100, and PL-12 are bedside point-of-care assays [9, 42–44].

Additionally, genetic testing has become more accessible, faster, and available, making it a potentially more practical option [38]. Genetic testing can be conducted directly during hospitalization for ACS as it is independent of the patient's current therapy [38]. However, its fundamental disadvantage is that genetics is only a determining factor in the response to clopidogrel, as the integration of genetics with clinical variables (e.g., ABCD-GENE score) can improve accuracy and better identify patients with reduced clopidogrel response [31]. Some of the new genetic tests that have emerged include the Genomadix CYP2C19 cube, Verigene, and ST Q3 [45].

One trial investigated a genotype-guided de-escalation strategy (Table 21.2). The POPular Genetics trial randomized 2,488 patients with STEMI undergoing PCI to receive either a $P2Y_{12}$ inhibitor based on early CYP2C19 genotyping or standard DAPT with either ticagrelor or prasugrel for 12 months [46]. The genotype-guided strategy was non-inferior to standard DAPT in terms of NACE (absolute difference, −0.7%; 95% CI, −2.0–0.7; $P < 0.001$ for non-inferiority) and resulted in a lower incidence of bleeding (mostly minor), defined according to Platelet Inhibition and Patient Outcomes (PLATO) criteria, without significant differences in ischemic/thrombotic outcomes. However, the trial had some limitations, including a lower-than-anticipated incidence of the co-primary combined endpoint affecting the power of the comparison, and a non-inferiority design with a primary endpoint that included both ischemic and bleeding outcomes.

Another approach to de-escalation is PFT-guided dose or drug adjustment, and two trials have tested this strategy (Table 21.2). The ANTARCTIC study investigated the effect of PFT-guided DAPT compared to standard DAPT with prasugrel 5 mg in 877 elderly patients with ACS undergoing PCI [47]. Patients randomized to the guided group underwent PFT (and dose adjustment if necessary) in two steps at days 14 and 28 after PCI. There was no significant difference between treatments in the primary NACE endpoint (HR, 1.00; 95% CI, 0.78–1.29; $P = 0.98$ for superiority). There were also no significant differences in the ischemic/thrombotic components of the primary endpoint, as well as in major, minor, or combined major and minor bleeds. However, it is important to underline that the relatively small sample size and the selected nature of the population represent an important limitation of this trial and limit its generalizability to other ethnicities and age groups.

In the TROPICAL ACS trial, 2,610 patients with STEMI or NSTEMI undergoing PCI were randomized to early de-escalation of DAPT guided by PFT or standard DAPT [48]. In the de-escalation group, patients received 1 week of DAPT with prasugrel (10 mg or 5 mg per day) at discharge, followed by 1 week of DAPT with clopidogrel (75 mg per day). Then, based on PFT results at 2 weeks from discharge, patients with high platelet reactivity were switched back to prasugrel, while patients without high platelet reactivity continued with clopidogrel. De-escalation was non-inferior in reducing combined thrombotic and bleeding events compared to standard DAPT; however, it did not meet the criteria for superiority (HR, 0.81; 95% CI, 0.62–1.06; $P = 0.0004$ for non-inferiority; $P = 0.12$ for superiority). It also resulted in a reduction in the composite of BARC bleeding type 2 or higher and the composite of all bleedings, mostly driven by minimal and minor bleeds; however this reduction was not statistically significant. Among the limitations, some have argued that this study used a relatively generous non-inferiority margin (1.30). Furthermore, the findings do not specifically apply to patients with high bleeding risk, who are generally candidates for clopidogrel and were therefore excluded from randomization. Finally, as in previous studies, only European patients were enrolled, which limits their generalization to other ethnic groups.

Table 21.2 Trials of guided de-escalation

	Antarctic	Tropical ACS	Popular genetics
Study design	Open-label, assessor-blinded, multicenter, superiority, randomized	Open-label, assessor-blinded, multicenter, non-inferiority, randomized	Open-label, assessor-blinded, multicenter, non-inferiority (primary efficacy endpoint) and superiority (primary safety endpoint), randomized
No. of patients	877	2,610	2,488
Population	ACS undergoing PCI	AMI undergoing PCI	STEMI undergoing primary PCI
Strategy	PFT-guided dose or drug adjustment from prasugrel 5 mg to prasugrel 10 mg in HPR patients, to clopidogrel in LPR patients or continuation with prasugrel 5 mg in patients with on-target inhibition at day 14 and 28 after PCI	PFT-guided switch from clopidogrel to prasugrel in HPR patients or continuation with clopidogrel in no-HPR patients at day 14 after discharge	Genotype-guided choice of P2Y12 inhibitor (ticagrelor or prasugrel in carriers of CYP2C19*2 or CYP2C19*3 LoF alleles, clopidogrel in noncarriers)
Control group	DAPT with prasugrel 5 mg and aspirin	DAPT with prasugrel and aspirin	DAPT with prasugrel or ticagrelor and aspirin
Primary endpoints	Cardiovascular death, MI, stroke, stent thrombosis, urgent revascularization, or BARC type 2, 3, or 5	Cardiovascular death, MI, stroke, or BARC type 2 or higher	All-cause death, MI, stent thrombosis, stroke, or PLATO major bleeding; PLATO major or minor bleeding
Follow-up	12 months from randomization	12 months from randomization	12 months from randomization
Result	HR, 1.00; 95% CI, 0.78–1.29; *P* for superiority = 0.98	HR, 0.81; 95% CI, 0.62–1.06; *P* for non-inferiority = 0.0004; P for superiority = 0.12	Absolute difference, −0.7%; 95% CI, −2.0–0.7; *P* for non-inferiority <0.001 (NACE); HR, 0.78; 95% CI, 0.61–0.98; *P* = 0.04 (bleeding)

Abbreviations: *ACS* acute coronary syndrome, *AMI* acute myocardial infarction, *BARC* Bleeding Academic Research Consortium, *CI* confidence interval, *DAPT* dual antiplatelet therapy, *HPR* high on-treatment platelet reactivity, *HR* hazard ratio, *LoF* loss-of-function, *LPR* low on-treatment platelet reactivity, *MI* myocardial infarction, *NACE* net adverse cardiac events, *PCI* percutaneous coronary intervention, *PFT* platelet function testing, *PLATO* platelet inhibition and patient outcomes, *STEMI* ST-segment elevation myocardial infarction

These results were confirmed by a meta-analysis of 15 trials which considered 61,898 patients with ACS. Compared with clopidogrel-based DAPT, the incidence of MACE was significantly lower with the guided de-escalation (incidence rate ratio [IRR], 0.80; 95% CI, 0.65–0.98); conversely, bleeding was significantly increased with standard DAPT but not with the guided approach (IRR, 1.22; 95% CI, 0.96–1.55) [49]. In a sub-analysis, the guided approach was associated with a marginally significant reduction of MACE compared with ticagrelor-based DAPT; however, this significant reduction was not observed when compared with prasugrel-based DAPT. These findings align with a preceding meta-analysis of 14 studies, which compared identical groups and concluded that the guided approach reduced both MACE and any bleeding events, particularly minor bleeding [50].

Ultimately, the main limitation of PFT-guided de-escalation is the delay in the initiation of guided therapy due to the need for patients to already be on clopidogrel before performing the PFT followed by the switch to a potent $P2Y_{12}$ inhibitor in the case of high platelet reactivity during treatment with clopidogrel; this caveat can delay the start of optimal therapy and therefore expose the patient to a greater ischemic risk in the period in which this risk is higher. Added to this issue is the availability of the necessary assays to implement the tests, which are not currently usable on a large scale, and the complexity of managing antiplatelet therapy with the need for undertaking different switches in case of high platelet reactivity or low platelet reactivity, as highlighted in ANTARCTIC, which make this strategy attractive but difficult to implement in daily clinical practice.

21.4 Conclusions

De-escalating antiplatelet therapy is gaining traction as an alternative to the standard DAPT for patients with ACS. The rationale behind de-escalation is to reduce the strength of antithrombotic treatments when the risk of bleeding outweighs the risk of ischemic events. This approach aims to curtail bleeding incidents without heightening the risk of ischemia. However, there are several knowledge gaps in this field. The comparative effectiveness and safety of unguided versus guided de-escalation remain uncertain. Moreover, the practical implementation of guided de-escalation in clinical practice is hindered by the availability of the necessary tests for routine use. Also, existing major studies did not address specific patient populations, such as those at high risk for ischemic events or bleeding. Consequently, the suitability of de-escalation in these contexts is still unclear. Presently, the most promising approach seems to be unguided de-escalation around 1 month after the initial procedure in patients unsuitable for potent platelet inhibition, with the aim to reducing the risk of bleeding. This approach offers comparable effectiveness to guided de-escalation while significantly reducing the bleeding rate. Additionally, it can be more straightforwardly and intuitively incorporated into clinical practice, even in settings where platelet function tests or genetic testing are not widely available.

References

1. Angiolillo DJ, Galli M, Collet JP, Kastrati A, O'Donoghue ML. Antiplatelet therapy after percutaneous coronary intervention. EuroIntervention. 2022;17(17):e1371–e96. https://doi.org/10.4244/eij-d-21-00904.
2. Lawton JS, Tamis-Holland JE, Bangalore S, Bates ER, Beckie TM, Bischoff JM, et al. 2021 ACC/AHA/SCAI guideline for coronary artery revascularization: executive summary: a report of the American College of Cardiology/American Heart Association Joint Committee on Clinical Practice Guidelines. Circulation. 2022;145(3):e4–e17. https://doi.org/10.1161/cir.0000000000001039.
3. Wiviott SD, Braunwald E, McCabe CH, Montalescot G, Ruzyllo W, Gottlieb S, et al. Prasugrel versus clopidogrel in patients with acute coronary syndromes. N Engl J Med. 2007;357(20):2001–15. https://doi.org/10.1056/NEJMoa0706482.
4. Wallentin L, Becker RC, Budaj A, Cannon CP, Emanuelsson H, Held C, et al. Ticagrelor versus clopidogrel in patients with acute coronary syndromes. N Engl J Med. 2009;361(11):1045–57. https://doi.org/10.1056/NEJMoa0904327.
5. Byrne RA, Rossello X, Coughlan JJ, Barbato E, Berry C, Chieffo A, et al. 2023 ESC Guidelines for the management of acute coronary syndromes: developed by the task force on the management of acute coronary syndromes of the European Society of Cardiology (ESC). Eur Heart J. 2023;44:3720. https://doi.org/10.1093/eurheartj/ehad191.
6. Valgimigli M, Bueno H, Byrne RA, Collet J-P, Costa F, Jeppsson A, et al. 2017 ESC focused update on dual antiplatelet therapy in coronary artery disease developed in collaboration with EACTS: the Task Force for dual antiplatelet therapy in coronary artery disease of the European Society of Cardiology (ESC) and of the European Association for Cardio-Thoracic Surgery (EACTS). Eur Heart J. 2017;39(3):213–60. https://doi.org/10.1093/eurheartj/ehx419.
7. Costa F, van Klaveren D, James S, Heg D, Räber L, Feres F, et al. Derivation and validation of the predicting bleeding complications in patients undergoing stent implantation and subsequent dual antiplatelet therapy (PRECISE-DAPT) score: a pooled analysis of individual-patient datasets from clinical trials. Lancet. 2017;389(10073):1025–34. https://doi.org/10.1016/s0140-6736(17)30397-5.
8. Urban P, Mehran R, Colleran R, Angiolillo DJ, Byrne RA, Capodanno D, et al. Defining high bleeding risk in patients undergoing percutaneous coronary intervention: a consensus document from the Academic Research Consortium for High Bleeding Risk. Eur Heart J. 2019;40(31):2632–53. https://doi.org/10.1093/eurheartj/ehz372.
9. Sibbing D, Aradi D, Alexopoulos D, Ten Berg J, Bhatt DL, Bonello L, et al. Updated expert consensus statement on platelet function and genetic

testing for guiding P2Y(12) receptor inhibitor treatment in percutaneous coronary intervention. JACC Cardiovasc Interv. 2019;12(16):1521–37. https://doi.org/10.1016/j.jcin.2019.03.034.
10. Becker RC, Bassand JP, Budaj A, Wojdyla DM, James SK, Cornel JH, et al. Bleeding complications with the P2Y12 receptor antagonists clopidogrel and ticagrelor in the PLATelet inhibition and patient Outcomes (PLATO) trial. Eur Heart J. 2011;32(23):2933–44. https://doi.org/10.1093/eurheartj/ehr422.
11. Antman EM, Wiviott SD, Murphy SA, Voitk J, Hasin Y, Widimsky P, et al. Early and late benefits of prasugrel in patients with acute coronary syndromes undergoing percutaneous coronary intervention: a TRITON-TIMI 38 (TRial to Assess Improvement in Therapeutic Outcomes by Optimizing Platelet InhibitioN with Prasugrel-Thrombolysis In Myocardial Infarction) analysis. J Am Coll Cardiol. 2008;51(21):2028–33. https://doi.org/10.1016/j.jacc.2008.04.002.
12. Angiolillo DJ, Rollini F, Storey RF, Bhatt DL, James S, Schneider DJ, et al. International expert consensus on switching platelet P2Y(12) receptor-inhibiting therapies. Circulation. 2017;136(20):1955–75. https://doi.org/10.1161/circulationaha.117.031164.
13. Galli M, Angiolillo DJ. De-escalation of antiplatelet therapy in acute coronary syndromes: why, how and when? Front Cardiovasc Med. 2022;9:975969. https://doi.org/10.3389/fcvm.2022.975969.
14. van der Sangen NMR, Rozemeijer R, Chan Pin Yin D, Valgimigli M, Windecker S, James SK, et al. Patient-tailored antithrombotic therapy following percutaneous coronary intervention. Eur Heart J. 2021;42(10):1038–46. https://doi.org/10.1093/eurheartj/ehaa1097.
15. Mazzone PM, Angiolillo DJ, Capodanno D. Approaches to de-escalation of antiplatelet treatment in stabilized post-myocardial infarction patients with high ischemic risk. Expert Rev Cardiovasc Ther. 2022;20(10):839–49. https://doi.org/10.1080/14779072.2022.2137492.
16. Laudani C, Greco A, Occhipinti G, Ingala S, Calderone D, Scalia L, et al. Short duration of DAPT versus de-escalation after percutaneous coronary intervention for acute coronary syndromes. JACC Cardiovasc Interv. 2022;15(3):268–77. https://doi.org/10.1016/j.jcin.2021.11.028.
17. Kuno T, Watanabe A, Shoji S, Fujisaki T, Ueyama H, Takagi H, et al. Short-term DAPT and DAPT de-escalation strategies for patients with acute coronary syndromes: a systematic review and network meta-analysis. Circ Cardiovasc Interv. 16(9):e013242. https://doi.org/10.1161/CIRCINTERVENTIONS.123.013242.
18. Capodanno D, Mehran R, Krucoff MW, Baber U, Bhatt DL, Capranzano P, et al. Defining strategies of modulation of antiplatelet therapy in patients with coronary artery disease: a consensus document from the Academic Research Consortium. Circulation. 2023;147(25):1933–44. https://doi.org/10.1161/CIRCULATIONAHA.123.064473.
19. Kang J, Rizas KD, Park KW, Chung J, van den Broek W, Claassens DMF, et al. Dual antiplatelet therapy de-escalation in acute coronary syndrome: an individual patient meta-analysis. Eur Heart J. 2023. https://doi.org/10.1093/eurheartj/ehac829.
20. Moon JY, Franchi F, Rollini F, Angiolillo DJ. Evolution of coronary stent technology and implications for duration of dual antiplatelet therapy. Prog Cardiovasc Dis. 2018;60(4–5):478–90. https://doi.org/10.1016/j.pcad.2017.12.004.
21. Valgimigli M, Costa F, Lokhnygina Y, Clare RM, Wallentin L, Moliterno DJ, et al. Trade-off of myocardial infarction vs. bleeding types on mortality after acute coronary syndrome: lessons from the Thrombin Receptor Antagonist for Clinical Event Reduction in Acute Coronary Syndrome (TRACER) randomized trial. Eur Heart J. 2017;38(11):804–10. https://doi.org/10.1093/eurheartj/ehw525.
22. Capodanno D, Bhatt DL, Gibson CM, James S, Kimura T, Mehran R, et al. Bleeding avoidance strategies in percutaneous coronary intervention. Nat Rev Cardiol. 2022;19(2):117–32. https://doi.org/10.1038/s41569-021-00598-1.
23. Cuisset T, Deharo P, Quilici J, Johnson TW, Deffarges S, Bassez C, et al. Benefit of switching dual antiplatelet therapy after acute coronary syndrome: the TOPIC (timing of platelet inhibition after acute coronary syndrome) randomized study. Eur Heart J. 2017;38(41):3070–8. https://doi.org/10.1093/eurheartj/ehx175.
24. Kim CJ, Park MW, Kim MC, Choo EH, Hwang BH, Lee KY, et al. Unguided de-escalation from ticagrelor to clopidogrel in stabilised patients with acute myocardial infarction undergoing percutaneous coronary intervention (TALOS-AMI): an investigator-initiated, open-label, multicentre, non-inferiority, randomised trial. Lancet. 2021;398(10308):1305–16. https://doi.org/10.1016/s0140-6736(21)01445-8.
25. Kim HS, Kang J, Hwang D, Han JK, Yang HM, Kang HJ, et al. Prasugrel-based de-escalation of dual antiplatelet therapy after percutaneous coronary intervention in patients with acute coronary syndrome (HOST-REDUCE-POLYTECH-ACS): an open-label, multicentre, non-inferiority randomised trial. Lancet. 2020;396(10257):1079–89. https://doi.org/10.1016/s0140-6736(20)31791-8.
26. De Luca L, D'Ascenzo F, Musumeci G, Saia F, Parodi G, Varbella F, et al. Incidence and outcome of switching of oral platelet P2Y12 receptor inhibitors in patients with acute coronary syndromes undergoing percutaneous coronary intervention: the SCOPE registry. EuroIntervention. 2017;13(4):459–66. https://doi.org/10.4244/eij-d-17-00092.
27. Franchi F, Rollini F, Rios JR, Rivas A, Agarwal M, Kureti M, et al. Pharmacodynamic effects of switching from ticagrelor to clopidogrel in patients with coronary artery disease. Circulation. 2018;137(23):2450–62. https://doi.org/10.1161/CIRCULATIONAHA.118.033983.

28. Kerneis M, Silvain J, Abtan J, Cayla G, O'Connor SA, Barthélémy O, et al. Switching acute coronary syndrome patients from prasugrel to clopidogrel. JACC Cardiovasc Interv. 2013;6(2):158–65. https://doi.org/10.1016/j.jcin.2012.09.012.
29. Kuno T, Fujisaki T, Shoji S, Sahashi Y, Tsugawa Y, Iwagami M, et al. Comparison of unguided de-escalation versus guided selection of dual antiplatelet therapy after acute coronary syndrome: a systematic review and network meta-analysis. Circ Cardiovasc Interv. 2022;15(8):e011990. https://doi.org/10.1161/circinterventions.122.011990.
30. Capodanno D, Angiolillo DJ, Lennon RJ, Goodman SG, Kim SW, O'Cochlain F, et al. ABCD-GENE score and clinical outcomes following percutaneous coronary intervention: insights from the TAILOR-PCI trial. J Am Heart Assoc. 2022;11(4):e024156. https://doi.org/10.1161/jaha.121.024156.
31. Angiolillo DJ, Capodanno D, Danchin N, Simon T, Bergmeijer TO, Ten Berg JM, et al. Derivation, validation, and prognostic utility of a prediction rule for nonresponse to clopidogrel: the ABCD-GENE score. JACC Cardiovasc Interv. 2020;13(5):606–17. https://doi.org/10.1016/j.jcin.2020.01.226.
32. Capodanno D, Alfonso F, Levine GN, Valgimigli M, Angiolillo DJ. ACC/AHA versus ESC guidelines on dual antiplatelet therapy: JACC guideline comparison. J Am Coll Cardiol. 2018;72(23 Pt A):2915–31. https://doi.org/10.1016/j.jacc.2018.09.057.
33. Shuldiner AR, O'Connell JR, Bliden KP, Gandhi A, Ryan K, Horenstein RB, et al. Association of cytochrome P450 2C19 genotype with the antiplatelet effect and clinical efficacy of clopidogrel therapy. JAMA. 2009;302(8):849–57. https://doi.org/10.1001/jama.2009.1232.
34. Gurbel PA, Bliden KP, Hiatt BL, O'Connor CM. Clopidogrel for coronary stenting: response variability, drug resistance, and the effect of pretreatment platelet reactivity. Circulation. 2003;107(23):2908–13. https://doi.org/10.1161/01.Cir.0000072771.11429.83.
35. Mega JL, Simon T, Collet JP, Anderson JL, Antman EM, Bliden K, et al. Reduced-function CYP2C19 genotype and risk of adverse clinical outcomes among patients treated with clopidogrel predominantly for PCI: a meta-analysis. JAMA. 2010;304(16):1821–30. https://doi.org/10.1001/jama.2010.1543.
36. Simon T, Verstuyft C, Mary-Krause M, Quteineh L, Drouet E, Méneveau N, et al. Genetic determinants of response to clopidogrel and cardiovascular events. N Engl J Med. 2009;360(4):363–75. https://doi.org/10.1056/NEJMoa0808227.
37. Hochholzer W, Trenk D, Fromm MF, Valina CM, Stratz C, Bestehorn HP, et al. Impact of cytochrome P450 2C19 loss-of-function polymorphism and of major demographic characteristics on residual platelet function after loading and maintenance treatment with clopidogrel in patients undergoing elective coronary stent placement. J Am Coll Cardiol. 2010;55(22):2427–34. https://doi.org/10.1016/j.jacc.2010.02.031.
38. Galli M, Franchi F, Rollini F, Cavallari LH, Capodanno D, Crea F, et al. Genetic testing in patients undergoing percutaneous coronary intervention: rationale, evidence and practical recommendations. Expert Rev Clin Pharmacol. 2021;14(8):963–78. https://doi.org/10.1080/17512433.2021.1927709.
39. Mega JL, Close SL, Wiviott SD, Shen L, Hockett RD, Brandt JT, et al. Cytochrome p-450 polymorphisms and response to clopidogrel. N Engl J Med. 2009;360(4):354–62. https://doi.org/10.1056/NEJMoa0809171.
40. Levine GN, Jeong YH, Goto S, Anderson JL, Huo Y, Mega JL, et al. Expert consensus document: World Heart Federation expert consensus statement on antiplatelet therapy in East Asian patients with ACS or undergoing PCI. Nat Rev Cardiol. 2014;11(10):597–606. https://doi.org/10.1038/nrcardio.2014.104.
41. Kim HK, Tantry US, Smith SC Jr, Jeong MH, Park SJ, Kim MH, et al. The East Asian paradox: an updated position statement on the challenges to the current antithrombotic strategy in patients with cardiovascular disease. Thromb Haemost. 2021;121(4):422–32. https://doi.org/10.1055/s-0040-1718729.
42. Angiolillo DJ. Dual antiplatelet therapy guided by platelet function testing. Lancet. 2017;390(10104):1718–20. https://doi.org/10.1016/s0140-6736(17)32279-1.
43. Galli M, Franchi F, Rollini F, Angiolillo DJ. Role of platelet function and genetic testing in patients undergoing percutaneous coronary intervention. Trends Cardiovasc Med. 2023;33(3):133–8. https://doi.org/10.1016/j.tcm.2021.12.007.
44. Jeong YH, Bliden KP, Antonino MJ, Park KS, Tantry US, Gurbel PA. Usefulness of the VerifyNow P2Y12 assay to evaluate the antiplatelet effects of ticagrelor and clopidogrel therapies. Am Heart J. 2012;164(1):35–42. https://doi.org/10.1016/j.ahj.2012.03.022.
45. Pakala R, Waksman R. Currently available methods for platelet function analysis: advantages and disadvantages. Cardiovasc Revasc Med. 2011;12(5):312–22. https://doi.org/10.1016/j.carrev.2010.09.005.
46. Claassens DMF, Vos GJA, Bergmeijer TO, Hermanides RS, van't Hof AWJ, van der Harst P, et al. A genotype-guided strategy for oral P2Y(12) inhibitors in primary PCI. N Engl J Med. 2019;381(17):1621–31. https://doi.org/10.1056/NEJMoa1907096.
47. Cayla G, Cuisset T, Silvain J, Leclercq F, Manzo-Silberman S, Saint-Etienne C, et al. Platelet function monitoring to adjust antiplatelet therapy in elderly patients stented for an acute coronary syndrome (ANTARCTIC): an open-label, blinded-endpoint, randomised controlled superiority trial. Lancet. 2016;388(10055):2015–22. https://doi.org/10.1016/s0140-6736(16)31323-x.
48. Sibbing D, Aradi D, Jacobshagen C, Gross L, Trenk D, Geisler T, et al. Guided de-escalation of antiplatelet

treatment in patients with acute coronary syndrome undergoing percutaneous coronary intervention (TROPICAL-ACS): a randomised, open-label, multicentre trial. Lancet. 2017;390(10104):1747–57. https://doi.org/10.1016/s0140-6736(17)32155-4.
49. Galli M, Benenati S, Franchi F, Rollini F, Capodanno D, Biondi-Zoccai G, et al. Comparative effects of guided vs. potent P2Y12 inhibitor therapy in acute coronary syndrome: a network meta-analysis of 61 898 patients from 15 randomized trials. Eur Heart J. 2022;43(10):959–67. https://doi.org/10.1093/eurheartj/ehab836.
50. Galli M, Benenati S, Capodanno D, Franchi F, Rollini F, D'Amario D, et al. Guided versus standard antiplatelet therapy in patients undergoing percutaneous coronary intervention: a systematic review and meta-analysis. Lancet. 2021;397(10283):1470–83. https://doi.org/10.1016/s0140-6736(21)00533-x.

22 Single Antiplatelet Therapy After DCB Angioplasty

Sylwia Iwanczyk, Wojciech Wańha, and Bernardo Cortese

Over the past decade, there has been substantial progress in the treatment of coronary heart disease, both in terms of device technology and pharmacotherapy. An individualized approach to antithrombotic treatment, including assessment of the risk of bleeding and ischemic events, has become crucial. In the face of abundant evidence of a significant deterioration of prognosis with highly increased mortality (up to sevenfold) in patients after a bleeding event, great emphasis is placed on shortening complex antithrombotic therapy after percutaneous coronary intervention (PCI) [1]. However, the final decision regarding the duration of treatment should be based on the stratification of the risk of ischemic events, primarily stent thrombosis, in the prevention of which dual antiplatelet therapy (DAPT) is of paramount importance.

Antiplatelet treatment approaches after PCI largely depend on the type of revascularization and distinct patients' manifestations. DAPT with aspirin and the addition of a P2Y12 platelet receptor inhibitor is the cornerstone of pharmacotherapy of patients undergoing PCI to prevent thrombotic complications within the stent during the healing process, and secondly, the progression of atherosclerosis by stabilization of atherosclerotic plaques. Reducing the risk of late and very late ST has been achieved in new-generation drug-eluting stents (DES) by coatings with subsequently less toxic antiproliferative drugs and more biocompatible polymer, as well as thinner stent struts made of modern alloys [2, 3]. However, ST remains a dreaded complication after stent implantation, with a mortality rate between 5% and 45% [4, 5]. Numerous risk factors significantly increase the risk of its occurrence, while the premature discontinuation of DAPT in the first 30 days after stent implantation is the strongest predictor for early ST [3, 6]. Among procedure-related factors, suboptimal angiographic findings, including stent underexpansion or undersizing or malapposition, evaginations, and stent fracture, are of decisive importance.

The new technique of PCI with a drug-coated balloon (DCB) is a treatment strategy for coronary artery disease (CAD) based on the fast and

S. Iwanczyk
Department of Cardiology, Poznan University of Medical Sciences, Poznañ, Poland

W. Wańha
Division of Cardiology and Structural Heart Diseases, Medical University of Silesia, Katowice, Poland

B. Cortese (✉)
University Hospitals Harrington Heart & Vascular Institute, Cleveland, OH, USA

Fondazione Ricerca e Innovazione Cardiovascolare, Milan, Italy

DCB Academy, Milan, Italy

B. Cortese, S. Rigattieri (eds.), *High Bleeding Risk Patients in Interventional Cardiology*, https://doi.org/10.1007/978-3-031-87302-7_22

consistent transfer of antiproliferative drugs into the vessel wall without leaving the stent platform [7]. DCBs have emerged as an alternative to DES for the treatment of in-stent restenosis and de novo lesions in small coronary arteries, especially in high-bleeding risk (HBR) patients. Delivery of an antiproliferative drug to the coronary artery wall without implanting a metal stent significantly reduces the risk of thrombosis. The features of DCB include the possibility of positive vessel remodeling in the absence of a stent, the theoretical lack of risk of stent thrombosis, and the possibility of shortening DAPT [8]. On the other side, the lack of a metal scaffold potentially pronounces the permanent exposure of subendothelial, platelet-activating molecules in DCB-PCI that can trigger vessel thrombosis.

Moreover, suboptimal vessel flow with angiographic evidence of extensive dissections following DCB treatment could potentially be harmful without DAPT. According to current European Society of Cardiology (ESC) guidelines, DES or DCB is recommended in patients undergoing PCI in ISR. However, the value of DCB in patients with de novo coronary artery lesions has been established in several subsequent clinical trials.

Although the risk of acute vessel occlusion remains, the role of antiplatelet therapy in other mechanisms is still uncertain [7]. Therefore, shortening the duration of DAPT after DCB therapy appears to be justified. Notably, no dedicated study to assess the optimal DAPT duration after DCB has been performed. The ESC guidelines recommend a 6-month duration of DAPT for the treatment of ISR without differentiating between DES and DCB-only PCI [9]. However, retrospective trials have demonstrated the safety of 1-month DAPT after DCB-only PCI [10], the most commonly used regimen. The absence of a stent platform reduces the risk of thrombosis; therefore, the single antiplatelet therapy (SAPT) might be safe for those types of revascularization. However, which antiplatelet agent would be best for SAPT following PCI with DCB still remains unclear.

High-bleeding risk (HBR) patients may particularly benefit from SAPT, significantly reducing the risk of major bleeding events and improving survival. The presence of bleeding is associated with poor outcomes in patients with acute coronary syndromes (ACS) and chronic coronary syndrome (CCS) treated with PCI [11, 12]. Notably, preexisting anemia is relatively frequent in patients presenting with ACS, occurring in 19–30% of currently treated patients [13]. Moreover, elderly patients presenting with ST-segment myocardial infarction (STEMI) have an exceptionally high incidence of anemia, which is reported in 43% of cases [14].

However, only a few scientific reports have been published based on retrospective analyses. Cortese et al. retrospectively analyzed 107 patients who underwent PCI with DCB for de novo coronary lesions followed by SAPT from the time of angioplasty due to HBR or active bleeding and compared the clinical outcome to a group of DCB patients treated with DAPT [15]. After 1 year, the primary endpoint of major adverse cardiac events (MACE) and all its components, including cardiac death, myocardial infarction, and target lesion revascularization, were not significantly different between SAPT and DAPT groups (10% versus 9%, $P = 0.78$). Still, a reduction in the cumulative rate of 2–5 BARC bleedings was observed in the SAPT group (9% versus 6%, $P = 0.04$). After adjusting for confounding factors through multivariate analysis, bleeding diathesis, DAPT, and anticoagulant use were predictors of BARC bleeding, whereas bleeding diathesis and acute coronary syndromes were predictors of MACE. This retrospective analysis allows us to hypothesize that a DCB strategy followed by SAPT should be considered in a fragile patient population with native coronary artery disease and HBR.

The study by Rasanen et al. aimed to assess the efficacy and safety of PCI using DCB, followed by a regimen consisting of only SAPT [16]. Almost all treated lesions were de novo (96%), and the majority (58%) were located in large coronary arteries (≥3.0 mm). Most (87%) of the patients were at HBR with at least one major or two minor Academic Research Consortium (ARC) risk factors for bleeding. The study included both patients with stable coronary artery disease and ACS (42.4% and 57.6% of patients, respectively). The clinical outcomes

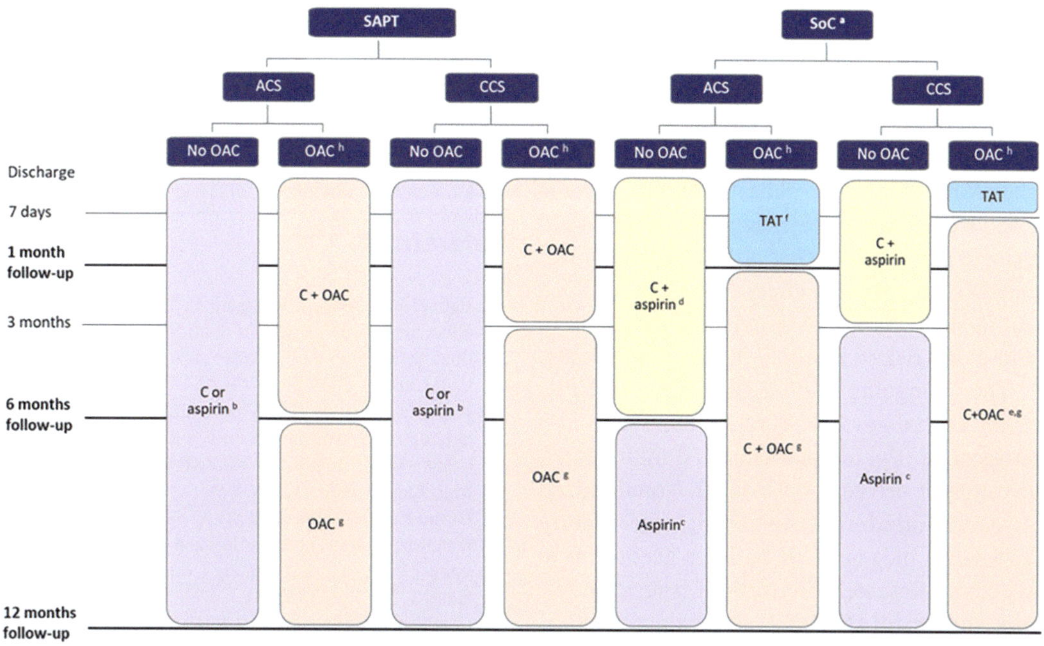

Fig. 22.1 Antithrombotic flowchart of the ongoing PICCOLETO IV-EPIC multi-national RCT

revealed a low rate of overall MACE at 12 and 24 months, respectively, 4.7% and 8.1%. Moreover, the differences in MACE and BARC 2–5 bleeding rates in patients with or without OAC or periprocedural DAPT were statistically insignificant. The procedure appeared safe without acute or subacute vascular occlusions after discharge. Within 2 months after PCI, the hospitalization rate for urgent revascularization was 2.9% (2.7% in stable CAD and 3.0% in ACS patients). The rate of ischemia-driven target lesion revascularization (TLR) was low in both groups: 3.0% in the ACS group and 0% in the stable CAD group at 12 months. Similarly, the myocardial infarction (MI) rate was low at 12 and 24 months (1.2% and 1.7%, respectively). The frequency of significant bleeding (BARC 2–5) was 10.5% at 12 months, while only 2.3% of the patients experienced severe bleeding (BARC 3–5).

Interestingly, many RCTs and registry studies have shown that the rate of acute vascular occlusion after DCB-only treatment in de novo lesions and DAPT treatment is very low, ranging from 0% to 0.5% [17–19]. In comparison, the incidence of acute stent thrombosis in DES trials of the HBR population varies from 0.5% to 2.0% [20, 21]. Thereafter, experts on DCB technology recognize the DCB approach followed by SAPT as a safe and effective treatment method in HBR patients.

More recently, a new kid came out of the blocks in DCB technologies, the sirolimus-coated balloon. The largest prospective study performed with this technology is the EASTBOURNE multicenter study. A prespecified post hoc analysis of this registry compared the 12-month outcomes among 2123 patients prescribed either SAPT (n = 113, 5.8%) or DAPT (n = 1826, 94.1%) and showed a comparable rate of TLR as a primary endpoint in the treatment of de novo lesions, with a rate of 7.7% for SAPT and 5.6% for DAPT (p = 0.6) (Fig. 22.1). Similarly, there was no difference in the secondary endpoint of MACE (all-cause mortality, TLR, and MI) between the SAPT and DAPT regimens (11.2% [n = 12] vs. 8.9% [n = 162], p = 0.4), including subgroups of de novo (56.3%, n = 1091) and in-stent restenosis (47.7%, n = 848) (Fig. 22.1). Notably, during the 12-month follow-up, no acute occlusive events occurred in the SAPT group, and no cases of TLR were recorded within a month following the index procedure. The patients treated with SAPT experienced more 3–5 BARC bleeding events at 12-month follow-up compared to patients treated with DAPT (2.9% [$n = 3$] vs. 0.6% [$n = 10$], $p = 0.027$), probably reflecting a greater fragility of patients in this group. Therefore, the post hoc analysis of the EASTBOURNE registry suggests that the use of a single antiplatelet agent after PCI with sirolimus-DCB is safe and effective in both de novo and in-stent restenosis lesions and may help to control the risk of bleeding in selected patients.

The ongoing PICCOLETO IV-EPIC (ClinicalTrial.gov: NCT06535568) study is a prospective, international, multicenter, investigator-driven, open-label, randomized (1:1), non-inferiority clinical trial. 560 elderly (>74 years old) or HBR patients according to Academic Research Consortium criteria undergone successful DCB-only PCI in native coronary artery disease within vessels diameter between 2.0 and 4.0 mm will be randomized in a 1:1 fashion between SAPT (experimental arm) and DAPT (comparative arm). Patients in the experimental arm will receive aspirin or clopidogrel. In the comparative arm, patients will be treated according to the standard of care. The primary endpoint is MACE defined as a cumulative endpoint [total mortality, TVR (target vessel revascularization), spontaneous myocardial infarction (MI)] at 12 months. The co-primary endpoint is BARC 2–5 bleedings. The PICCOLETO IV-EPIC trial is powered for non-inferiority for the primary and superiority for the co-primary endpoint. Primary analysis will be performed by intention to treat, secondary by as treated. Randomization will occur after successful PCI without stent implantation and patients are being enrolled in Spain, Italy, Belgium, and Luxemburg. The antithrombotic flowchart of this study is reported in the figure.

In summary, the choice of any antiplatelet therapy regimen after PCI requires a deep assessment of the risk of bleeding and ischemic events. The *DCB approach* reduces the risk of ischemic complications, potentially enabling de-escalation of antiplatelet therapy. Although there is only limited data confirming the safety and effectiveness of SAPT in patients treated with DCB, the initial results are promising and further randomized clinical trials (RCT) will shed light on this novel therapeutic option.

References

1. Palmerini T, Bacchi Reggiani L, Della Riva D, et al. Bleeding-related deaths in relation to the duration of dual-antiplatelet therapy after coronary stenting. J Am Coll Cardiol. 2017;69:2011–22.
2. Kedhi E, Joesoef KS, McFadden E, et al. Second-generation everolimus-eluting and paclitaxel-eluting stents in real-life practice (COMPARE): a randomised trial. Lancet. 2010;375:201–9.
3. Byrne RA, Joner M, Kastrati A. Stent thrombosis and restenosis: what have we learned and where are we going? The Andreas Grüntzig Lecture ESC 2014. Eur Heart J. 2015;36:3320–31.
4. Claessen BE, Henriques JP, Jaffer FA, Mehran R, Piek JJ, Dangas GD. Stent thrombosis: a clinical perspective. JACC Cardiovasc Interv. 2014;7:1081–92.
5. Lemesle G, Tricot O, Meurice T, et al. Incident myocardial infarction and very late stent thrombosis in outpatients with stable coronary artery disease. J Am Coll Cardiol. 2017;69:2149–56.
6. Généreux P, Rutledge DR, Palmerini T, et al. Stent thrombosis and dual antiplatelet therapy interruption with everolimus-eluting stents: insights from the Xience V Coronary Stent System trials. Circ Cardiovasc Interv. 2015;8:e001362.
7. Cortese B, Silva-Orrego P, Agostoni P, Buccheri D, Piraino D, Andolina G, Seregni R. Effect of drug-coated balloons in native coronary arterydisease left with a dissection. JACC Cardiovasc Interv. 2015;8:2003–9.
8. Jeger RV, Farah A, Ohlow MA, et al. Drug- coated balloons for small coronary artery disease (BASKET-SMALL 2): an open-label randomised non-inferiority trial. Lancet. 2018;392:849–56.
9. Valgimigli M, Bueno H, Byrne RA, et al. 2017 ESC focused update on dual antiplatelet therapy in coronary artery disease developed in collaboration with EACTS. Eur Heart J. 2018;39(3):213–60.
10. Corballis NH, Wickramarachchi U, Vassiliou VS, Eccleshall SC. Duration of dual antiplatelet therapy in elective drug-coated balloon angioplasty. Catheter Cardiovasc Interv. 2020;96(5):1016–20.
11. Anker SD, Voors A, Okonko D, et al. Prevalence, incidence, and prognostic value of anaemia in patients after an acute myocardial infarction: data from the OPTIMAAL trial. Eur Heart J. 2009;30:1331–9.
12. Bassand JP, Afzal R, Eikelboom J, et al. Relationship between baseline haemoglobin and major bleeding complications in acute coronary syndromes. Eur Heart J. 2010;31:50–8.

13. Sabatine MS, Morrow DA, Giugliano RP, et al. Association of hemoglobin levels with clinical outcomes in acute coronary syndromes. Circulation. 2005;111:2042–9.
14. Wu WC, Rathore SS, Wang Y, Radford MJ, Krumholz HM. Blood transfusion in elderly patients with acute myocardial infarction. N Engl J Med. 2001;345:1230–6.
15. Cortese B, Serruys PW. Single-antiplatelet treatment after coronary angioplasty with drug-coated balloon. J Am Heart Assoc. 2023;12(6):e028413. https://doi.org/10.1161/JAHA.122.028413. Epub 2023 Mar 9. PMID: 36892083; PMCID: PMC10111529.
16. Räsänen A, Kärkkäinen JM, Eranti A, Eränen J, Rissanen TT. Percutaneous coronary intervention with drug-coated balloon-only strategy combined with single antiplatelet treatment in patients at high bleeding risk: single center experience of a novel concept. Catheter Cardiovasc Interv. 2023;101(3):569–78.
17. Wöhrle J, Zadura M, Möbius-Winkler S, et al. SeQuent please world wide registry. J Am Coll Cardiol. 2012;60(18):1733–8.
18. Uskela S, Kärkkäinen JM, Eränen J, et al. Percutaneous coronary intervention with drug-coated balloon-only strategy in stable coronary artery disease and in acute coronary syndromes: an all-comers registry study. Catheter Cardiovasc Interv. 2019;93(5):893–900.
19. Rissanen TT, Uskela S, Eränen J, et al. Drug-coated balloon for treatment of de-novo coronary artery lesions in patients with high bleeding risk (DEBUT): a single-blind, randomised, non-inferiority trial. Lancet. 2019;394(10194):230–9.
20. Urban P, Meredith IT, Abizaid A, et al. Polymer-free drug-coated coronary stents in patients at high bleeding risk. N Engl J Med. 2015;373(21):2038–47.
21. Smits PC, Frigoli E, Tijssen J, et al. Abbreviated antiplatelet therapy in patients at high bleeding risk with or without oral anticoagulant therapy after coronary stenting: an open-label, randomized, controlled trial. Circulation. 2021;144:1196–211.

23 Triple or Double Antithrombotic Therapy in Atrial Fibrillation Patients Treated with Stents

Alessandro Sciahbasi and Simona Minardi

Patients treated with percutaneous coronary interventions (PCI) are exposed to a double risk related to the possible acute post-angioplasty thrombosis and to the haemorrhagic complications linked to aggressive antithrombotic therapy. Management of this delicate risks' balance becomes even harder when an indication for oral anticoagulant therapy (OAT) coexists, and it is estimated that 5–8% of patients who undergo PCI have an indication for OAT [1]. The most frequent indication for OAT is the prevention of cardioembolic stroke in patients suffering from atrial fibrillation (AF), a common arrhythmia that shared some predisposing risk factors with coronary artery disease (CAD). Almost one-third of patients with AF also suffer for CAD and 70% of OAT indication in patients with CAD is due to concomitant AF [2–4]. Moreover, in the context of acute coronary syndromes (ACS), the risk of AF is increased of [illegible]0–77% [5, 6]. The coexistence of CAD and AF is also burdened by poorer prognosis: in the setting of ACS, this association has been correlated with a mortality rate at least twice higher than that of patient affected by isolated AF or ACS [7]. The reason for this worse prognosis is multifactorial: for example AF patients with ACS often have more pre-existing comorbidities and the acute condition increases the haemodynamic burden [8]. Furthermore, especially in the past, these patients tended to be less treated invasively and pharmacologically [9] even though a more aggressive strategy could improve their outcome. De Luca et al. in an analysis of the national association of Italian hospital cardiologists (ANMCO) registry demonstrated that by increasing the number of coronary angiographies and PCI in patients with concomitant AF and ACS, regardless of presentation with or without ST-elevation, there was a substantial reduction of in-hospital mortality [10]. These observations underline the extreme importance of the therapeutic strategy, interventional and pharmacological, for the management of patients in the acute and long-term period.

A. Sciahbasi (✉)
Interventional Cardiology, Sandro Pertini Hospital – ASL RM2, Rome, Italy

S. Minardi
Cardiology Unit, Spaziani Hospital, Frosinone, Italy

23.1 Management of Concomitant Thrombotic Risks

Dual antiplatelet therapy constitutes the cornerstone of the treatment of ACS and chronic coronary syndromes (CCS) treated with PCI since 1995–1996 [11–13]. However, the scenario changes when, not infrequently, these patients also suffer for AF or any other condition requiring OAT such as need for prevention and treatment of pulmonary embolism, deep vein

B. Cortese, S. Rigattieri (eds.), *High Bleeding Risk Patients in Interventional Cardiology*,
https://doi.org/10.1007/978-3-031-87302-7_23

thrombosis, surgical implantation of mechanical heart valves, or left ventricular thrombosis. In these conditions, the ideal therapeutic option to prevent vein thrombosis or cardioembolic phenomena is OAT, since these thrombi are mainly promoted by stasis and made of fibrin, without contribution from platelet activation [14–16]. DAPT is less effective in this context while, as above-mentioned, it is the preferred treatment for coronary thrombosis, where platelet activation represents the main mechanism for thrombus formation associated with plaque rupture and stent placement [13]. Consequently, triple antithrombotic therapy (TAT, a combination of dual antiplatelet and OAT) was introduced in these patients in order to afford coronary and systemic thrombotic risks.

The association of DAPT with an OAT, initially implemented on a deductive basis, was subsequently supported by literature data: in 2010, the first consensus document was published with the recommendation to use TAT with vitamin K antagonist (VKA), aspirin, and clopidogrel in patients undergoing PCI and concomitant AF [17]. It was immediately clear, however, that TAT is associated with a significant increase in bleeding at follow-up (FU), which affects the net benefit of the therapy as confirmed by Lamberts et al. in 2012: TAT was associated with a high risk of bleeding without safe therapeutic window [18].

The fear of haemorrhagic complications pushed on to the tendency to reduce the dosage of anticoagulant drugs, with possible compromise of the efficacy profile, and has led the various authors to design further trials comparing TAT with dual antithrombotic therapy (DAT, a combination of dual antiplatelet and OAT), in the post-PCI period.

23.2 Literature Supporting Dual Antithrombotic Therapy

The first study testing the possible use of DAT in patients requiring OAT and undergoing PCI was the WOEST trial (What is the Optimal anticoagulation and anticoagulant therapy in patients with oral anticoagulation and coronary StenTing) (Fig. 23.1) [19]. The study has been conducted on a population of almost 500 patients, randomized to DAT or TAT using VKA as oral anticoagulant. The primary endpoint of the study was the safety of a DAT strategy in term of total bleedings that were reduced by more than 60% in the group treated with DAT compared to TAT. No significant differences in terms of efficacy (reduction of ischaemic events) were observed even though the small sample size of the study limited the value of this analysis.

The WOEST trial was followed by the ISAR-TRIPLE [20] (Triple Therapy in Patients on Oral Anticoagulation After Drug Eluting Stent Implantation) study, a randomized trial comparing 6-week TAT (followed by DAT) with 6-month TAT. The study demonstrated a significant reduction of bleeding events in the 6-week group confirming the important role of a short TAT.

Subsequently, with the advent of direct oral anticoagulants (DOAC), that were associated with a reduced bleeding risk and at least a comparable efficacy compared to VKA, four randomized clinical trials (RCTs) were performed to compare TAT and DAT with the four DOAC commercially available (apixaban, dabigatran, edoxaban, and rivaroxaban).

The PIONEER-AF-PCI has been the first RCT conducted on patients with non-valvular AF (NVAF) undergoing PCI using the DOAC rivaroxaban. More than 2000 patients were randomized 1:1:1 to three treatments: rivaroxaban 15 mg/day together with a P2Y12 receptor inhibitor vs. rivaroxaban 2.5 mg twice daily together with DAPT vs. standard TAT with VKA. The primary safety endpoint, consisting of clinically relevant bleeding, was reduced in the two groups treated with rivaroxaban compared to VKA, without significant differences in term of cardiovascular death and ischaemic events among the three groups. An important limitation of this study was the use of DOAC at dosages (15 mg daily and 2.5 mg twice a day) of unproven efficacy in the prevention of cardioembolism during AF [21].

The RE-DUAL PCI trial randomized 2700 patients suffering from non-valvular AF and undergoing PCI with stent implantation into three groups: dabigatran 150 mg/bid plus a P2Y12

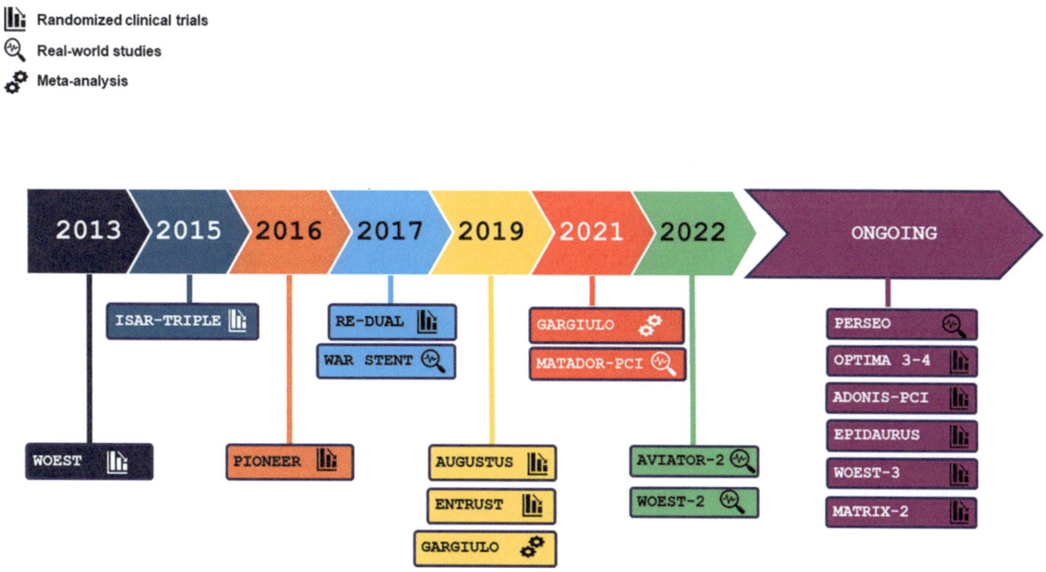

Fig. 23.1 Clinical studies supporting antithrombotic therapy in patients with atrial fibrillation undergoing percutaneous coronary interventions

inhibitor (mainly clopidogrel) vs dabigatran 110 mg/bid plus a P2Y12 inhibitor vs standard TAT strategy with VKA plus DAPT. The study showed a reduction in haemorrhagic events in both groups treated with dabigatran in DAT compared to the group treated with VKA in TAT with the 110 mg dabigatran dosage associated with less bleeding than the 150 mg dosage. Regarding ischaemic events, no statistically significant differences were observed between the three groups, but the rate of stent thrombosis (ST) in the group treated with dabigatran 110 mg in DAT was almost double compared to the groups treated with dabigatran 150 mg in DAT and VKA in TAT (1.5% vs 0.8% vs 0.9%. $P = 0.98$) [22].

The third RCT was the ENTRUST-AF PCI trial that compared the DOAC edoxaban in association with a P2Y12 inhibitor (DAT strategy) vs a TAT strategy using VKA in association with DAPT. The dosage of edoxaban was 60 mg, except for patients with weight <60 kg and/or glomerular filtration rate (GFR) between 15 and 50 ml/min and/or under treatment with potent inhibitors of P-glycoprotein, in which the dose was reduced to 30 mg daily. The study provided non-inferiority results between the two groups (edoxaban in DAT vs VKA in TAT), but compared to the PIONEER AF and the REDUAL PCI, the study failed to show a significant advantage of DAT compared to TAT in term of major and clinically relevant bleedings [23].

These three studies [21–23] had concordant results, demonstrating that DAT with DOACs significantly reduces the risk of bleeding compared to TAT with VKA, without compromising the benefit in terms of protection from ischaemic events. However, a limitation of these trials was that they did not demonstrate whether the benefits in term of reduced bleeding were due to the strategy (DAT vs TAT) or to the drug used (DOAC vs VKA) as the arm on DAT using VKA was lacking.

Overcoming this limit, the AUGUSTUS trial was finally published (not chronologically as it was shortly before ENTRUST), which had a 2 × 2 factorial design used to compare apixaban with VKA, each in a DAT vs TAT strategy. The results demonstrated that apixaban causes a reduction in haemorrhagic events compared to VKA and that the addition of aspirin is associated with an increase in bleeding compared to placebo, without a significant difference in the incidence of ischaemic events [24]. Major limitations of this study were the short FU (limited to only

6 months) and the patient selection that included either patients who underwent to PCI or patients with ACS managed medically.

In all these RCTs, the primary endpoint was represented by haemorrhagic events; therefore, they were not powered to evaluate differences in thrombotic events, and thus, they failed to provide conclusive data regarding the effectiveness in terms of ischaemic events of a DAT regimen compared to TAT. To partially overcome this limitation, multiple meta-analyses have been performed, and one of these has been conducted on over 10,000 patients (DAT: 5496 patients vs TAT: 4738 patients). The meta-analysis confirmed that a DAT regimen significantly reduces bleeding compared to TAT but only a DAT with DOAC can significantly reduce intracranial bleeding. Moreover, there were no significant differences between DAT and TAT for all-cause death, major adverse cardiac events (MACE), or stroke, but DAT regimen was associated with a significantly higher risk of ST (1.0% vs 0.6%; RR: 1.59, 95% CI: 1.01–2.50; $p = 0.04$; $I^2 = 0\%$) and a borderline higher risk of MI (3.6% vs 3.0% RR: 1.22, 95% CI: 0.99–1.52; $p = 0.07$; $I^2 = 0\%$) [25]. The same results were also confirmed when the safety and efficacy of DAT and TAT were explored according to clinical presentation: DAT regimen significantly reduced bleedings irrespective of the clinical presentation, including intracranial haemorrhages, and there were no differences for all-cause death, MACE, or stroke but MI and ST were more frequent in DAT compared to TAT [26].

23.3 Guideline Recommendations

In 2020, the ESC guidelines on the management of AF were published, defining the indications on antithrombotic therapy management even in the setting of patients who simultaneously present both AF and CAD [27].

According to the guidelines, in patients with AF and ACS, a strategy of TAT in the in-hospital phase or in any case for a duration ≤1 week is indicated by default, with subsequent suspension of an antiplatelet, preferably aspirin, and continuation of DAT with DOAC/VKA and a P2Y12, preferably clopidogrel since the use of prasugrel or ticagrelor has been associated with a greater risk of major bleeding [28–31], for at least 12 months (Class I-B) [27]. TAT with aspirin, clopidogrel, and oral anticoagulant can be prolonged beyond 1 week when the risk of stent thrombosis is considered higher than the bleeding risk and maintained for no longer than 1 month (Class IIa-C) [27].

Similarly, in patients with AF and CCS undergoing PCI, TAT is indicated by default for a period ≤1 week post-procedure (Class I-B), then continuing with DAT for a maximum of 6 months. If the ischaemic risk is considered higher than the haemorrhagic risk, TAT can be extended for up to 1 month, then suspending an antiplatelet agent, according to a time program that should be specified in the discharge letter (Class IIa-C) [27].

In order to reduce the risk of bleeding, the lower dosage of rivaroxaban 15 mg or dabigatran 110 mg should be considered for the duration of TAT, even in the absence of clinical criteria for dose reduction (Class IIa-B). Moreover, for those patients on TAT with VKA, the INR range should be maintained between 2.0 and 2.5 with a TTR >70% in order to limit the risk of bleeding (Class IIa-B) [27].

While the evaluation of the bleeding risk mainly relies on HAS-BLED score, (identifying patients at high risk of bleeding with a HAS-BLED ≥3), the definition of the coronary ischaemic risk is more complex. Multiple clinical elements linked to the patient (severe chronic kidney disease, diabetes, prior stent thrombosis on antiplatelet therapy, left ventricle ejection fraction <40%) and to technical elements related to the revascularization procedure (at least three stents implanted, at least three lesion treated, bifurcation with two stents implanted, stenting of the last remaining patent vessel, total stent length >60 mm, treatment of chronic total occlusion) have been associated with higher risk [32]. However, it is unclear whether these criteria can guide the decision-making about TAT strategy since subgroup analyses of several trials failed to identify a specific profile favoured by TAT rather than by DAT.

Globally, what emerges from these guidelines is the need to personalize therapy based on the patient's profile, balancing the ischaemic and the haemorrhagic risk and choosing the most suitable strategy in terms of either drugs or duration of treatment.

23.4 Real-World Data

"Real-life" data come from observational studies comparing DAT with TAT, mainly in national and international registries.

A first prospective observational study has been conducted in Italy from November 2008 to June 2010 (Fig. 23.1) showing that DAT was prescribed in only 5% of patients [33]. Subsequently, the AVIATOR-2 registry, a multicentre prospective study enrolling 514 AF patients who underwent PCI between June 2015 and August 2016, confirmed the low rate of DAT therapy that was limited to just 12.8% of patients. Aspirin was the antiplatelet cut out in 50% of de-escalation from TAT to DAT. No significant differences were observed in the primary outcome of 1-year major adverse cardiac or cerebrovascular events (MACCE) (TAT 14.1% vs DAT 12.7; $p = 0.25$) and Bleeding Academic Research Consortium (BARC) 2, 3 or 5 (14.7% vs 7.9%, respectively; $p = 0.89$) [34].

From August 2018 and December 2019, another Italian prospective, observational, nationwide registry enrolled 598 patients treated with PCI for ACS and concomitant AF. The study, called MATADOR-PCI (Management of Antithrombotic TherApy in Patients with Chronic or DevelOping AtRial Fibrillation During Hopsitalization for PCI), showed that 155 (26.4%) patients were discharged on DAPT, 381 (64.8%) on TAT, and only 52 (8.8%) on DAT. Further observations were that the commonest anticoagulant therapies were DOACs (62.1%), clopidogrel was the most frequently used oral P2Y12 receptor inhibitor, while ticagrelor and prasugrel were prescribed in 2.3% and 13.5% of patients on TAT or DAT, respectively. However, no data on outcomes are available [35].

In 2022, the WOEST-2 (dual versus triple antithrombotic therapy after percutaneous coronary intervention) study analysed 1075 patients undergoing PCI who had concomitant OAT indication, and at 1-year FU, net clinical events did not differ between the two strategies. DAT was associated with a significant decrease in clinically relevant bleeding, BARC type 2 and 3, compared to TAT (16.8% vs 23.6%. $p = 0.003$), whereas MACCE rate, including all-cause death, MI, ST, ischaemic stroke, and transient ischaemic attack, was higher in patients on DAT (12.4% vs 9.6%. $p = 0.17$) even though the difference was not statistically significant [36].

23.5 Antiplatelet Choice and Timing for Interruption

Dual antiplatelet therapy with aspirin and P2Y12 inhibitor is the recommended treatment in people with ACS or who undergo PCI [11–13]. The randomized Platelet Inhibition and Platelet Oucomes (PLATO) and the Therapeutic Outcomes by Optimizing Platelet Inhibition with Prasugrel-Thrombolysis in Myocardial Infarction (TRITON-TIMI 38) trials established the superiority of DAPT with ticagrelor or prasugrel compared with clopidogrel in reducing the risk of recurrent ischaemic events in patients with ACS [37, 38]. However, the greater potency of new P2Y12 inhibitors comes at the expense of increased bleeding risk, and the use of prasugrel or ticagrelor is not endorsed by guidelines in the context of TAT (Class III-C). Nevertheless, even though in a reduced percentage of cases, these drugs have been used in the setting of a DAT strategy in 5.6% of patients in the PIONEER AF-PCI, in 6.2% in the AUGUSTUS, in 7.6% in the ENTRUST AF-PCI, and in 12% in the REDUAL PCI without alarming events. Besides, a recent registry-based nationwide study analysed 2259 patients with AF undergoing PCI for ACS from 2011 to 2019. Clopidogrel was the P2Y12 inhibitor prescribed in 85% of patients at discharge while ticagrelor and prasugrel in the remaining 15%. With the limits of a retrospective registry, the results were interesting: the risk of

MACE was significantly lower in patients treated with ticagrelor–prasugrel compared to patients treated with clopidogrel (16.4% vs 19.4% RR: 0.84, 95% CI:0.70–0.98; $p = 0.02$) without difference in bleeding events (5.5% vs 5.1%; RR: 1.07; 95% CI:0.73-1-41; $p = 0.69$) [39]. Consequently, the association of OAC and ticagrelor/prasugrel in patients at very high thrombotic risk could be an option even though this strategy should be confirmed in dedicated studies.

When an antiplatelet is required to be stopped, in general, the aspirin is selected, leaving DAT with clopidogrel. This association results by the original design of the first comparison study between DAT and TAT (the WOEST Trial), by which aspirin interruption was preferred. Subsequent trials followed this strategy, but no studies have explored clopidogrel rather than aspirin interruption.

What is the optimal timing for de-escalation from TAT to DAT is still uncertain. Current European guidelines recommend TAT for up to 1 week, even though a more precise duration is not suggested due to the lack of evidence. In the famous four RCTs, a variable window for randomization was allowed, and this means that at least a short course of TAT was administered until the randomization. The median time to randomization was 1 day in the PIONEER and the RE-DUAL trials, 6 days in the AUGUSTUS study, and 1.9 days in the ENTRUST trial [21–24]. Given the irreversible inhibition of cyclooxygenase-1 enzyme by aspirin and the median life of platelets of 7–10 days [40], some authors investigated the safety of discontinuation aspirin on the first day post-PCI [41]. Von Stein et al. enrolled 322 patients undergoing PCI and requiring OAT: patients were divided in group 1 that received aspirin only during the procedure or before and group 2 that received aspirin ≥1 day post-PCI. The results showed that immediate post-procedural DAT (discontinuation of aspirin) did not increase the rate of in-hospital ischaemic events compared to TAT.

According to guidelines DAT duration after PCI should be 6 months in CAD patients and up to 12 months in ACS setting. Then, antiplatelet therapy should be interrupted and OAC continued. Few trials investigated long-term antithrombotic therapy for AF patients treated with PCI [42, 43]. The OAC-ALONE [43] and the AFIRE trials [42] were both prematurely terminated, the first due to the slow enrolment and failure to demonstrate the non-inferiority of OAC alone to DAT in terms of the composite of all-cause death, stoke, MI, and systemic embolism at 1 year and the second because of increased mortality in the DAT group.

23.6 Ongoing Studies and Future Prospectives

Still today, a lot of trials and registries about management of patients treated with PCI who had a concomitant indication to OAT are ongoing. One of these is the Italian PERcutaneous coronary intErventions in Patients Treated with Oral Anticoagulant Therapy (PERSEO) registry [44], a multicentre, prospective, observational study evaluation the safety and efficacy of DOACs versus VKA both in DAT and TAT in over 1000 patients at 1-year FU. The registry has completed enrolment and FU, and its results are expected soon.

An interesting multicentre RCT (70 centres nationwide in China) (OPTIMA 3-4, NCT03234114) is enrolling 3746 patients with non-valvular AF and concomitant ACS undergoing new-generation drug-eluting stent implantation and contains two sub-studies. OPTIMA-3 sub-study will randomize 1:1 2274 patients to receive TAT with warfarin as anticoagulant and targeted INR 2.0–3.0, clopidogrel 75 mg and aspirin 100 mg for 1 month or 6 months, and then quit aspirin till 12 months after PCI. Primary composite endpoint will be a composite of cardiovascular death, MI, ischaemic stroke, systemic embolism, and unplanned revascularization up to 12 months. Differently the OPTIMA-4 will investigate the association of DOAC with a more potent P2Y12 inhibitor: 1427 patients will be randomized 1:1 to a DAT with dabigatran 110 mg twice daily and ticagrelor 90 mg twice daily or with clopidogrel 75 mg once a day for 12 months after PCI. The primary safety endpoint will be major bleedings at 12 months whereas the primary efficacy endpoint will be a composite of cardiovascular death, MI, ischaemic stroke, systemic thromboembolism, and unplanned revascularization. In the same field, the ADONIS-PCI (Dual Antithrombotic Therapy With Dabigatran and Ticagrelor in Patients With ACS and Non-valvular AF Undergoing PCI, NCT04695106) is a prospective RCT aimed to demonstrate that DAT including reduced dose ticagrelor and dabigatran is at least non-inferior regarding bleeding risk and ischaemic protection, compared to the standard TAT in patients with AF and ACS, treated with PCI. More than 2000 patients will be randomized 1:1 to receive dual therapy with dabigatran (150 mg twice daily or 110 mg twice daily) and ticagrelor (90 mg twice daily for 1 month, followed by 60 mg twice daily up to 12 months) or TAT with dabigatran (150 mg or 110 mg twice daily) plus clopidogrel (75 mg daily) plus aspirin (75 mg daily) followed by dual therapy depending on the bleeding and ischaemic risk. Finally, the EPIDAURUS (Escalated Single Platelet Inhibition for One Month Plus NOAC in Patients With Atrial Fibrillation and ACS Undergoing PCI- NCT04981041) trial will assess safety of 1 month DAT with DOAC and prasugrel or ticagrelor followed by standard DAT with clopidogrel and DOAC in terms of clinically relevant bleeding and cardiovascular events at 6 months.

Another field of research is the possibility to temporarily skip the OAT therapy immediately after PCI. In this setting, the WOEST-3 (What is the Optimal Antithrombotic Strategy in Patients with Atrial Fibrillation Undergoing PCI? NCT 04436978) trial is a multicentre, open-label, randomized controlled study investigating the safety and efficacy of 1-month DAPT compared to guideline-directed therapy. The hypothesis is that in the first month post-PCI, where the risk of both bleeding and stent thrombosis is greatest, the use of short course of DAPT without OAT is superior in bleeding and non-inferior in preventing ischaemic events. The primary safety endpoint will be major or clinically relevant non-major bleeding at 6 weeks after PCI whereas the primary efficacy endpoint will be a composite of all-cause death, MI, stroke, systemic embolism, or ST at 6 weeks after PCI. With the same rational, there is the MATRIX-2 (Monotherapy With P2Y12 Inhibitors in Patients With Atrial fIbrillation Undergoing Supraflex Stent Implantation-NCT05955365) trial, a multicentre RCT on 3010 AF patients with indication for long-term oral anticoagulation who have undergone successful PCI with a sirolimus-eluting stent implantation. Patients will be randomized 1:1 ratio to the standard of care strategy or a monotherapy with any of the commercially available oral P2Y12 inhibitors immediately discontinuing aspirin and DOAC. After 1 month, the P2Y12 inhibitor will be stopped and treatment with a commercially available DOAC will be initiated for the duration of 11 months (Fig. 23.2).

Over the last years, persistent drawbacks with existing antithrombotic drugs, first of all increased bleeding risk, have prompted the search for other molecules aiming to preventing thrombosis with minimal interferences on haemostasis [45, 46]. In particular, it was observed that people with congenital factor XI (FXI) deficiency have a lower risk of thrombotic events without increasing bleeding and FXI inhibition was identified as a therapeutic target in cardiovascular settings [45–48] developing a number of drugs able to inhibit these factors. Several Phase 2 RCTs investigated treatment with FXI inhibitors in patients undergoing major orthopaedic surgery and patients with AF with promising results [49]. The FXI inhibitor asundexian has also been tested as TAT strategy in patients with acute MI undergoing PCI [50] showing a good safety (no increased of bleeding has been observed but no advantage in term of ischaemic events). According with these results, the FXI inhibitors represent an interesting potential treatment of patients with concomitant myocardial infarction and AF, but future studies as the OCEANIC AF (NCT05643573, prematurely interrupted) and the LIBREXIA-AF (NCT05757869, ongoing) will clarify their possible role.

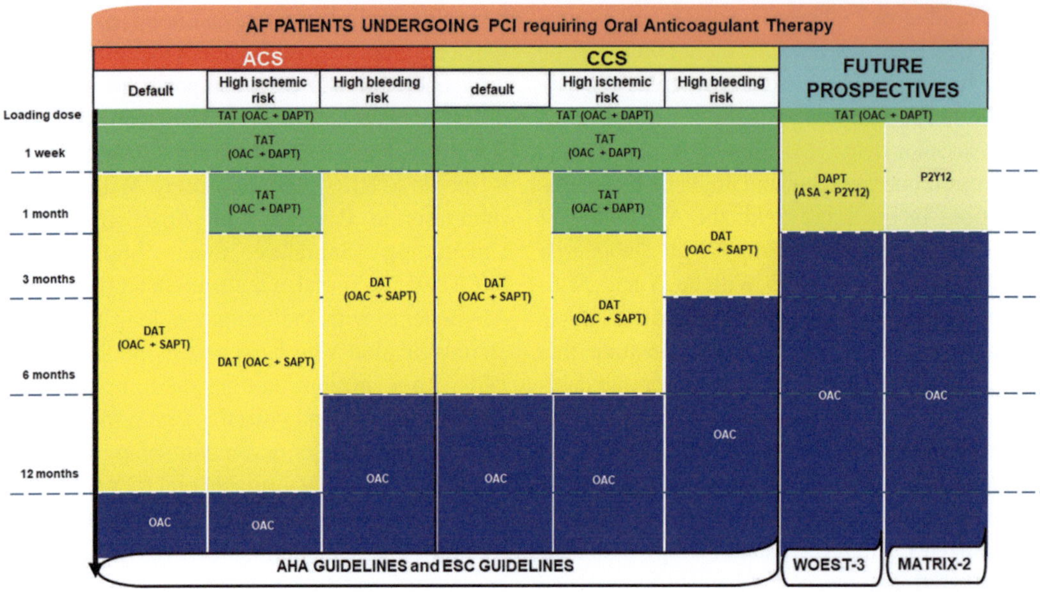

Fig. 23.2 Current and future antithrombotic strategies in patients with atrial fibrillation undergoing percutaneous coronary interventions

23.7 Conclusion

Patients treated with PCI and concomitant indication for oral antithrombotic treatment face two thrombotic risks that require different therapeutic management. Indeed, for acute stent thrombosis prevention, the ideal treatment is dual antiplatelet therapy instead of anticoagulant therapy that is optimal to avoid venous thrombosis. Triple antithrombotic therapy, born from the fusion of dual antiplatelet and oral anticoagulant therapy, is aimed to prevent both risks but is often associated with a significant rise in bleeding events, losing therefore its effectiveness. Balancing ischaemic and haemorrhagic risk in these patients is the harder challenge of antithrombotic therapy. European guidelines suggest some standard strategies (Fig. 23.2), allowing flexible case-by-case adaptations, about choice of drugs, association, and timing of interruption, based on the individual patient profile. The current trend is to prefer direct oral anticoagulant and aspirin early interruption and shorten the combination therapy as much as possible according to the ischaemic risk. Lots of trials and registries are continuously published making the topic constantly evolving.

References

1. Kralev S, Schneider K, Lang S, Süselbeck T, Borggrefe M. Incidence and severity of coronary artery disease in patients with atrial fibrillation undergoing first-time coronary angiography. PLoS One. 2011;6:e24964.
2. Rubboli A, Colletta M, Valencia J, Capecchi A, Franco N, Zanolla L, et al. Periprocedural management and in-hospital outcome of patients with indication for oral anticoagulation undergoing coronary artery stenting. J Interv Cardiol. 2009;22:390–7.
3. Wang TY, Robinson LA, Ou FS, Roe MT, Ohman EM, Gibler WB, et al. Discharge antithrombotic strategies among patients with acute coronary syndrome previously on warfarin anticoagulation: physician practice in the CRUSADE registry. Am Heart J. 2008;155:361–8.
4. Rossini R, Musumeci G, Lettieri C, Molfese M, Mihalcsik L, Mantovani P, et al. Long-term outcomes in patients undergoing coronary stenting on dual oral antiplatelet treatment requiring oral anticoagulant therapy. Am J Cardiol. 2008;102:1618–23.
5. Krijthe BP, Leening MJG, Heeringa J, Kors JA, Hofman A, Franco OH, et al. Unrecognized myocardial infarction and risk of atrial fibrillation: the Rotterdam Study. Int J Cardiol. 2013;168:1453–7.
6. González-Pacheco H, Márquez MF, Arias-Mendoza A, Álvarez-Sangabriel A, Eid-Lidt G, González-Hermosillo A, et al. Clinical features and in-hospital mortality associated with different types of atrial fibrillation in patients with acute coronary syndrome with and without ST elevation. J Cardiol. 2015;66:148–54.

7. De Luca L, Rubboli A, Lettino M, Tubaro M, Leonardi S, Casella G, et al. ANMCO Position paper: antithrombotic treatment of patients with atrial fibrillation undergoing intracoronary stenting and/or acute coronary syndromes. G Ital Cardiol. 2022;23:379–95.
8. Angeli F, Reboldi G, Garofoli M, Ramundo E, Poltronieri C, Mazzotta G, et al. Atrial fibrillation and mortality in patients with acute myocardial infarction: a systematic overview and meta-analysis. Curr Cardiol Rep. 2012;14:601–10.
9. Schmitt J, Duray G, Gersh BJ, Hohnloser SH. Atrial fibrillation in acute myocardial infarction: a systematic review of the incidence, clinical features and prognostic implications. Eur Heart J. 2009;30:1038–45.
10. De Luca L, Casella G, Rubboli A, Gonzini L, Lucci D, Boccanelli A, et al. Recent trends in management and outcome of patients with acute coronary syndromes and atrial fibrillation. Int J Cardiol. 2017;248:369–75.
11. Colombo A, Hall P, Nakamura S, Almagor Y, Maiello L, Martini G, et al. Intracoronary stenting without anticoagulation accomplished with intravascular ultrasound guidance. Circulation. 1995;91:1676–88.
12. Schömig A, Neumann FJ, Kastrati A, Schühlen H, Blasini R, Hadamitzky M, et al. A randomized comparison of antiplatelet and anticoagulant therapy after the placement of coronary-artery stents. N Engl J Med. 1996;334:1084–9.
13. Valgimigli M, Bueno H, Byrne RA, Collet JP, Costa F, Jeppsson A, et al. 2017 ESC focused update on dual antiplatelet therapy in coronary artery disease developed in collaboration with EACTS. Eur Heart J. 2018;39:213–60.
14. ACTIVE Writing Group of the ACTIVE Investigators, Connolly S, Pogue J, Hart R, Pfeffer M, Hohnloser S, Chrolavicius S, Pfeffer M, Hohnloser S, Yusuf S. Clopidogrel plus aspirin versus oral anticoagulation for atrial fibrillation in the Atrial fibrillation Clopidogrel Trial with Irbesartan for prevention of Vascular Events (ACTIVE W): a randomised controlled trial. Lancet. 2006;367:1903–12.
15. Sjalander S, Sjalander A, Svensson PJ, Friberg L. Atrial fibrillation patients do not benefit from acetylsalicylic acid. Europace. 2014;16:631–8.
16. Mant J, Hobbs FR, Fletcher K, Roalfe A, Fitzmaurice D, Lip GY, et al. Warfarin versus aspirin for stroke prevention in an elderly community population with atrial fibrillation (the Birmingham Atrial Fibrillation Treatment of the Aged Study, BAFTA): a randomised controlled trial. Lancet. 2007;370:493–503.
17. Lip GYH, Huber K, Andreotti F, Arnesen H, Airaksinen JK, Cuisset T, et al. Antithrombotic management of atrial fibrillation patients presenting with acute coronary syndrome and/or undergoing coronary stenting: executive summary—a Consensus Document of the European Society of Cardiology Working Group on Thrombosis, endorsed by the European Heart Rhythm Association (EHRA) and the European Association of Percutaneous Cardiovascular Interventions (EAPCI). Eur Heart J. 2010;31:1311–8.
18. Lamberts M, Olesen JB, Ruwald MH, Hansen CM, Karasoy D, Kristensen SL, et al. Bleeding after initiation of multiple antithrombotic drugs, including triple therapy, in atrial fibrillation patients following myocardial infarction and coronary intervention. Circulation. 2012;126:1185–93.
19. Dewilde WJ, Oirbans T, Verheugt FW, Kelder JC, De Smet BJ, Herrman JP, et al. Use of clopidogrel with or without aspirin in patients taking oral anticoagulant therapy and undergoing percutaneous coronary intervention: an open-label, randomised, controlled trial. Lancet. 2013;381:1107–15.
20. Fiedler KA, Maeng M, Mehilli J, Schulz-Schüpke S, Byrne RA, Sibbing D, et al. Duration of triple therapy in patients requiring oral anticoagulation after drug-eluting stent implantation. J Am Coll Cardiol. 2015;65:1619–29.
21. Gibson CM, Mehran R, Bode C, Halperin J, Verheugt FW, Wildgoose P, et al. Prevention of bleeding in patients with atrial fibrillation undergoing PCI. N Engl J Med. 2016;375:2423–34.
22. Cannon CP, Bhatt DL, Oldgren J, Lip GYH, Ellis SG, Kimura T, et al. Dual antithrombotic therapy with dabigatran after PCI in atrial fibrillation. N Engl J Med. 2017;377:1513–24.
23. Vranckx P, Valgimigli M, Eckardt L, Tijssen J, Lewalter T, Gargiulo G, et al. Edoxaban-based versus vitamin K antagonist-based antithrombotic regimen after successful coronary stenting in patients with atrial fibrillation (ENTRUST-AF PCI): a randomised, open-label, phase 3b trial. Lancet. 2019;394:1335–43.
24. Lopes RD, Heizer G, Aronson R, Vora AN, Massaro T, Mehran R, et al. Antithrombotic therapy after acute coronary syndrome or PCI in atrial fibrillation. N Engl J Med. 2019;380:1509–24.
25. Gargiulo G, Goette A, Tijssen J, Eckardt L, Lewalter T, Vranckx P, et al. Safety and efficacy outcomes of double vs. triple antithrombotic therapy in patients with atrial fibrillation following percutaneous coronary intervention: a systematic review and meta-analysis of non-vitamin K antagonist oral anticoagulant-based randomized clinical trials. Eur Heart J. 2019;40:3757–67.
26. Gargiulo G, Cannon CP, Gibson CM, Goette A, Lopes RD, Oldgren J, et al. Safety and efficacy of double vs. triple antithrombotic therapy in patients with atrial fibrillation with or without acute coronary syndrome undergoing percutaneous coronary intervention: a collaborative meta-analysis of non-vitamin K antagonist oral anticoagulant-based randomized clinical trials. Eur Heart J Cardiovasc Pharmacother. 2021;7:50–60.
27. Hindricks G, Potpara T, Dagres N, Arbelo E, Bax JJ, Blomström-Lundqvist C, et al. 2020 ESC Guidelines for the diagnosis and management of atrial fibrillation developed in collaboration with the European Association for Cardio-Thoracic Surgery (EACTS). Eur Heart J. 2021;42:373–498.
28. Andreou I, Briasoulis A, Pappas C, Ikonomidis I, Alexopoulos D. Ticagrelor versus clopidogrel as part of dual or triple antithrombotic therapy: a systematic

review and meta-analysis. Cardiovasc Drugs Ther. 2018;32:287–94.

29. Fu A, Singh K, Abunassar J, Malhotra N, Le May M, Labinaz M, et al. Ticagrelor in triple antithrombotic therapy: predictors of ischemic and bleeding complications. Clin Cardiol. 2016;39:19–23.
30. Jackson LR, Ju C, Zettler M, Messenger JC, Cohen DJ, Stone GW, et al. Outcomes of patients with acute myocardial infarction undergoing percutaneous coronary intervention receiving an oral anticoagulant and dual antiplatelet therapy. JACC Cardiovasc Interv. 2015;8:1880–9.
31. Sarafoff N, Martischnig A, Wealer J, Mayer K, Mehilli J, Sibbing D, et al. Triple therapy with aspirin, prasugrel, and vitamin K antagonists in patients with drug-eluting stent implantation and an indication for oral anticoagulation. J Am Coll Cardiol. 2013;61:2060–6.
32. Byrne RA, Rossello X, Coughlan JJ, Barbato E, Berry C, Chieffo A, et al. 2023 ESC Guidelines for the management of acute coronary syndromes. Eur Heart J. 2023;44:3720–826.
33. Rubboli A, Saia F, Sciahbasi A, Leone AM, Palmieri C, Bacchi-Reggiani ML, et al. Twelve-month outcome of patients with an established indication for oral anticoagulation undergoing coronary artery stenting and stratified by the baseline risk of bleeding. Cardiovasc Revasc Med. 2017;18:425–30.
34. Chandrasekhar J, Baber U, Sartori S, Goel R, Nicolas J, Vogel B, et al. Antithrombotic strategy variability in atrial fibrillation and obstructive coronary disease revascularised with percutaneous coronary intervention: primary results from the AVIATOR 2 international registry. EuroIntervention. 2022;18:e656–65.
35. De Luca L, Bolognese L, Rubboli A, Vetrano A, Callerame M, Rivetti L, et al. Combinations of antithrombotic therapies prescribed after percutaneous coronary intervention in patients with acute coronary syndromes and atrial fibrillation: data from the nationwide MATADOR-PCI registry. Eur Heart J Cardiovasc Pharmacother. 2021;7:e45–7.
36. Bor WB, de Veer AJW, Olie RO, Rikken SR, Chan Pin Yin DCPY, Herrman JPH, et al. Dual versus triple antithrombotic therapy after percutaneous coronary intervention: the prospective multicentre WOEST 2 Study. EuroIntervention. 2022;18:e303–13.
37. Wallentin L, Becker RC, Budaj A, Cannon CP, Emanuelsson H, Held C, et al. Ticagrelor versus clopidogrel in patients with acute coronary syndromes. N Engl J Med. 2009;361:1045–57.
38. Wiviott SD, Braunwald E, McCabe CH, Montalescot G, Ruzyllo W, Gottlieb S, et al. Prasugrel versus clopidogrel in patients with acute coronary syndromes. N Engl J Med. 2007;357:2001–15.
39. Godtfredsen SJ, Kragholm KH, Kristensen AMD, Bekfani T, Sørensen R, Sessa M, et al. Ticagrelor or prasugrel vs. clopidogrel in patients with atrial fibrillation undergoing percutaneous coronary intervention for myocardial infarction. Eur Heart J Open. 2023;4(1):oead134.
40. Funk CD, Funk LB, Kennedy ME, Pong AS, Fitzgerald GA. Human platelet/erythroleukemia cell prostaglandin G/H synthase: cDNA cloning, expression, and gene chromosomal assignment. FASEB J. 1991;5:2304–12.
41. von Stein P, Seitz L, Wienemann H, Hohmann C, Baar T, Baldus S, et al. Early in-hospital discontinuation of aspirin on the first post-procedural day after percutaneous coronary stent implantation in patients on direct oral anticoagulation. Front Cardiovasc Med. 2023;13:10.
42. Yasuda S, Kaikita K, Akao M, Ako J, Matoba T, Nakamura M, et al. Antithrombotic therapy for atrial fibrillation with stable coronary disease. N Engl J Med. 2019;381:1103–13.
43. Matsumura-Nakano Y, Shizuta S, Komasa A, Morimoto T, Masuda H, Shiomi H, et al. Open-label randomized trial comparing oral anticoagulation with and without single antiplatelet therapy in patients with atrial fibrillation and stable coronary artery disease beyond 1 year after coronary stent implantation. Circulation. 2019;29(139):604–16.
44. Sciahbasi A, Gargiulo G, Talarico GP, Cesaro A, Zilio F, De Rosa S, et al. Design of the PERSEO Registry on the management of patients treated with oral anticoagulants and coronary stent. J Cardiovasc Med. 2022;23:738–43.
45. Greco A, Laudani C, Spagnolo M, Agnello F, Faro DC, Finocchiaro S, et al. Pharmacology and clinical development of factor XI inhibitors. Circulation. 2023;147:897–913.
46. Muscente F, De Caterina R. The new in anticoagulation: factor XI inhibitors. Eur Heart J Suppl. 2023;25(Supplement_B):B65–8.
47. Harrington J, Piccini JP, Alexander JH, Granger CB, Patel MR. Clinical evaluation of factor XIa inhibitor drugs. J Am Coll Cardiol. 2023;81:771–9.
48. Santagata D, Donadini MP, Ageno W. Factor XI inhibitors for the prevention of cardiovascular disease: a new therapeutic approach on the horizon? Blood Rev. 2023;62:101119.
49. De Caterina R, Prisco D, Eikelboom JW. Factor XI inhibitors: cardiovascular perspectives. Eur Heart J. 2023;44:280–92.
50. Rao SV, Kirsch B, Bhatt DL, Budaj A, Coppolecchia R, Eikelboom J, et al. A multicenter, phase 2, randomized, placebo-controlled, double-blind, parallel-group, dose-finding trial of the oral factor XIa inhibitor asundexian to prevent adverse cardiovascular outcomes after acute myocardial infarction. Circulation. 2022;146:1196–206.

24 Management and Prognostic Implications of Bleeding Post-TAVI

Hamza Lodhi, Guilherme Attizzani, and Anene Ukaigwe

Abbreviations

AS	Aortic stenosis
BARC	Bleeding Academic Research Consortium
BEV	Balloon-expandable valve
PCI	Percutaneous coronary intervention
SAVR	Surgical aortic valve replacement
SEV	Self-expanding valve
TAVI	Transcatheter aortic valve implant
VARC	Valve Academic Research Consortium

Objectives

1. Changing trends in bleeding complications post-TAVI
2. Prognostic implications of bleeding post-TAVI
3. Predictors of bleeding complications post-TAVI
4. Prevention and management of bleeding post-TAVI

H. Lodhi · G. Attizzani · A. Ukaigwe (✉)
Harrington Heart and Vascular Institute, University Hospitals Cleveland Medical Center, Cleveland, OH, USA
e-mail: Hamza.Lodhi@AlignedCardio.com; Guilherme.Attizzani@UHhospitals.org; Anene.Ukaigwe@UHhospitals.org

24.1 Introduction

Since the acceptance of transcatheter aortic valve implantation (TAVI) as standard of care procedure for severe aortic stenosis in all risk categories, the volumes have increased along with interest in optimization of technique and safety. Among the considerations for the procedure is the balance between thrombogenicity and bleeding risks associated with the procedure. These aspects are considered in all transcatheter interventions; however, the TAVI procedure is unique due to higher comorbidity burden of patient population, large bore arterial access, prevalence of thrombocytopenia, and risk for acquired von Williebrand factor (vWF) deficiency. This patient population has a higher prevalence of PAD, as compared to patients undergoing elective PCI. For instance, the prevalence of PAD in the PCI arm of ISCHEMIA trial was 4.5% compared to TAVI arms of PARTNER 3 trial where it was 6.9% and Evolut Low-Risk trial which had 7.5%. Indeed, the overall bleeding post-TAVI in the trial setting is much higher than PCI. Low-risk TAVI trials have shown 1-year major or life-threatening bleeding rate of 7.7% in PARTNER 3 and 3.2% Evolut Low-Risk trial; these numbers are higher than what has been shown in majority of PCI trials, where bleeding rates have consistently been <2%. CENTER-2 study

B. Cortese, S. Rigattieri (eds.), *High Bleeding Risk Patients in Interventional Cardiology*,
https://doi.org/10.1007/978-3-031-87302-7_24

looked at data from 10 large centers, in contemporary, non-trial setting and reported 30-day post-TAVI bleeding rates of 5.5% between 2019 and 2022.

Post-TAVI bleeding can be divided into two categories. Early, which is up to 30 days after TAVI, is predominantly influenced by immediately post-procedure bleeding which is related to intra-procedural anticoagulation, access site, methods, and success of closure. Late, which is beyond 30 days, is determined by overall patient profile and includes post-TAVR antithrombotic therapy. One important common dominator in post-TAVI bleeding patients is atrial fibrillation, which is widely prevalent in the patient population undergoing TAVI. Mentias et al. looked at data from Medicare claims of 72,660 patients undergoing non-apical TAVI between 2014 and 2016 and reported prevalence of pre-existing atrial fibrillation in 40.7% and new incidence of atrial fibrillation to be 6.8%. The presence of atrial fibrillation mandates the use of oral anticoagulants which further contribute to both short-term and long-term risk of bleeding post-procedure.

24.2 Definitions

All TAVI trials reported bleeding events as their endpoints. However, there was some difference in definitions and endpoint selection when it came to bleeding; for instance, PARTNER 3 trial reported both major and life-threatening or disabling bleeding as its endpoint compared to Evolut Low-Risk trial where only life-threatening or disabling bleeding was reported. This could potentially explain the apparent significant differences in the 30-day and 1-year bleeding outcomes between the two trials. In addition, previous VARC-2 definitions of minor, major, life-threatening, or disabling bleeding were not considered granular enough to accurately represent the consequences of those bleeding events, especially because the surgical aortic valve replacement-related events where higher intra-procedural blood loss is normally expected used the same definitions. Therefore, VARC-3 guidelines updated the bleeding definition as shown in Table 24.1. This update is expected to improve standardization of bleeding definitions for

Table 24.1 VARC-3 definition of bleeding post-TAVI or SAVR

Type	Criteria	BARC classification
Type 1	Overt bleeding that does not require surgical or percutaneous intervention	BARC 2
	Overt bleeding requiring a transfusion of 1 unit of whole blood/red blood cells	BARC 3a
Type 2	Overt bleeding requiring a transfusion of 2–4 units of whole blood/red blood cells	BARC 3a
	Overt bleeding associated with a hemoglobin drop of >3 g/dL but <5 g/dL	BARC 3a
Type 3	Overt bleeding in a critical organ	BARC 3b and 3c
	Overt bleeding causing hypovolemic shock or severe hypotension	BARC 3b
	Overt bleeding requiring reoperation, surgical exploration, or re-intervention	BARC 3b and 4
	Post-thoracotomy chest tube output ≥2 L within a 24-h period	BARC 4
	Overt bleeding requiring a transfusion of ≥5 units of whole blood/red blood cells	BARC 3a
	Overt bleeding associated with a hemoglobin drop ≥5 g/dL	BARC 3b
Type 4	Overt bleeding leading to death	BARC 5a and 5b
	Probable: clinical suspicion	BARC 5a
	Definite: confirmed by autopsy or imaging	BARC 5b

post-TAVI events. In addition, VARC-3 also differentiates between overt bleeding with an obvious source and concealed bleeding where a source cannot be identified.

24.3 Temporal Changes in Bleeding Trends Post-TAVI

Since the early publication of TAVI data in the high-risk population, there has been a significant change in the overall bleeding event rates as this procedure has been refined over the years. This is evident in the bleeding rates reported in these trials (Table 24.2); each subsequent publication has significant reduction in vascular complications which mirrors the associated bleeding events overall. One of the important evolutions has been reduction in the sheath size for both self-expanding valve (SEVs) and balloon-expandable valve (BEVs). For SEVs, the sheath size in both high-risk (US CoreValve Trial) and intermediate-risk (SURTAVI) trials was 18 F; however, in low-risk trial (Evolut Low-Risk), the new sheath sizes ranged from 14 to 18 F. In the BEVs, they evolved from 22 to 24 F in the high-risk trials (Partner 1A/B), 16–20 F in intermediate-risk trial (Partner 2), and 14–16 F in the low-risk trial (Partner 3). Although it should be noted that for BEV, the E-sheath is expandable and its size increases by 5–5.5 F at its max as the valve advances through it, in the ex vivo studies.

Similar to the trials, a downtrend in vascular and bleeding complications has been noted in the TVT registry data as well. Sherwood et al. [1] reported data from TVT registry analyzing bleeding and vascular complications trends between 2011 and 2016. They explored data from 34,893 patients from 445 centers. They observed a downward trend in both vascular and bleeding complications from around 18–20% in 2011 to 7–8% in 2016.

As the number of TAVI procedures is increasing, so is the frequency of alternate TAVI. Overall data on outcomes for alternate access TAVI is still limited. Chamandi et al. studied a cohort of 329 patients with alternate access TAVI (transapical/transaortic [228] and transcarotid [101]) and reported major or life-threatening of 14% with transaortic/transapical combined subgroup vs 4% in the transcarotid group. A study by Lederman et al. looked at data from 344 patients undergoing transcaval (238 pts) and transaxillary (106 pt) TAVI and reported major or life-threatening bleeding rates of 10% and 13%, respectively, with these approaches.

24.4 Prognostic Implications of Bleeding Post-TAVI

Post-TAVI bleeding has profound prognostic implications. A study from Piccolo et al. [2] ($n = 926$), looked at data from the Swiss TAVR registry from 2007 to 2014. Bleeding was noted to have occurred in 30% of the patients 5 years from the procedure. There was nearly equal proportion of access site and nonaccess site bleed-

Table 24.2 Bleeding and vascular complications in BEVs and SEVs trials

	Bleeding rates[a]		Vascular complications[+]	
Trial	30 days (%)	1 year (%)	30 days (%)	1 year (%)
Partner 1	16.8	22.3	16.2	16.8
Partner 2	10.4	15.2	7.9	8.4
Partner 3	3.6	7.7	2.2	2.8
US CoreValve	13.6	16.6	5.9	6.2
SURTAVI	12.2	NR	6.0	NR
Evolut low-risk	2.4	3.2	3.8	3.8

[a]Major, life-threatening, or disabling bleeding; *NR* not reported; [+]Major vascular complications

ing. In the patients undergoing transfemoral TAVI, they showed that patients with access site bleeding had increased all-cause mortality by 1.3-fold as compared to no bleeding at 5 years. The findings were similar in non-access site bleeding as well where all-cause mortality increased by twofold as compared to no bleeding at 5 years. In fact, non-access site bleeding was associated with a significantly higher risk for mortality as compared to access site bleeding by approximately 1.5-fold. Increased mortality risk was noted in case of life-threatening or major bleeding. There was a trend toward increased mortality noted in the minor bleeding subgroup as well. The gastrointestinal tract (GI) was the most common source of nonaccess site bleeding. All the access site bleeding occurred within 30 days while 40% of the nonaccess site bleeding happened more than 30 days post-TAVI.

Genereux et al. [3] used data from PARTNER trial registry ($n = 2401$) and found that late bleeding post-TAVI occurred in 5.9% between 30 days and 1 year. The median time of occurrence was 132 days post-TAVI. GI bleeding was the most common source of bleeding followed by intracranial bleeding. These patients were more likely to be men, hypertensive, and baseline atrial fibrillation. The multivariable model showed that moderate to severe paravalvular leak (PVL), atrial fibrillation, higher left ventricle (LV) mass, and low hemoglobin predicted late bleeding post-TAVI. The patients who had late major bleeding complications post-TAVI had almost fourfold increased mortality. It also increased the risk of stroke and rehospitalization.

24.5 Predictors of Bleeding Post-TAVI

There have been multiple factors which have been shown to predict bleeding events after TAVI. These predictors typically have similar trends as seen in other cardiac catheterization laboratory procedures.

Age has been well established in most risk scores as a factor predicting bleeding. Similarly increased frailty is a strong predictor of bleeding. A study by Bendayan et al. looked at 1195 patients and showed that each additional point on the Essential Frailty Toolset (EFT) increased odds ratio (OR) of bleeding by 1.30. Vlastra et al. used data from CENTER registry (12,381 patients) and showed 50% higher incidence of major or life-threatening bleeding in women (6.7% vs 4.4%) in patient undergoing transfemoral TAVI. Another major predictor of post-TAVI bleeding is underlying renal disease. Gupta et al. looked at a large sample from National Inpatient Sample (41,025 pts) and showed OR of major bleeding of 1.35 with CKD. Peripheral arterial disease was shown to have a hazard ratio of 1.18 for bleeding in a study from STS registry data by Fanaroff et al. (19, 660 pt) undergoing transfemoral TAVI. Atrial fibrillation has a high prevalence in patients undergoing TAVI. A large meta-analysis (158,220 pts) by Nso et al. showed OR of 2.06 of bleeding complications post-TAVI in patients with preexisting atrial fibrillation.

In addition to patient characteristics, there are procedural factors which increase the bleeding events. This includes French size of the sheath used in a particular patient, which has been reduced over the years as mentioned earlier. Similarly, as previously indicated, alternate access TAVI is associated with about twofold increase in the risk of bleeding as compared to transfemoral TAVI, with only exception being transcarotid TAVI which appears to have similar bleeding events. The secondary access-related bleeding burden is also not negligible in patients undergoing TAVI. A multicenter study by Junquera et al. (4949 pts) showed major or life-threatening bleeding related to secondary access sites of 1.0% for transfemoral vs 0% for transradial access [4].

In the PREDICT-TAVR study, Navarese et al. [5] used 5185 patients from the Italian RISPEVA registry to train a model (AUC 0.80) to predict bleeding post-TAVI and validated the model to 5043 in the POL-TAVI registry (AUC 0.78). This helped identify the risk factors and establish a bleeding prediction score based on them with a range of <1% to >12% risk of 30-day post-TAVI bleeding (Tables 24.3 and 24.4).

One of the most important factors in risk of post-TAVI bleeding is the choice of anti-

Table 24.3 PREDICT-TAVR score variables

Variables	Scores	Description
OAT	0–2	No = 0; yes = 2
Hb (g/dL)	0–10	7–15 g/dL continuous range; 1 point for each unit drop in Hb
CFA diameter (mm)	0–3	4–9 continuous range; 0.5 point for each mm change in size
DAPT	0–2	No = 0; yes = 2
Serum iron (mcg/dL)	0–5	0–180 continuous range; 0.5 points for every 20-unit change in serum iron
CrCl (mL/min)	0–3	10–120; 0.5 point (appr) for every 20- to 30-unit change in CrCl

OAT oral anticoagulant treatment, *Hb* hemoglobin, *CFA* common femoral artery, *DAPT* dual antiplatelet therapy, *CrCl* creatinine clearance

Table 24.4 PREDICT-TAVR score stratification

Total score	Risk
≤8	Low
>8 and ≤10	Moderate
>10 and ≤12	High
>12	Very high

thrombotic therapy. Since the initial TAVI trials where dual antiplatelet therapy (DAPT) was used as a standard post-procedure, several trials have established the feasibility of single antiplatelet therapy (SAPT). Most worth mentioning in this regard is the POPular TAVI trial which had multiple cohorts to study the efficacy and adverse events associated with various combinations of antiplatelet and anticoagulant agents. One cohort of the trial compared SAPT vs DAPT for the first 3 months followed by SAPT alone post-TAVI, $n = 665$. At 1 year "all bleeding" occurred in 15.1% in SAPT group vs 26.6% in DAPT group. There was no difference in ischemic events between the two groups. In another cohort of this trial, oral anticoagulation (OAC) alone was compared with OAC and clopidogrel for 3 months post-TAVI, in patients with independent indication of OAC, $n = 313$. At 1 year, "all bleeding" occurred in 21.7% of patients in OAC group vs 34.6% of patients in OAC and clopidogrel group. Again, there was no difference in ischemic events. Therefore, current evidence has moved the practice of post-TAVI antiplatelet therapy to SAPT and in patients with indication of oral anticoagulation to use OAC alone without any antiplatelet therapy. This is represented in 2021 European Society of Cardiology (ESC) guidelines.

24.6 Prevention and Management of Bleeding Post-TAVI

Comprehensive procedural planning is necessary to avoid bleeding in the TAVI patients. This includes understanding the baseline characteristics of the patient to assess for baseline bleeding risk, based on demographics and anatomical features. It is important to hold OAC appropriately before the procedure. In rare cases, bridging with enoxaparin may be needed. Typically, unfractionated heparin is used intra-procedure which is successfully reversed with protamine at the end of the procedure. Minimalistic post-TAVI antithrombotic therapy is applied which includes SAPT in most patients and OAC alone in patients in whom OAC is otherwise indicated.

Many of the risk factors for bleeding post-TAVI are not modifiable (e.g., age, gender, and CKD). One of the most important preventable bleedings is related to access site. Transfemoral approach while performing TAVI has the most well-established safety data. To obtain safe femoral access, computed tomography (CT) images are used to identify the optimum CFA access site. This includes the evaluation of the size of the vessel, location of bifurcation, calcium distribution, tortuosity, and any complications from previous pre-TAVI diagnostic cardiac catheterization. Thereafter, fluoroscopic and ultrasound guidance is used along with micropuncture needle to get access. Ultrasound guidance is particularly important in calcified vessels to ensure healthy segment puncture to avoid vessel injury and closure device failure. Afterward, the soft micropuncture dilator or the sheath can be used to obtain angiography of the access site before upsizing to the bigger sheath. For the primary access site, the most common method is the use of Perclose suture-mediated closure device (Abbott Medical Laboratories, IL, USA) which is used in "pre-close" fashion to allow for closure of the arteriotomy after the sheath removal. Typically, two Perclose sutures are deployed before large bore sheath insertion. Some institutions use one Perclose (pre-close) and use an 8-Fr Angio-seal (Terumo Interventional Systems, NJ, USA) in the end. Using radial artery as a secondary access site has also been shown to reduce bleeding. Similarly, using pacing via LV wire instead of transvenous pacemaker may also slightly reduce bleeding events [6].

In case of closure failure or vessel injury, the approaches include manual hold, balloon occlusion at the arteriotomy site using the secondary access, or covered stent deployment from the secondary access site, to prevent bleeding. In rare cases, surgical cutdown may be needed to obtain hemostasis. All the standard measures used in case of bleeding from any source are utilized as well.

24.7 Conclusion

Post-TAVI bleeding portends a poor prognosis. Overall incidence is on the decline due to refinement of procedural techniques. Optimization of access technique and antithrombotic therapy use post-TAVI are the most important modifiable factors to prevent post-TAVI bleeding.

Suggested Readings and References

1. Sherwood MW, Xiang K, Matsouaka R, Li Z, Vemulapalli S, Vora AN, et al. Incidence, temporal trends, and associated outcomes of vascular and bleeding complications in patients undergoing transfemoral transcatheter aortic valve replacement: insights from the Society of Thoracic Surgeons/American College of Cardiology Transcatheter Valve Therapies Registry. Circ Cardiovasc Interv. 2020;13(1):e008227.
2. Piccolo R, Pilgrim T, Franzone A, Valgimigli M, Haynes A, Asami M, et al. Frequency, timing, and impact of access-site and non-access-site bleeding on mortality among patients undergoing transcatheter aortic valve replacement. JACC Cardiovasc Interv. 2017;10(14):1436–46.
3. Genereux P, Cohen DJ, Mack M, Rodes-Cabau J, Yadav M, Xu K, et al. Incidence, predictors, and prognostic impact of late bleeding complications after transcatheter aortic valve replacement. J Am Coll Cardiol. 2014;64(24):2605–15.
4. Mangieri A, Montalto C, Poletti E, Sticchi A, Crimi G, Giannini F, et al. Thrombotic versus bleeding risk after transcatheter aortic valve replacement: JACC review topic of the week. J Am Coll Cardiol. 2019;74(16):2088–101.
5. Navarese EP, Zhang Z, Kubica J, Andreotti F, Farinaccio A, Bartorelli AL, et al. Development and validation of a practical model to identify patients at risk of bleeding after TAVR. JACC Cardiovasc Interv. 2021;14(11):1196–206.
6. Avvedimento M, Nuche J, Farjat-Pasos JI, Rodes-Cabau J. Bleeding events after transcatheter aortic valve replacement: JACC state-of-the-art review. J Am Coll Cardiol. 2023;81(7):684–702.

Part V

Management and Prognostic Implications of Bleedings in HBR Patients

25 High Bleeding Risk in Complex High Risk and Indicated Patient

Manel Sabaté

25.1 Definition of Complex High Risk and Indicated Patient

Patients with severe and extensive coronary artery disease in combination of comorbidities and specific haemodynamic features portend a high risk of clinical events (Fig. 25.1). In this complex scenario, coronary artery bypass graft (CABG) is usually offered, but, in many instances, the comorbid condition of the patient may preclude the surgical approach. Percutaneous coronary intervention (PCI), as a less invasive approach than CABG, may be then deemed indicated after a heart team discussion [1]. In this clinical context, PCI is challenging requiring complex techniques and the implantation of multiple stents. Outcomes of PCI may be tarnished by the occurrence of clinical complications directly (i.e. stent thrombosis, periprocedural myocardial infarction) or indirectly related to the procedure (i.e. acute kidney injury, bleeding complications, etc.). Although the definition of complex PCI may slightly vary among trials [2, 3], the current consensus is to include at least one of the following characteristics: 3 vessels treated, ≥3 lesions treated, total stent length >60 mm, bifurcation with 2 stents implanted, use of any atherectomy device, left main as target vessel, surgical bypass graft or chronic total occlusion as target lesions [4]. These features have been previously associated with an increased ischaemic risk after PCI [5–8].

It is the combination of complex PCI in patients with comorbidities and complicated heart disease what defines a complex high risk and indicated patient (CHIP) [9]. In this scenario, a CHIP-PCI score was defined from the BCIS (British Cardiovascular Intervention Society) database [10]. From a total of 313,054 patients, seven patient factors (age >80 years, female sex, previous stroke, previous myocardial infarction, peripheral vascular disease, ejection fraction <30% and chronic kidney disease) and six procedural factors (rotational atherectomy, left main PCI, three-vessel PCI, dual arterial access, planned LV mechanical support and total lesion length >60 mm) were independently associated with adverse in-hospital major adverse coronary or cerebrovascular events. These factors were used to construct a score and a cut-off value of 5 or more was proposed to define a CHIP case [10].

Remarkably, important patient comorbidities are also components of the high bleeding risk (HBR) scores. As a matter of fact, any major criteria of HBR defined by the Academic Research Consortium (ARC) [11] are a comorbid condition, and, consequently, a patient with HBR requiring complex PCI can be considered per se a CHIP. Furthermore, major bleeding risk also

M. Sabaté (✉)
Interventional Cardiology Department, Cardiovascular Institute, Hospital Clínic, Barcelona, Spain
e-mail: MASABATE@clinic.cat

B. Cortese, S. Rigattieri (eds.), *High Bleeding Risk Patients in Interventional Cardiology*,
https://doi.org/10.1007/978-3-031-87302-7_25

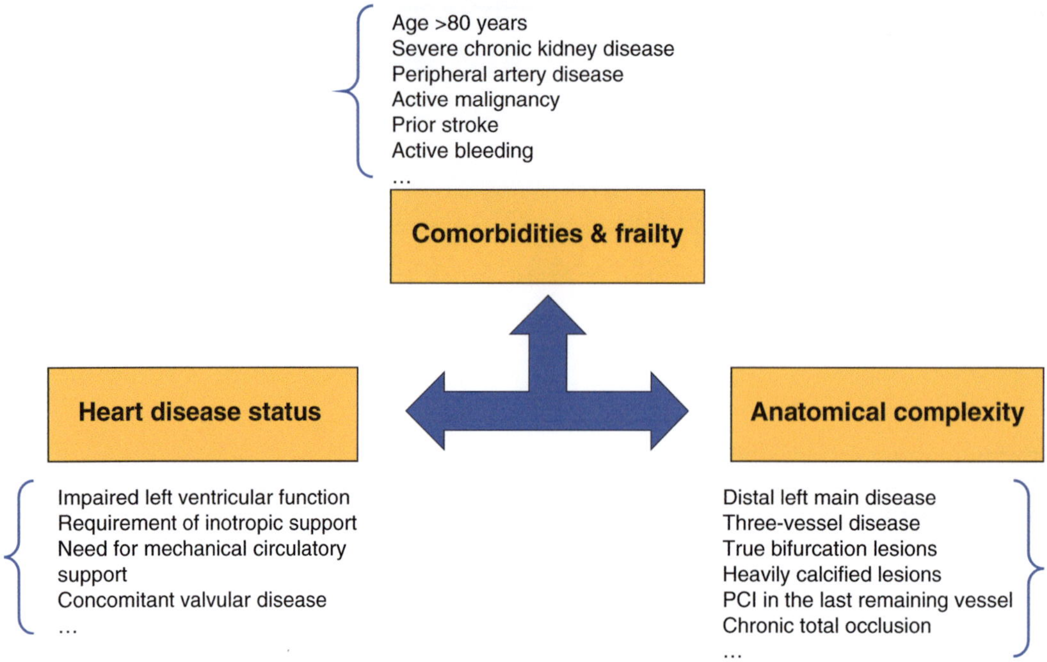

Fig. 25.1 Diagram illustrating three interconnected factors in assessing patient risk: "Comorbidities & Frailty," "Heart Disease Status," and "Anatomical Complexity. Arrows indicate the interrelation between these factors

Table 25.1 Major Academic Research Consortium (ARC) criteria for HBR after PCI and periprocedural risk during CHIP PCI

HBR-ARC major criteria[a]	Risk during CHIP procedures
Anticipated use of long-term oral anticoagulation	+
Severe or end-stage CKD (eGFR <30 mL/min)	+++
Haemoglobin <11 g/dL	+++
Spontaneous bleeding requiring hospitalization or transfusion in the past 6 months or at any time, if recurrent	++
Moderate or severe baseline thrombocytopenia (platelet count <100 × 109/L)	++
Chronic bleeding diathesis	++
Liver cirrhosis with portal hypertension	++
Active malignancy (excluding nonmelanoma skin cancer) within the past 12 months	+
Previous spontaneous ICH (at any time); previous traumatic ICH within the past 12 months; presence of a bAVM; moderate or severe ischaemic stroke within the past 6 months	++
Nondeferrable major surgery on DAPT	+
Recent major surgery or major trauma within 30 days before PCI	+

HBR high bleeding risk, *ARC* Academic Research Consortium, *CHIP* complex higher risk indicated patient, *CKD* chronic kidney disease, *eGFR* estimated glomerular filtration rate, *ICH* intracerebral haemorrhage, *bAVM* brain arteriovenous malformation, *DAPT* dual antiplatelet therapy, *PCI* percutaneous coronary intervention
[a]See Ref. [11]

increases as the above-mentioned CHIP score increases [10]. However, there are some other comorbid conditions included in the CHIP score (i.e. peripheral artery disease) that are not directly related with HBR. In addition, the degree of the periprocedural risk of each of the major criteria defined by ARC-HBR may be variable during complex PCI (Table 25.1). As an example, the periprocedural risk of treating a patient with severe chronic kidney disease or severe anaemia is much higher than that of patient with active malignancy in the past 12 months. Therefore, some comorbidities associated with HBR may be more impactful on clinical outcomes than others during complex PCI.

25.2 Clinical Outcomes Following CHIP Procedures

Percutaneous treatment of CHIP confers an increased risk of complications. These can be categorized as cardiac and noncardiac (Table 25.2). Complex PCI requires the use of higher number of stents in difficult anatomies (i.e. bifurcation, calcified vessels, chronic total occlusions). As compared with noncomplex PCI, complex treatments usually need larger bore sheaths, additional non-radial access sites, increased contrast volume and greater dose of heparin; require more resources (intravascular imaging, ablative techniques, microcatheters, specific wires…); and are exposed to longer procedural times and higher radiation dose. Consequently, periprocedural risk of events is increased. Classically, rates of MACE following complex PCI are higher than those of noncomplex PCI [4]. One study involved 998 complex PCIs, and those performed in CHIP showed higher rate of in-hospital major complications than those in non-CHIP. The use of immunosuppressive drugs (OR 3.040, 95% CI 1.251–7.386, p = 0.014), unstable haemodynamics (OR 5.753, 95% CI 1.217–27.201, p = 0.027) and frailty (OR 2.039, 95% CI 1.108–3.751, p = 0.022) were identified as independent predictors of in-hospital complications among CHIP [12].

At long-term follow-up, the outcomes of CHIP procedures were also found to be worse than those of non-CHIP [13]. In that study, predictors of events during follow-up include active malignancy, pulmonary disease, haemodialysis, unstable haemodynamics, left ventricular ejection fraction and valvular disease [13].

Table 25.2 Complications during or following CHIP procedures

Cardiac complications	Noncardiac complications
Stent thrombosis	Access site-related vascular complications
In-stent restenosis	Access site-related bleedings
Stent fracture	Non-access site-related bleedings
Coronary perforation	Contrast-induced nephropathy
Distal embolization	Post-procedural thrombocytopenia
Periprocedural myocardial infarction	Ischaemic or haemorrhagic stroke
Malignant arrhythmias	Infections secondary to orotracheal intubation
Heart failure decompensation	Other infections
Acute pulmonary oedema	Non-cardiovascular death
Cardiovascular death	

Brener et al. demonstrated that PCI performed in CHIP presented a 2.5-fold higher risk of 1-year mortality and that four factors were found independently associated with 1-year mortality: >80 years, dialysis, low ejection fraction and treatment of multiple lesions [14].

25.3 Mechanical Circulatory Support in CHIP-PCI

Percutaneous treatment of complex lesions in patients with reduced left ventricular function may expose them to an extreme periprocedural risk. In such scenario, the use of mechanical circulatory support devices is haemodynamically appealing. However, evidence of clinical benefit is scarce.

The use of intra-aortic balloon pump (IABP) in high-risk PCI in patients with depressed ejection fraction was addressed in the BCIS-1 (Balloon Pump–Assisted Coronary Intervention Study) randomized controlled trial [15]. A total of 301 patients were randomized 1:1 to elective IABP balloon pump insertion vs no planned IABP. The primary endpoint (major adverse cardiac or cardiovascular events at hospital discharge) did not differed between groups (15.2% of the elective IABP and 16.0% of the no planned IABP groups, $p = 0.85$). However, major or minor bleeding and access site complications tended to occur more often in the elective IABP group ($p = 0.06$ for both events).

The use of the transaortic microaxial pump (Impella™) was tested in the PROTECT II trial (A Prospective, Randomized Clinical Trial of Hemodynamic Support With Impella™ 2.5 Versus Intra-Aortic Balloon Pump in Patients Undergoing High-Risk Percutaneous Coronary Intervention) [16]. A total of 452 patients were randomized 1:1 to either Impella™ 2.5 vs IABP. The primary endpoint (30-day major adverse events) was not statistically different between groups: 35.1% for Impella™ 2.5 versus 40.1% for IABP, $p = 0.227$ in the intent-to-treat (ITT) population. As hypothesis-generating, at 90 days, a trend towards decreased major adverse events was observed in Impella™ 2.5–supported patients in the ITT comparison with IABP: 40.6% versus 49.3%, $p = 0.066$. However, more strokes/TIA and vascular surgical repairs were observed in the Impella™ 2.5 arm [16]. Despite the lack of robust evidence, the Italian Society of Interventional Cardiology Working Group Endorsed by Spanish and Portuguese Interventional Cardiology Societies issued a clinical expert consensus document on the use of percutaneous left ventricular assist support devices during CHIP-PCI [17]. The panel strongly recommended the use of Impella™ for PCI to unprotected distal left main with SYNTAX score ≥33 and severe left ventricular dysfunction (ejection fraction <35%). In this context, Impella™ use should be evaluated based on patient characteristics and clinical conditions assessed by a multidisciplinary team.

Finally, the use of extracorporeal membrane oxygenation (ECMO) in the context of high-risk PCI remains anecdotal.

25.4 Antithrombotic Regime After CHIP Procedures

Dual antiplatelet therapy (DAPT) is the mainstay after PCI. Current guidelines consider the clinical condition of the patient (stable coronary artery disease or acute coronary syndrome) and risk of bleeding to establish the duration of the DAPT regime. Specifically, in acute coronary syndromes, DAPT duration can be reduced from the established 1 year to 6 months in HBR patients. In chronic coronary syndromes, it can be reduced from 6 months to 3 or even 1 month in HBR patients [18]. Conversely, DAPT should be prolonged beyond 1 year in high ischaemic risk patients and without an increased risk of major or life-threatening bleeding based on the results of PrEvention with TicaGrelor of SecondAry Thrombotic Events in High-RiSk Patients with Prior AcUte Coronary Syndrome—Thrombolysis In Myocardial Infarction Study Group (PEGASUS-TIMI) 54 and Dual Antiplatelet Therapy (DAPT) trials [18, 19]. Along the same way, based on the Cardiovascular Outcomes for People Using Anticoagulation Strategies (COMPASS) trial, the addition of Factor Xa inhibition with a very low dose of rivaroxaban (2.5 mg b.i.d.) to aspirin should be considered as an option for maintenance treatment beyond 12 months post-acute coronary syndrome (ACS) in patients at high thrombotic risk and without an increased risk of major or life-threatening bleeding [18, 19]. Technical and clinical factors defining high thrombotic risk are presented in Table 25.3. These factors also define a complex PCI. While patients deemed at high ischaemic risk and low bleeding risk would benefit from prolonged DAPT (≥12 months), and patients at HBR and low ischaemic risk would benefit from shortening duration of DAPT, it remains challenging to deal with patients with both at high thrombotic and HBR. (Fig. 25.2) In this CHIP scenario, physicians should individualize the DAPT regime, prioritizing the safety of the patient.

Table 25.3 High thrombotic risk factors after PCI

Risk enhancers	Technical aspects
Diabetes mellitus requiring medication	At least three stents implanted
History of recurrent myocardial infarction	At least three lesions treated
Any multivessel CAD	Total stent length >60 mm
Premature (<45 years) or accelerated (new lesion within a 2-year timeframe) CAD	History of complex revascularization (left main, bifurcation stenting with ≥2 stents implanted, chronic total occlusion, stenting of last patent vessel)
Concomitant systemic inflammatory disease (e.g. human immunodeficiency virus, systemic lupus erythematosus, chronic arthritis)	History of stent thrombosis on antiplatelet treatment
Polyvascular disease (CAD plus PAD) CKD with eGFR 15–59 mL/min/1.73 m^2	

Adapted from Ref. [19]

CAD coronary artery disease, *PAD* peripheral artery disease, *CKD* chronic kidney disease, *eGFR* estimated glomerular filtration rate

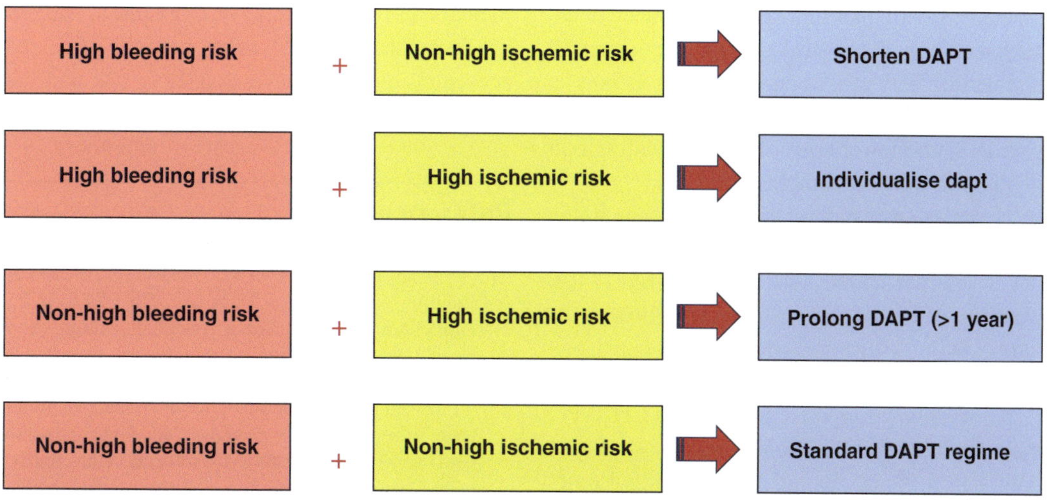

Fig. 25.2 Flowchart for DAPT (Dual Antiplatelet Therapy) decision-making based on bleeding and ischemic risks. Four scenarios: 1) Highbleeding risk and non-high ischemic risk suggest shortening DAPT. 2) High bleeding and ischemic risks require individualizedDAPT. 3) Non-high bleeding and high ischemic risks recommend prolonging DAPT beyond one year. 4) Non-high bleedingand ischemic risks follow a standard DAPT regimen.

25.5 Strategies to Reduce Bleeding in CHIP

Several studies evaluated the safety of shortening the duration of DAPT in complex PCI. A post hoc analysis of the Global Leaders trial evaluated the impact of an experimental strategy (23-month ticagrelor monotherapy following 1-month DAPT) vs. a reference regimen (12-month aspirin monotherapy following 12-month DAPT) after complex PCI [2]. In the complex PCI group, the monotherapy arm demonstrated a reduction in the primary endpoint of all-cause mortality and myocardial infarction at 2 years (3.5% vs. 5.4%, HR: 0.64; 95% CI: 0.48–0.85; $p = 0.002$). Interestingly, the risk of BARC Type 3 or 5 bleeding did not differ significantly between the two regimes [2]. In the post hoc assessment of complex PCI in the Ticagrelor with Aspirin or Alone in High-Risk Patients after Coronary Intervention (TWILIGHT) trial, ticagrelor plus placebo resulted in lower rates of the primary endpoint of

BARC type 2, 3 or 5 bleeding (4.2% vs. 7.7%; HR 0.54; 95% CI: 0.38–0.76), with no differences in ischaemic outcomes: death, myocardial infarction or stroke (3.8% vs. 4.9%; HR: 0.77; 95% CI: 0.52–1.15) [3]. In the Management of High Bleeding Risk Patients Post Bioresorbable Polymer-Coated Stent Implantation With an Abbreviated Versus Standard DAPT Regimen (MASTER-DAPT) trial, DAPT discontinuation was associated with similar ischaemic events and lower bleeding rates compared with standard DAPT, regardless of the PCI complexity [20]. In a recent meta-analysis involving five trials, 31,627 patients, of whom 8328 (26.3%) underwent complex PCI, P2Y12 inhibitor monotherapy compared with standard DAPT was associated with a similar risk of all-cause death, stent thrombosis and stroke, with no evidence for interaction between complex and noncomplex PCI; a reduction in myocardial infarction in complex PCI; and lower rates of major bleeding both in complex and noncomplex PCI [21].

However, we should take into account that patients included in the above-mentioned trials are rather selected as they were randomized if they were free of events at 1 or 3 months following the index PCI. Therefore, population considered CHIP may not be fully represented in those trials.

Another way to reduce bleeding in CHIP-PCI may include DAPT de-escalation strategies. Although it is not recommended during the first month after PCI in acute coronary syndrome patients, de-escalation from a potent P2Y12 inhibitor (prasugrel or ticagrelor) to clopidogrel may be considered according to the recent 2023 European Society of Cardiology Guidelines on acute coronary syndromes [19].

The use of intravascular imaging may improve outcomes in complex PCI. The Randomized Controlled Trial of Intravascular Imaging Guidance Versus Angiography-Guidance on Clinical Outcomes After Complex Percutaneous Coronary Intervention (RENOVATE-COMPLEX-PCI) demonstrated that intravascular imaging-guided PCI reduced the composite endpoint of death from cardiac causes, target-vessel-related myocardial infarction or clinically driven target-vessel revascularization as compared to angiography-guided PCI [22]. In the same way, a meta-analysis involving 16 trials and 7814 patients, intravascular imaging-guided PCI reduced the risk of major adverse cardiac events, stent thrombosis, target-lesion revascularization and target-vessel revascularization. In complex lesion subsets, there was a trend towards a reduction in all-cause death for imaging-guided PCI compared with angiography-guided PCI [23].

In summary, CHIP-PCI requires a refined technique with the use of intravascular imaging, performed by skilled interventionalist. It is therefore advocated to organize in each centre a specialized team of interventionalists with adequate cognitive and technical skills to manage these patients and anatomies [24]. Decision to shorten or de-escalate DAPT must be individualized according to the residual ischaemic risk and the components of the HBR score.

References

1. Neumann FJ, Sousa-Uva M, Ahlsson A, Alfonso F, Banning AP, Benedetto U, et al. 2018 ESC/EACTS Guidelines on myocardial revascularization. Eur Heart J. 2019;40:87–165.
2. Serruys PW, Takahashi K, Chichareon P, Kogame N, Tomaniak M, Modolo R, et al. Impact of long-term ticagrelor monotherapy following 1-month dual antiplatelet therapy in patients who underwent complex percutaneous coronary intervention: insights from the Global Leaders trial. Eur Heart J. 2019;40(31):2595–604.
3. Dangas G, Baber U, Sharma S, Giustino G, Mehta S, Cohen DJ, et al. Ticagrelor with or without aspirin after complex PCI. J Am Coll Cardiol. 2020;75(19):2414–24.
4. Giustino G, Chieffo A, Palmerini T, Valgimigli M, Feres F, Abizaid A, et al. Efficacy and safety of dual antiplatelet therapy after complex PCI. J Am Coll Cardiol. 2016;68(17):1851–64.
5. Suh J, Park DW, Lee JY, Jung IH, Lee SW, Kim YH, et al. The relationship and threshold of stent length with regard to risk of stent thrombosis after drug-eluting stent implantation. J Am Coll Cardiol Intv. 2010;3:383–9.
6. Brilakis ES, Banerjee S, Karmpaliotis D, Lombardi WL, Tsai TT, Shunk KA, et al. Procedural outcomes of chronic total occlusion percutaneous coronary intervention: a report from the NCDR (National Cardiovascular Data Registry). J Am Coll Cardiol Intv. 2015;8:245–53.

7. Park TK, Park YH, Song YB, Oh JH, Chun WJ, Kang GH, et al. Long-term clinical outcomes of true and non-true bifurcation lesions according to Medina classification-results from the COBIS (COronary BIfurcation Stent) II registry. Circ J. 2015;79(9):1954–62.
8. Song YB, Hahn JY, Yang JH, Choi SH, Choi JH, Lee SH, et al. Differential prognostic impact of treatment strategy among patients with left main versus non-left main bifurcation lesions undergoing percutaneous coronary intervention: results from the COBIS (Coronary Bifurcation Stenting) Registry II. JACC Cardiovasc Interv. 2014;7:255–63.
9. Fujimoto Y, Sakakura K, Fujita H. Complex and high-risk intervention in indicated patients (CHIP) in contemporary clinical practice. Cardiovasc Interv Ther. 2023;38(3):269–74.
10. Protty M, Sharp ASP, Gallagher S, Farooq V, Spratt JC, Ludman P, et al. Defining percutaneous coronary intervention complexity and risk: an analysis of the United Kingdom BCIS Database 2006–2016. JACC Cardiovasc Interv. 2022;15:39–49.
11. Urban P, Mehran R, Colleran R, Angiolillo DJ, Byrne RA, Capodanno D, et al. Defining high bleeding risk in patients undergoing percutaneous coronary intervention: a consensus document from the Academic Research Consortium for High Bleeding Risk. Eur Heart J. 2019;40:2632–53.
12. Fujimoto Y, Sakakura K, Jinnouchi H, Taniguchi Y, Tsukui T, Watanabe Y, et al. Comparison of outcomes of elective percutaneous coronary intervention between complex and high-risk intervention in indicated patients (CHIP) versus non-CHIP. J Atheroscler Thromb. 2023;30:1229–41.
13. Fujimoto Y, Sakakura K, Jinnouchi H, Taniguchi Y, Tsukui T, Watanabe Y, et al. Comparison of long-term clinical outcomes of elective percutaneous coronary intervention between complex and high-risk intervention in indicated patients (CHIP) versus non-CHIP. Am J Cardiol. 2023;194:1–8.
14. Brener SJ, Cunn GJ, Desai PH, Faroqui M, Ha LD, Handa G, et al. A novel risk score to predict one-year mortality in patients undergoing complex high-risk indicated percutaneous coronary intervention (CHIP-PCI). J Invasive Cardiol. 2021;33:E253–8.
15. Perera D, Stables R, Thomas M, Booth J, Pitt M, Blackman D, et al. Elective intra-aortic balloon counterpulsation during high-risk percutaneous coronary intervention: a randomized controlled trial. JAMA. 2010;304:867–74.
16. O'Neill WW, Kleiman NS, Moses J, Henriques JP, Dixon S, Massaro J, et al. A prospective, randomized clinical trial of hemodynamic support with Impella 2.5 versus intra-aortic balloon pump in patients undergoing high-risk percutaneous coronary intervention: the PROTECT II study. Circulation. 2012;126:1717–27.
17. Chieffo A, Burzotta F, Pappalardo F, Briguori C, Garbo R, Masiero G, et al. Clinical expert consensus document on the use of percutaneous left ventricular assist support devices during complex high-risk indicated PCI: Italian Society of Interventional Cardiology Working Group Endorsed by Spanish and Portuguese Interventional Cardiology Societies. Int J Cardiol. 2019;293:84–90.
18. Valgimigli M, Bueno H, Byrne RA, Collet JP, Costa F, Jeppsson A, et al. 2017 ESC focused update on dual antiplatelet therapy in coronary artery disease developed in collaboration with EACTS: the Task Force for dual antiplatelet therapy in coronary artery disease of the European Society of Cardiology (ESC) and of the European Association for Cardio-Thoracic Surgery (EACTS). Eur Heart J. 2018;39(3):213–60.
19. Byrne RA, Rossello X, Coughlan JJ, Barbato E, Berry C, Chieffo A, et al. 2023 ESC Guidelines for the management of acute coronary syndromes. Eur Heart J. 2023;44(38):3720–826.
20. Valgimigli M, Smits PC, Frigoli E, Bongiovanni D, Tijssen J, Hovasse T, et al. Duration of antiplatelet therapy after complex percutaneous coronary intervention in patients at high bleeding risk: a MASTER DAPT trial sub-analysis. Eur Heart J. 2022;43(33):3100–14.
21. Oliva A, Castiello DS, Franzone A, Condorelli G, Colombo A, Esposito G, et al. P2Y12 inhibitors monotherapy in patients undergoing complex vs non-complex percutaneous coronary intervention: a meta-analysis of randomized trials. Am Heart J. 2023;255:71–81.
22. Lee JM, Choi KH, Song YB, Lee JY, Lee SJ, Lee SY, et al. Intravascular imaging-guided or angiography-guided complex PCI. N Engl J Med. 2023;388(18):1668–79.
23. Sreenivasan J, Reddy RK, Jamil Y, Malik A, Chamie D, Howard JP, et al. Intravascular imaging-guided versus angiography-guided percutaneous coronary intervention: a systematic review and meta-analysis of randomized trials. J Am Heart Assoc. 2024;13(2):e031111.
24. Kirtane AJ, Doshi D, Leon MB, Lasala JM, Ohman EM, O'Neill WW, et al. Treatment of higher-risk patients with an indication for revascularization: evolution within the field of contemporary percutaneous coronary intervention. Circulation. 2016;134:422–31.

Antithrombotic Therapy After Transcatheter Aortic Valve Implantation or Left Atrial Appendage Occlusion

26

Ilan Merdler, Brian C. Case, and Ron Waksman

26.1 Introduction

Transcatheter aortic valve implantation (TAVI) introduces a unique clinical scenario characterized by patients who are at an increased risk of both thrombosis and hemorrhage [1]. These complications include a 0.5–5% incidence of stroke and a substantial 9–17% incidence of major bleeding (MB) at 30 days [2–4]. Not only do bleeding events have a negative impact on clinical outcomes, but they also carry substantial consequences for patients' quality of life [5–8]. The ongoing debate in this context revolves around identifying the most effective approach to manage antithrombotic therapy, particularly with the aim of averting clinical and subclinical valve thrombosis and potential valve degeneration without increasing the patient's overall risk of bleeding complications.

Atrial fibrillation (AF) is the most prevalent cardiac arrhythmia, with its incidence and prevalence steadily increasing. In the general population, AF affects approximately 2% of individuals, and its prevalence rises with age, carrying a lifetime risk of around 15% [9, 10]. Importantly, AF serves as an independent risk factor for ischemic strokes and thromboembolic events, leading to significantly elevated mortality rates, substantial morbidity, and severe disabilities [11]. The annual stroke rate among AF patients hovers around 5%, with at least 20% of all ischemic strokes attributed to AF [12]. Oral anticoagulation (OAC) therapy plays a central role in managing AF patients at heightened risk of stroke, with the CHA_2DS_2-VASc score being the recommended tool for assessing thromboembolic risk [13].

The use of left atrial appendage occlusion (LAAO) devices stands out as a mechanical alternative to mitigate cardioembolic risks in AF patients, especially those patients with an increased risk of bleeding. This approach is supported by compelling evidence indicating that over 90% of thrombi in nonvalvular AF cases originate in the left atrial appendage (LAA) [14, 15]. LAAO substantially reduces the risk of life-threatening bleeding events and has demonstrated notable safety and efficacy, resulting in ischemic stroke rates as low as 1.1% [16]. However, a key challenge post-LAAO revolves around the potential formation of thrombi on the device's surface, necessitating post-procedural antithrombotic therapy.

The definition of "high bleeding risk" is itself a subject of ongoing debate, influenced by factors such as renal failure, prior bleeding episodes, liver cirrhosis, hematological abnormalities, and the use of medications such as nonsteroidal anti-

I. Merdler · B. C. Case · R. Waksman (✉)
Section of Interventional Cardiology, MedStar Washington Hospital Center, Washington, DC, USA
e-mail: ilan.merdler@medstar.net; Brian.C.Case@medstar.net; ron.waksman@medstar.net

B. Cortese, S. Rigattieri (eds.), *High Bleeding Risk Patients in Interventional Cardiology*, https://doi.org/10.1007/978-3-031-87302-7_26

inflammatory drugs or steroids [17]. This chapter aims to delve into the intricate realm of identifying high-bleeding-risk patients in the context of TAVI and LAAO. The initial section discusses TAVI, and the subsequent section relates to LAAO.

26.2 TAVI

In this section, we will begin by elucidating the underlying biological mechanisms and outlining the imperative requirements for antithrombotic therapy post-TAVI. Subsequently, we will discuss the identification of patients susceptible to high bleeding risk following this procedure and the methods for their identification. Lastly, we will synthesize the insights gleaned from published literature concerning antithrombotic treatment for such patients.

26.2.1 TAVI-Related Thrombosis

26.2.1.1 Mechanism

As blood moves through the newly implanted aortic valve, the positioning of the valve leaflets disrupts flow into the neo sinus, causing abnormally slow flow [18, 19]. Materials introduced by the valve can also lead to clots [20]. Some evidence suggests these materials act as a starting point for clot formation and speed up the process. Regarding damage to the blood vessel lining, there is no proof that the TAVI stent may cause more harm to the lining than the conditions associated with severe aortic stenosis. Thrombus formation in TAVI is also linked to changes in blood chemistry, and biomarkers related to blood clotting have been observed to increase immediately after the implantation [21]. Platelet microparticles and changes in platelet counts may further contribute to the development of blood clots [22].

26.2.1.2 Clinical and Subclinical Presentations of Thrombosis Post-TAVI

Thrombotic events following TAVI can be grouped into two primary categories: those that manifest with symptoms (clinical) and those that occur without noticeable symptoms (asymptomatic/subclinical). These categories can be further divided into local events, such as leaflet thrombosis, and systemic events, such as stroke.

The cumulative occurrence of symptomatic leaflet thrombosis after TAVI falls within the range of 0.6–2.8%, and the development of valve leaflet thrombosis has been linked to two adverse consequences—hemodynamic valve deterioration and an increased risk of stroke [23, 24]. Stroke, arguably the most dreaded ischemic/embolic complication following TAVI, manifests in approximately 7% of patients [25]. Post-TAVI strokes can be further categorized as acute, subacute, and late. Periprocedural stroke, occurring within 24 h of the procedure, is often the result of embolization of tissue-derived debris, stemming from the mechanical interplay between the device and the calcified aortic valves. Subacute strokes, emerging between 1 and 30 days, may be attributed to the onset of new AF, which is detected in roughly 10% of patients during their initial hospitalization. Late strokes, affecting patients from 30 days to a year after the procedure, have connections with preexisting AF, prevalent in about one-third of those undergoing TAVI, as well as systemic atherosclerosis.

In parallel with symptomatic presentations, the adoption of TAVI has unveiled an intriguing phenomenon—subclinical leaflet thrombosis, commonly referred to as hypoattenuated leaflet thickening (HALT). Studies have reported the incidence of HALT ranging from 4% to as high as 32% [26]. The timing of HALT's onset remains a mystery, with instances of HALT appearing as early as 3–5 days following TAVI, and its incidence increasing over the course of a year. The primary concern surrounding subclinical leaflet thrombosis centers on the heightened risks of thromboembolism, stroke, and transient ischemic attacks. Research has produced mixed outcomes, with some studies establishing a link between HALT and an increased risk of transient ischemic attacks [27–29]. However, the majority of research endeavors have not revealed a significant impact on clinical outcomes, including mortality and stroke.

26.2.2 TAVI Patients at High Risk of Bleeding

Given the above-described inherent risks, the administration of post-TAVI antithrombotic therapy is crucial. However, it is essential to acknowledge that all currently available antithrombotic therapies inevitably come with a risk of bleeding. This poses a particular challenge in the context of TAVI because patients undergoing this procedure often present with multiple comorbidities, which are well documented to further elevate the risk of bleeding. It is also important to note that bleeding following TAVI is linked to unfavorable clinical outcomes and increased mortality [30, 31]. Consequently, the pressing need remains to establish the optimal antithrombotic therapy and determine the appropriate duration of treatment. This section aims to explore the methods for recognizing patients who are at an elevated risk of bleeding after undergoing TAVI [32].

26.2.2.1 Factors Leading to Bleeding (Fig. 26.1)

Patients diagnosed with severe aortic stenosis are at a higher risk of experiencing spontaneous bleeding, mainly because of their advanced age [33]. However, various specific risk factors for bleeding have been identified in regard to TAVI. Several studies have independently identified prior stroke, kidney dysfunction, the use of transapical access, and preexisting atrial fibrillation as predictors of post-TAVI bleeding [34, 35]. A meta-analysis has shown that a history of peripheral vascular disease (PVD) and preexisting anemia significantly increases the likelihood of bleeding [36]. TAVI also has specific blood-related factors, such as acquired reversible von Willebrand factor (vWF) deficiency and acquired thrombocytopenia, which have been associated with aortic stenosis and post-TAVI bleeding [4, 37, 38]. The unfolding of vWF multimers, especially due to turbulent blood flow through the narrowed valve, impairs their role in primary hemostasis and platelet activation, contributing to gastrointestinal bleeding, often observed in Heyde's syndrome. Acquired thrombocytopenia after TAVI may result from various factors, such as increased platelet consumption due to immune reactions, shear stress, and other mechanisms [39]. Although the link between acquired thrombocytopenia and a higher risk of short-term complications, including increased bleeding, has been inconsistently reported, it remains a significant concern.

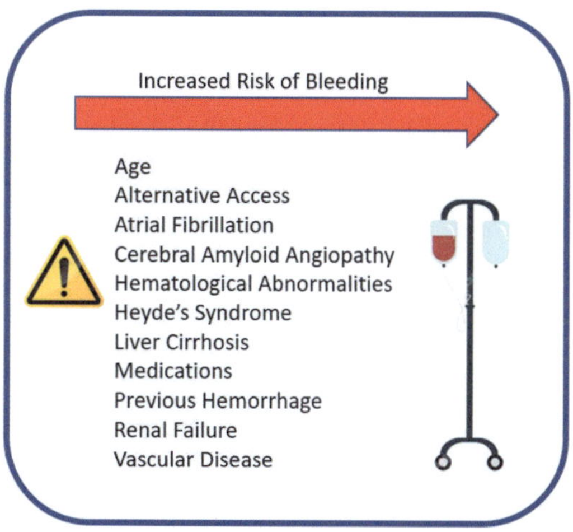

Fig. 26.1 Factors associated with the risk of bleeding in TAVI patients

26.2.2.2 Onset of Bleeding

The timing of bleeding is related to the etiology. Periprocedural bleeding occurs shortly after TAVI, is primarily linked to vascular complications at puncture sites or cardiac injuries such as pericardial tamponade, and escalates the risk of mortality [3]. Technical advancements, including the use of smaller sheaths and expanded transfemoral access, have led to a gradual reduction in procedural bleeding rates. To minimize the risk of vascular complications in high-risk patient subgroups (e.g., those with small artery size, severe calcification, a higher sheath-to-vessel ratio, or severe obesity), technical improvements such as the use of ultrasound guidance for vascular access are advisable. Late-onset bleeding, occurring more than 30 days after TAVI, significantly raises the risk of mortality during a 12-month follow-up period [40]. This type of later-onset bleeding is predominantly gastrointestinal (40.8%) and neurological (15.5%) and is influenced by patients' susceptibility to bleeding

Table 26.1 Bleeding-related risk scores and their components

Risk score	Components
HAS-BLED [41]	Hypertension, renal disease, liver disease, stroke history, prior major bleeding or predisposition to bleeding, labile INR
ARC-HBR [17][a]	Long-term OAC, renal failure, anemia, recent bleeding, low platelet count, chronic bleeding disorders, liver cirrhosis, active malignancy, recent major surgery or trauma, advanced age, ischemic stroke, NSAIDs, or steroids
PREDICT-TAVR [43][b]	Hemoglobin, serum iron, creatinine clearance, common femoral artery diameter, dual antiplatelet therapy, anticoagulation therapy

OAC oral anticoagulation, *NSAIDs* nonsteroidal anti-inflammatory drugs
[a]Based on major and minor criteria
[b]Based on deep-learning models

and their long-term antithrombotic and anticoagulant regimens [4].

26.2.2.3 Risk Scores

Several risk scores (Table 26.1) have been used to identify patients at risk of MB following TAVI. One of the established tools is the HAS-BLED score [41], originally designed to predict 1-year bleeding in AF patients [42]. Studies exploring this score's applicability in patients receiving dual or triple antithrombotic therapy for acute coronary syndrome have demonstrated moderate accuracy. However, the score's performance in predicting bleeding post-TAVI was inconsistent [36]. Another well-investigated risk score is the Academic Research Consortium for High Bleeding Risk (ARC-HBR) criteria, which also showed mixed results in studies. In recent times, researchers have ventured into the realm of deep learning to predict late MB after transcatheter aortic valve replacement (TAVR). One notable innovation brought by this is the PREDICT-TAVR score, comprising six components (blood hemoglobin, serum iron, creatinine clearance, common femoral artery diameter, dual antiplatelet therapy [DAPT], and anticoagulant therapy) [43]. The selection of variables was fine-tuned through recursive feature elimination and cross-validation to eliminate weaker components. These six items were derived from an extensive pool of 104 baseline variables obtained from 5185 consecutive patients undergoing transfemoral TAVI in the prospective RISPEVA (Registro Italiano GISE sull'Impianto di Valvola Aortica Percutanea) registry [44] between March 2012 and December 2019 and then validated in 5043 patients within the prospective POL-TAVI [45] (Polish Registry of Transcatheter Aortic Valve Implantation) between January 2013 and December 2019.

26.2.3 Medical Management and Guidelines for High-Risk Bleeding Patients

26.2.3.1 European and American Guidelines (Table 26.2)

According to the 2021 European guidelines for valvular disorders [46], for post-TAVI management, the use of OAC is recommended for life in TAVI patients who have other indications for OAC. Lifelong single antiplatelet therapy (SAPT) is suggested after TAVI for patients with no pre-existing indication for OAC. Both of these recommendations are classified as class I indications. On the other hand, routine use of OAC is discouraged after TAVI in patients without an existing OAC indication, which is classified as a class III indication. If the patient has had coronary stenting in the past 3 months or concomitant with the valve intervention, dual therapy consisting of OAC plus aspirin (or clopidogrel) is suggested for 1–6 months, depending on bleeding risk, followed by lifelong anticoagulation. These guidelines consider high bleeding risk as calculated by ARC-HBR criteria, but they do not provide specific recommendations for managing high-bleeding-risk patients. The optimal choice between clopidogrel and aspirin in patients undergoing TAVI without an OAC indication remains uncertain. The use of aspirin or an oral P2Y12 inhibitor is yet to be definitively determined. While clopidogrel is an option in the

Table 26.2 Recommendations for antithrombotic treatment after TAVI

	European Society of Cardiology (2021) [46]	The American College of Cardiology/American Heart Association (2020) [47]
Oral anticoagulation	OAC is recommended for life in TAVI patients who have other indications for OAC (Class I)	For those with other indication for OAC
Single antiplatelet therapy	Lifelong for patients with no preexisting indication for OAC (Class I)	Aspirin (75–100 mg daily) after TAVI for patients without other indications for oral anticoagulants (Class IIa)
Dual antiplatelet therapy	If the patient has had coronary stenting in the past 3 months or concomitant with the valve intervention, OAC plus SAPT is suggested for 1 to 6 months, depending on bleeding risk, followed by lifelong anticoagulation	Aspirin 75–100 mg plus clopidogrel 75 mg daily (Class IIb)

DAPT dual antiplatelet therapy, *OAC* oral anticoagulation, *SAPT* single antiplatelet therapy, *TAVI* transcatheter aortic valve implantation

guidelines, aspirin is commonly used when SAPT is indicated after TAVI. Also, there is no clear recommendation regarding which OAC is preferred. The American College of Cardiology (ACC)/American Heart Association guidelines from 2020 recommend SAPT with aspirin (75–100 mg daily) after TAVI for patients without other indications for oral anticoagulants, with a class IIa recommendation [47]. The use of DAPT (aspirin 75–100 mg plus clopidogrel 75 mg daily) for 3–6 months has been downgraded to a class IIb recommendation. This is a notable shift from previous years of recommending DAPT.

26.2.3.2 Results from Clinical Studies (Table 26.3)

The change in recommendations is supported by randomized controlled trials (RCTs) such as the ARTE trial [48] and Cohort A of the POPular TAVI trial [49], which showed no significant advantage of DAPT over SAPT for patients undergoing TAVI without an OAC indication. Instead, DAPT was associated with a higher rate of major or life-threatening bleeding events. An analysis of the PARTNER 2 cohort [50] suggested that OAC alone did not reduce the risk of stroke after TAVI, whereas antiplatelet therapy, with or without OAC, was more effective in preventing stroke. The use of direct oral anticoagulants (DOACs) instead of vitamin K antagonists (VKA) in TAVI patients is a subject of debate. In the GALILEO trial [51], which compared low-dose rivaroxaban plus aspirin to aspirin plus clopidogrel, the use of rivaroxaban was associated with higher rates of all-cause death, thromboembolic events, and MB compared to antiplatelet therapy. Similarly, in Stratum 2 of the ATLANTIS trial [52], apixaban resulted in higher all-cause and non-cardiovascular mortality compared to SAPT or DAPT in patients without an OAC indication. These results challenge the use of DOACs in this patient population. However, the ATLANTIS trial showed no superiority of apixaban over VKA in terms of the primary outcome. Additionally, the Society of Thoracic Surgeons/ACC Transcatheter Valve Therapy registry and a meta-analysis provided evidence suggesting the benefits of DOACs in terms of mortality and bleeding, although the results should be interpreted with caution [53].

26.2.4 Summary

The PREDICT-TAVI score provides a valuable tool for pinpointing patients at risk of bleeding after TAVI. Guidelines and research continue to recommend the use of at least aspirin following the procedure. Given the need for long-term treatment and the absence of definitive evidence for newer valves that might eliminate the need for any antithrombotic medications, the primary focus should be on effectively managing the underlying comorbidities that contribute to an elevated risk of bleeding.

Table 26.3 Summary of landmark trials

Trial	Device	Study purpose	Findings
ARTE [48]	TAVI	To compare aspirin plus clopidogrel with aspirin alone as antithrombotic treatment following TAVI for the prevention of ischemic events, bleeding events, and death	SAPT reduced the risk for major or life-threatening events while not increasing the risk for MI or stroke
ATLANTIS [52]	TAVI	To assess the efficacy and safety of apixaban compared with standard of care (antiplatelet therapy [APT] or OAC) among patients undergoing TAVI	Apixaban is not superior to standard of care (VKA if an indication for OAC; APT if no indication) among routine patients undergoing TAVI; valve leaflet thrombosis was lower with apixaban compared with APT, but this did not translate into an improvement in clinical outcomes Among patients without an indication for OAC, apixaban use resulted in higher non-cardiovascular mortality compared with APT use
GALILEO [51]	TAVI	To assess whether the direct factor Xa inhibitor rivaroxaban can prevent thromboembolic events after TAVI	In patients without an established indication for oral anticoagulation after successful TAVI, a treatment strategy including rivaroxaban at a dose of 10 mg daily was associated with a higher risk of death or thromboembolic complications and a higher risk of bleeding than an antiplatelet-based strategy
PARTNER 2 (sub-analysis) [50]	TAVI	To examine TAVI in intermediate risk patients	OAC alone did not reduce the risk of stroke after TAVI, whereas antiplatelet therapy, with or without OAC, was more effective in preventing stroke
POPular TAVI [49, 73]	TAVI	Cohort A—to examine the roles of anticoagulation alone or with an antiplatelet agent after TAVI	Cohort A—in patients undergoing TAVI who were receiving oral anticoagulation, the incidence of serious bleeding over a period of 1 month or 1 year was lower with oral anticoagulation alone than with oral anticoagulation plus clopidogrel
		Cohort B—the effect of single as compared with dual antiplatelet treatment on bleeding and thromboembolic events after TAVI	Cohort B—among patients undergoing TAVI who did not have an indication for oral anticoagulation, the incidence of bleeding and the composite of bleeding or thromboembolic events at 1 year were significantly less frequent with aspirin than with aspirin plus clopidogrel administered for 3 months
ADALA [72]	LAAO	To examine if low-dose apixaban tops DAPT after LAA closure	A low dose of a DOAC may be a better option than DAPT after LAAO—according to preliminary findings
ANDES [72]	LAAO	To compare short-term (8 weeks) anticoagulation therapy (DOAC) vs. antiplatelet therapy for the prevention of device thrombosis following transcatheter LAA	Ongoing
PREVAIL [71, 73]	LAAO	To assess the safety and efficacy of LAAO for stroke prevention in patients with AF compared with long-term warfarin therapy	LAAO was noninferior to warfarin for ischemic stroke prevention
PROTECT-AF [69, 70]	LAAO	To determine whether percutaneous left atrial appendage closure with a filter device (Watchman) was noninferior to warfarin for stroke prevention in atrial fibrillation	Left atrial appendage closure is noninferior to anticoagulation with warfarin

SAPT single antiplatelet therapy, *MI* myocardial infarction, *OAC* oral anticoagulants, *VKA* vitamin K antagonist, *TAVI* transcatheter aortic valve implantation, *LAA* left atrial appendage, LAAO left atrial appendage occlusion, *DAPT* dual antiplatelet therapy, *AF* atrial fibrillation

26.3 Left Atrial Appendage Occlusion

Percutaneous LAAO has emerged as a promising alternative to OAC for selected patients with nonvalvular AF, especially those with high bleeding risk. LAAO devices mechanically exclude the LAA from the systemic circulation, significantly reducing the risk of AF-related strokes. However, these patients face an increased risk of thromboembolic stroke, primarily attributed to clot formation and embolization from the LAA.

26.3.1 Introducing LAAO and Antithrombotic Treatment

In March 2015, the Watchman LAAO device (Boston Scientific, Marlborough, Massachusetts, USA) received approval from the US Food and Drug Administration (FDA) following two pivotal randomized controlled clinical trials that mandated the implementation of standardized post-procedure protocols, encompassing follow-up procedures, imaging assessments, and antithrombotic medications [54]. These protocols were carefully designed to minimize the risk of device-related thrombosis, along with associated thromboembolism and strokes. Consequently, these protocols were integrated into the FDA's approval process for the device [55].

In particular, patients who were randomized to undergo LAAO were discharged with a prescription for warfarin and aspirin (81–325 mg) for the initial 45 days following the implantation procedure. At the follow-up visit (scheduled for 45 days ± 2 weeks after the procedure), patients underwent transesophageal echocardiography (TEE). Based on the TEE results, if there was a peri-device leak exceeding 5 mm, patients were advised to continue taking warfarin and aspirin. On the other hand, if there was no significant leak, or the leak was 5 mm or less, patients transitioned to DAPT, consisting of daily clopidogrel (75 mg) and aspirin until the 6-month mark post-implantation. Subsequently, they continued with aspirin alone.

26.3.2 LAAO-Related Thrombus

Device-related thrombus (DRT) represents a significant concern within the realm of LAAO and can have far-reaching implications for the success of LAAO procedures. DRT occurs in approximately 3–4% of patients post-LAAO [56]. Various observational studies have shown that a history of stroke or transient ischemic attack, permanent AF, reduced ejection fraction, and vascular disease can be considered as factors that make one more susceptible to this condition [56]. An attempt has been made to formulate a risk-prediction scheme known as the DRT score [55]. This score was derived from an international registry of 711 patients, of whom 237 experienced DRT and 474 did not. From a pool of more than 40 potential risk factors considered in the logistic regression model, five factors were independently predictive of DRT: hypercoagulopathy, renal insufficiency, permanent AF, deep device implantation, and the presence of pericardial effusion (Fig. 26.2).

The question of whether the risk of DRT is device specific remains unresolved. In the Amulet IDE trial, the Amulet device exhibited a slightly lower DRT rate compared to the Watchman 2.5 device [57]. This was hypothesized to be associated with the larger neo-LAA that remains with a plug-based device as opposed to a disc-lobe device, as well as the differential impact of device design on healing and reendothelialization. Iterative LAAO device design also considers the risk of DRT. For example, the Watchman FLX device was developed with significantly less exposed metal screw surface to reduce the risk of DRT [55]. Device manufacturers are also exploring innovative preventative methods for DRT, such as the addition of antithrombotic device coatings to minimize the risk of thrombus formation on the device, similar to what has been employed with drug-coated stents.

The management and prevention of DRT continue to present a clinical dilemma. The choice of post-LAAO antithrombotic therapy in the aforementioned global registry did not appear to significantly affect the risk of DRT. In the Watchman trials and nested registries, the incidence of DRT

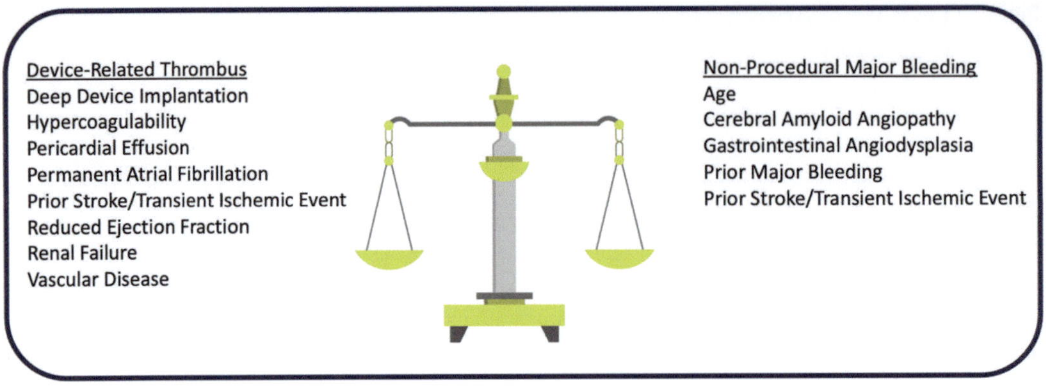

Fig. 26.2 The equilibrium between device-related thrombosis and non-procedural major hemorrhaging in LAAO patients

was higher when the post-LAAO regimen solely comprised antiplatelet therapy compared to anticoagulation (3.1% vs. 1.4%, $P = 0.018$) [58]. The National Cardiovascular Data Registry Left Atrial Appendage Occlusion registry [59] indicated that a short course of anticoagulation with warfarin or a DOAC following the procedure was linked to a lower incidence of major adverse events throughout the initial 6 months of follow-up.

Several problems remain unresolved. First, many patients referred for LAAO are not suitable candidates for intensified or prolonged anticoagulation regimens. This leaves them in a precarious situation, where they must balance the risk of embolic events with DRT against the risk of MB associated with the initiation or resumption of anticoagulation. Second, even among patients who receive anticoagulation, a sizable percentage (20–25%) continue to experience DRT [60], resulting in substantially higher morbidity and mortality. Furthermore, DRT recurrence rates are notably high, with a 35% recurrence rate [61] while patients are still on anticoagulation and a 50% recurrence rate when anticoagulation is discontinued [62]. Third, not all DRTs are equivalent, and managing large and/or highly mobile thrombi remains uncertain.

26.3.3 High Bleeding Risk in LAAO

In the context of LAAO, the goal is to employ the minimal possible antithrombotic and anticoagulation medications. While the incidence of MB tends to decline over time, a continual risk of MB persists, even when adhering to a restricted antithrombotic regimen, particularly within this high-bleeding-risk population. Notably, 23% of all MB events are attributed to the procedure, with a notable portion occurring during the periprocedural phase [63]. MB events associated with the procedure primarily stem from pericardial effusion [64], often accompanied by tamponade, and vascular complications. Key aspects for mitigation encompass thorough physician training, precise assessment of LAA anatomy using 3D imaging modalities, optimal device sizing, adherence to standardized implantation protocols, and scrupulous procedural anticoagulation. These measures aim to not only reduce acute procedure- or device-related MB events but also late pericardial effusions.

Several trials have tried to address the incidence of MB post-LAAO. The AMPLATZER Cardiac Plug registry [65], encompassing 1047 patients implanted with the first-generation AMPLATZER™ LAAO device (Abbott Vascular), observed an annualized rate of MB of 2.1%. The prospective 2-year follow-up of the EWOLUTION registry [66] involving 1020 patients implanted with the WATCHMAN™ found an annualized rate of non-procedural MB of 2.7%, excluding procedural bleeding events such as tamponade or vascular complications. Furthermore, a focused analysis within this trial, limited to 318 patients with a prior

Table 26.4 Recommendations for antithrombotic treatment after left atrial appendage occlusion in high bleeding risk [69]

Medication	Dose	Period	Comments
Aspirin	75–325 mg/day	Indefinitely	–
Oral anticoagulation	None	None	–
Clopidogrel	75 mg/day	1–6 months	Adequate sealing is less than 5 mm leak. Shorten as possible for high-risk.

MB history, revealed higher rates of non-procedural MB at 4.5% per year. A separate single-center registry by Weise et al., which included 298 patients undergoing LAAO with various devices, identified an elevated incidence of MB events during follow-up of 10.7% [67]. When including cardiac tamponades, the incidence surged to 14%. Notably, this population had a high mean HAS-BLED score of 3.5 ± 1 and a substantial proportion of patients with previous bleeding history (61%). This underscores the presence of high-risk patients who are prone to bleeding in these studies.

With regard to non-procedural MB events, gastrointestinal bleeding was described to be the predominant source. Prior stroke and pre-LAAO MB were shown to independently predict MB during follow-up post-LAAO, while age demonstrated borderline significance. This suggests that patients with a history of MB represent a population at a heightened risk of recurrent bleeding events after LAAO. They necessitate closer monitoring and an enhancement of strategies aimed at averting bleeding. However, it is important to acknowledge that certain bleeding conditions, such as gastrointestinal angiodysplasia and cerebral amyloid angiopathy, have a high likelihood of recurrence even after all antithrombotic treatments are discontinued. Turning to the clinical implications of non-procedural MB after LAAO, it is notable that bleeding complications are an independent predictor of all-cause mortality.

26.3.4 Antithrombotic Regimens

26.3.4.1 Guidelines

The 2020 European Society of Cardiology AF guidelines [68] recommend specific antithrombotic regimens for patients undergoing Watchman LAAO based on their risk profile (Table 26.4). For patients at high risk of bleeding, the guidelines recommend aspirin at a daily dose of 75–325 mg indefinitely without OAC. Additionally, patients can receive 75 mg/day of clopidogrel for 1–6 months to ensure adequate sealing of the LAA. In very high-risk situations, the use of clopidogrel can be shortened. Similar protocols are advised for Amplatzer or Amulet devices. There are no clear American guidelines on this topic.

26.3.4.2 Prominent Trials (Table 26.3)

The pivotal randomized trials PROTECT-AF [69] and PREVAIL [70, 71] were conducted before the era of DOACs. These trials primarily assessed the efficacy of LAAO in preventing ischemic events in patients who were not contraindicated for chronic anticoagulation. Following successful LAAO with the WATCHMAN device, patients received a combination of warfarin and 81 mg/day of aspirin for 45 days, followed by DAPT (aspirin 325 mg/day and clopidogrel 75 mg/day) for up to 6 months, and lifelong aspirin at 325 mg/day. This antithrombotic regimen, as mentioned previously, was subsequently approved by the FDA after WATCHMAN implantation. Subsequent registries offered further evidence supporting this regimen. A pooled analysis of patients who received the WATCHMAN implant in these trials identified a small percentage of DRT cases, with DRT being associated with an increased risk of stroke or systemic embolism. However, it is essential to note that a majority of ischemic events occurred in patients without recognized DRT. Concerning safety, the addition of an antiplatelet agent to VKA showed mixed results. After 5 years of follow-up in the

PROTECT-AF and PREVAIL trials, LAAO failed to reduce the rate of MB compared to VKA alone, largely due to procedural complications and the initial phase of the antithrombotic regimen. In real-world practice, VKA and aspirin combination therapy was linked to higher adverse events (primarily MB) compared to VKAs and DOACs alone. This led to a shift away from VKA therapy in favor of DOACs or alternative antithrombotic regimens. DOACs have demonstrated superiority over VKA in preventing ischemic events while reducing bleeding complications in nonvalvular AF. The introduction of the WATCHMAN FLX device, approved by the FDA, has further solidified DOAC use, replacing VKA in the antithrombotic regimen. Nonetheless, data on DOAC efficacy and safety following LAAO are limited and primarily derived from non-randomized studies. These studies have shown relatively low rates of DRT, stroke, and MB in the DOAC group. However, the optimal DOAC dosage after LAAO is still under investigation. The need for randomized clinical trials to assess the most suitable antithrombotic therapy after LAAO is evident. Two such trials, ANDES and ADALA, are currently comparing DOACs to DAPT after LAAO [72]. Nevertheless, DOAC use after LAAO remains an evolving area of research. DAPT is commonly used after LAAO, with European device labeling recommending a 3-month course of DAPT in cases where the standard PROTECT-AF study therapy is not feasible after WATCHMAN or Amulet implantation. This has become the dominant regimen in Europe, particularly for patients with high bleeding risk. However, there is a lack of randomized trials evaluating the clinical efficacy of DAPT after LAAO. While SAPT or no antithrombotic treatment after LAAO is used in specific cases to reduce bleeding risk, it should be employed selectively by an expert team considering individual risks. Finally, long-term antithrombotic strategies after LAAO are not well studied. There is ongoing research to determine the most appropriate approach for preventing both ischemic and hemorrhagic events in these patients, particularly considering the risk DRT. Patients with the highest bleeding risk and a low risk of ischemic complications may benefit from discontinuing antithrombotic therapy early after LAAO, although further research is needed to confirm this approach's safety and efficacy, and there are ongoing trials.

26.3.5 Summary

The choice of antithrombotic treatment type and duration after LAAO remains a topic of uncertainty, marked by considerable variation in regimens found in published studies. The inclusion of patients with bleeding risks spanning from low to extreme further compounds the ambiguity surrounding the selection of antithrombotic therapies. Prioritizing the avoidance of MB events should likely guide the selection of antithrombotic regimens for LAAO recipients, while considering risk factors associated with DRT. The most appropriate approach is one that is tailored, considering both bleeding risk and the risk of DRT-induced ischemic events.

Conflicts of Interest Ron Waksman reports serving on the advisory boards of Abbott Vascular, Boston Scientific, J Valve, Medtronic, Philips IGT, and Pi-Cardia Ltd.; being a consultant for Abbott Vascular, Biotronik, Boston Scientific, CardioMed LLC, Cordis, Medtronic, Philips IGT, Pi-Cardia Ltd., Swiss Interventional Systems/SIS Medical AG, and Transmural Systems Inc., and Venous MedTech; receiving institutional grant support from Amgen, Biotronik, Boston Scientific, Chiesi, Medtronic, and Philips IGT; and being an investor in MedAlliance, Pi-Cardia Ltd., and Transmural Systems.

References

1. Ranasinghe MP, Peter K, McFadyen JD. Thromboembolic and bleeding complications in transcatheter aortic valve implantation: insights on mechanisms, prophylaxis and therapy. J Clin Med. 2019;8:280.
2. Huded CP, Tuzcu EM, Krishnaswamy A, Mick SL, Kleiman NS, Svensson LG, et al. Association between transcatheter aortic valve replacement and early postprocedural stroke. JAMA. 2019;321:2306–15.
3. Avvedimento M, Nuche J, Farjat-Pasos JI, Rodés-Cabau J. Bleeding events after transcatheter aortic valve replacement: JACC state-of-the-art review. J Am Coll Cardiol. 2023;81:684–702.

4. Mangieri A, Montalto C, Poletti E, Sticchi A, Crimi G, Giannini F, et al. Thrombotic versus bleeding risk after transcatheter aortic valve replacement: JACC review topic of the week. J Am Coll Cardiol. 2019;74:2088–101.
5. Costa F, Cohen MG. Transfusion and mortality after transcatheter aortic valve replacement: association or causation? Circ Cardiovasc Interv. 2020;13:e010225.
6. Piccolo R, Pilgrim T, Franzone A, Valgimigli M, Haynes A, Asami M, et al. Frequency, timing, and impact of access-site and non-access-site bleeding on mortality among patients undergoing transcatheter aortic valve replacement. JACC Cardiovasc Interv. 2017;10:1436–46.
7. Arnold SV, Zhang Y, Baron SJ, McAndrew TC, Alu MC, Kodali SK, et al. Impact of short-term complications on mortality and quality of life after transcatheter aortic valve replacement. JACC Cardiovasc Interv. 2019;12:362–9.
8. Arnold SV, Cohen DJ, Dai D, Jones PG, Li F, Thomas L, et al. Predicting quality of life at 1 year after transcatheter aortic valve replacement in a real-world population. Circ Cardiovasc Qual Outcomes. 2018;11:e004693.
9. Kornej J, Börschel CS, Benjamin EJ, Schnabel RB. Epidemiology of atrial fibrillation in the 21st century: novel methods and new insights. Circ Res. 2020;127:4–20.
10. Staerk L, Sherer JA, Ko D, Benjamin EJ, Helm RH. Atrial fibrillation: epidemiology, pathophysiology, and clinical outcomes. Circ Res. 2017;120:1501–17.
11. Botto GL, Tortora G, Casale MC, Canevese FL, Brasca FAM. Impact of the pattern of atrial fibrillation on stroke risk and mortality. Arrhythm Electrophysiol Rev. 2021;10:68–76.
12. Alshehri AM. Stroke in atrial fibrillation: review of risk stratification and preventive therapy. J Family Community Med. 2019;26:92–7.
13. Lane DA, Lip GY. Use of the CHA(2)DS(2)-VASc and HAS-BLED scores to aid decision making for thromboprophylaxis in nonvalvular atrial fibrillation. Circulation. 2012;126:860–5.
14. Regazzoli D, Ancona F, Trevisi N, Guarracini F, Radinovic A, Oppizzi M, et al. Left atrial appendage: physiology, pathology, and role as a therapeutic target. Biomed Res Int. 2015;2015:205013.
15. Kong B, Liu Y, Huang H, Jiang H, Huang C. Left atrial appendage closure for thromboembolism prevention in patients with atrial fibrillation: advances and perspectives. J Thorac Dis. 2015;7:199–203.
16. Merella P, Lorenzoni G, Delitala AP, Sechi F, Decandia F, Viola G, et al. Left atrial appendage occlusion in high bleeding risk patients. J Interv Cardiol. 2019;2019:6704031.
17. Urban P, Mehran R, Colleran R, Angiolillo DJ, Byrne RA, Capodanno D, et al. Defining high bleeding risk in patients undergoing percutaneous coronary intervention. Circulation. 2019;140:240–61.
18. Ng ACT, Holmes DR, Mack MJ, Delgado V, Makkar R, Blanke P, et al. Leaflet immobility and thrombosis in transcatheter aortic valve replacement. Eur Heart J. 2020;41:3184–97.
19. Raghav V, Midha P, Sharma R, Babaliaros V, Yoganathan A. Transcatheter aortic valve thrombosis: a review of potential mechanisms. J R Soc Interface. 2021;18:20210599.
20. Sibilitz KL, Fukutomi M, Sondergaard L. Valve thrombosis after transcatheter aortic valve replacement-cause for concern? Ann Cardiothorac Surg. 2020;9:505–7.
21. Sedaghat A, Falkenberg N, Sinning JM, Kulka H, Hammerstingl C, Nickenig G, et al. TAVI induces an elevation of hemostasis-related biomarkers, which is not causative for post-TAVI thrombocytopenia. Int J Cardiol. 2016;221:719–25.
22. Jung C, Lichtenauer M, Figulla HR, Wernly B, Goebel B, Foerster M, et al. Microparticles in patients undergoing transcatheter aortic valve implantation (TAVI). Heart Vessel. 2017;32:458–66.
23. Yanagisawa R, Tanaka M, Yashima F, Arai T, Jinzaki M, Shimizu H, et al. Early and late leaflet thrombosis after transcatheter aortic valve replacement. Circ Cardiovasc Interv. 2019;12:e007349.
24. Marwan M, Mekkhala N, Göller M, Röther J, Bittner D, Schuhbaeck A, et al. Leaflet thrombosis following transcatheter aortic valve implantation. J Cardiovasc Comput Tomogr. 2018;12:8–13.
25. Lansky AJ, Ghare MI, Pietras C. Carotid disease and stroke after transcatheter aortic valve replacement. Circ Cardiovasc Interv. 2018;11:e006826.
26. Goel K, Lindman BR. Hypoattenuated leaflet thickening after transcatheter aortic valve replacement: expanding the evidence base but questions remain. Circ Cardiovasc Imaging. 2019;12:e010151.
27. Hein M, Schoechlin S, Schulz U, Minners J, Breitbart P, Lehane C, et al. Long-term follow-up of hypoattenuated leaflet thickening after transcatheter aortic valve replacement. JACC Cardiovasc Interv. 2022;15:1113–22.
28. Garcia S, Fukui M, Dworak MW, Okeson BK, Garberich R, Hashimoto G, et al. Clinical impact of hypoattenuating leaflet thickening after transcatheter aortic valve replacement. Circ Cardiovasc Interv. 2022;15:e011480.
29. Rashid HN, Michail M, Ramnarain J, Nasis A, Nicholls SJ, Cameron JD, et al. The impact of hypoattenuated leaflet thickening on haemodynamic valve deterioration following transcatheter aortic valve replacement. J Cardiovasc Comput Tomogr. 2022;16:168–73.
30. Arnold SV, Reynolds MR, Lei Y, Magnuson EA, Kirtane AJ, Kodali SK, et al. Predictors of poor outcomes after transcatheter aortic valve replacement: results from the PARTNER (Placement of Aortic Transcatheter Valve) trial. Circulation. 2014;129:2682–90.
31. VARC-3 Writing Committee, Généreux P, Piazza N, Alu MC, Nazif T, Hahn RT, et al. Valve Academic

Research Consortium 3: updated endpoint definitions for aortic valve clinical research. J Am Coll Cardiol. 2021;77:2717–46.
32. Merdler I, Rogers T, Case BC, Bhogal S, Reddy PK, Ben-Dor I, et al. Aspirin versus warfarin after transcatheter aortic valve replacement in low-risk patients: 2-year follow-up. Am J Cardiol. 2023;206:108–15.
33. Riva N, Smith DE, Lip GY, Lane DA. Advancing age and bleeding risk are the strongest barriers to anticoagulant prescription in atrial fibrillation. Age Ageing. 2011;40:653–5.
34. Natorska J, Mazur P, Undas A. Increased bleeding risk in patients with aortic valvular stenosis: from new mechanisms to new therapies. Thromb Res. 2016;139:85–9.
35. Wang J, Yu W, Jin Q, Li Y, Liu N, Hou X, et al. Risk factors for post-TAVI bleeding according to the VARC-2 bleeding definition and effect of the bleeding on short-term mortality: a meta-analysis. Can J Cardiol. 2017;33:525–34.
36. Albabtain MA, Arafat AA, Alonazi Z, Aluhaydan H, Alkharji M, Alsaleh R, et al. Risk of bleeding after transcatheter aortic valve replacement: impact of preoperative antithrombotic regimens. Braz J Cardiovasc Surg. 2022;37:836–42.
37. Horiuchi H, Doman T, Kokame K, Saiki Y, Matsumoto M. Acquired von Willebrand syndrome associated with cardiovascular diseases. J Atheroscler Thromb. 2019;26:303–14.
38. De Larochellière H, Puri R, Eikelboom JW, Rodés-Cabau J. Blood disorders in patients undergoing transcatheter aortic valve replacement: a review. JACC Cardiovasc Interv. 2019;12:1–11.
39. Dvir D, Généreux P, Barbash IM, Kodali S, Ben-Dor I, Williams M, et al. Acquired thrombocytopenia after transcatheter aortic valve replacement: clinical correlates and association with outcomes. Eur Heart J. 2014;35:2663–71.
40. Yamamoto M, Otsuka T, Shimura T, Yamaguchi R, Adachi Y, Kagase A, et al. Incidence, timing, and causes of late bleeding after TAVR in an Asian cohort. JACC Asia. 2022;2:622–32.
41. Clinical characteristics comprising the HAS-BLED bleeding risk score. Wolters Kluwer. https://www.uptodate.com/contents/image?imageKey=HEME%2F75259. Accessed 10 Oct 2023.
42. Zhu W, He W, Guo L, Wang X, Hong K. The HAS-BLED score for predicting major bleeding risk in anticoagulated patients with atrial fibrillation: a systematic review and meta-analysis. Clin Cardiol. 2015;38:555–61.
43. Navarese EP, Zhang Z, Kubica J, Andreotti F, Farinaccio A, Bartorelli AL, et al. Development and validation of a practical model to identify patients at risk of bleeding after TAVR. JACC Cardiovasc Interv. 2021;14:1196–206.
44. Pepe M, Corcione N, Petronio AS, Berti S, Iadanza A, Morello A, et al. Assessing the best prognostic score for transcatheter aortic valve implantation (from the RISPEVA Registry). Am J Cardiol. 2021;144:91–9.
45. Zembala-John J, Wilczek K, Tobota Z, Chodór P, Cieśla D, Jaźwiec T, et al. POL-TAVI – Polish Registry of Transcatheter Aortic Valve Implantation – simple tool, great value, rationale and design. Kardiochir Torakochirurgia Pol. 2016;13:309–15.
46. Vahanian A, Beyersdorf F, Praz F, Milojevic M, Baldus S, Bauersachs J, et al. 2021 ESC/EACTS Guidelines for the management of valvular heart disease. Eur Heart J. 2022;43:561–632.
47. Otto CM, Nishimura RA, Bonow RO, Carabello BA, Erwin JP 3rd, Gentile F, et al. 2020 ACC/AHA guideline for the management of patients with valvular heart disease: a report of the American College of Cardiology/American Heart Association Joint Committee on Clinical Practice Guidelines. Circulation. 2021;143:e72–e227.
48. Rodés-Cabau J, Masson JB, Welsh RC, Garcia Del Blanco B, Pelletier M, Webb JG, et al. Aspirin versus aspirin plus clopidogrel as antithrombotic treatment following transcatheter aortic valve replacement with a balloon-expandable valve: the ARTE (Aspirin versus aspirin + clopidogrel following transcatheter aortic valve implantation) randomized clinical trial. JACC Cardiovasc Interv. 2017;10:1357–65.
49. Brouwer J, Nijenhuis VJ, Delewi R, Hermanides RS, Holvoet W, Dubois CLF, et al. Aspirin with or without clopidogrel after transcatheter aortic-valve implantation. N Engl J Med. 2020;383:1447–57.
50. Leon MB, Smith CR, Mack MJ, Makkar RR, Svensson LG, Kodali SK, et al. Transcatheter or surgical aortic-valve replacement in intermediate-risk patients. N Engl J Med. 2016;374:1609–20.
51. Dangas GD, Tijssen JGP, Wohrle J, Sondergaard L, Gilard M, Mollmann H, et al. A controlled trial of rivaroxaban after transcatheter aortic-valve replacement. N Engl J Med. 2020;382:120–9.
52. Collet JP, Van Belle E, Thiele H, Berti S, Lhermusier T, Manigold T, et al. Apixaban vs. standard of care after transcatheter aortic valve implantation: the ATLANTIS trial. Eur Heart J. 2022;43:2783–97.
53. Tanawuttiwat T, Stebbins A, Marquis-Gravel G, Vemulapalli S, Kosinski AS, Cheng A. Use of direct oral anticoagulant and outcomes in patients with atrial fibrillation after transcatheter aortic valve replacement: insights from the STS/ACC TVT registry. J Am Heart Assoc. 2022;11:e023561.
54. Reddy VY, Gibson DN, Kar S, O'Neill W, Doshi SK, Horton RP, et al. Post-approval U.S. experience with left atrial appendage closure for stroke prevention in atrial fibrillation. J Am Coll Cardiol. 2017;69:253–61.
55. Alkhouli M, Ellis CR, Daniels M, Coylewright M, Nielsen-Kudsk JE, Holmes DR. Left atrial appendage occlusion: current advances and remaining challenges. JACC Adv. 2022;1:100136.
56. Simard T, Jung RG, Lehenbauer K, Piayda K, Pracoń R, Jackson GG, et al. Predictors of device-related thrombus following percutaneous left atrial appendage occlusion. J Am Coll Cardiol. 2021;78:297–313.
57. Lakkireddy D, Thaler D, Ellis CR, Swarup V, Sondergaard L, Carroll J, et al. Amplatzer amulet left

atrial appendage occluder versus watchman device for stroke prophylaxis (Amulet IDE): a randomized, controlled trial. Circulation. 2021;144:1543–52.

58. Li X, Jin Q, Zhang X. Closure device-related thrombosis after anticoagulation with dabigatran in patients undergoing percutaneous left atrial appendage closure: case reports and literature review. Front Pharmacol. 2020;11:563920.
59. Freeman JV, Varosy P, Price MJ, Slotwiner D, Kusumoto FM, Rammohan C, et al. The NCDR Left Atrial Appendage Occlusion Registry. J Am Coll Cardiol. 2020;75:1503–18.
60. Sedaghat A, Vij V, Al-Kassou B, Gloekler S, Galea R, Fürholz M, et al. Device-related thrombus after left atrial appendage closure: data on thrombus characteristics, treatment strategies, and clinical outcomes from the EUROC-DRT-Registry. Circ Cardiovasc Interv. 2021;14:e010195.
61. Asmarats L, Cruz-González I, Nombela-Franco L, Arzamendi D, Peral V, Nietlispach F, et al. Recurrence of device-related thrombus after percutaneous left atrial appendage closure. Circulation. 2019;140:1441–3.
62. Holmes DR Jr, Korsholm K, Rodés-Cabau J, Saw J, Berti S, Alkhouli MA. Left atrial appendage occlusion. EuroIntervention. 2023;18:e1038–e65.
63. López-Mínguez JR, Nogales-Asensio JM, Infante De Oliveira E, Santos L, Ruiz-Salmerón R, Arzamendi-Aizpurua D, et al. Major bleeding predictors in patients with left atrial appendage closure: the Iberian Registry II. J Clin Med. 2020;9:2295.
64. Yu Y, Chu H, Wang B, He B, Fu G. Pericardial effusion following percutaneous left atrial appendage closure using the LAmbre device. Front Cardiovasc Med. 2023;10:1188322.
65. Cruz-González I, González-Ferreiro R, Freixa X, Gafoor S, Shakir S, Omran H, et al. Left atrial appendage occlusion for stroke despite oral anticoagulation (resistant stroke). Results from the Amplatzer Cardiac Plug registry. Rev Esp Cardiol (Engl Ed). 2020;73:28–34.
66. Turagam MK, Reddy VY, Dukkipati SR. EWOLUTION of watchman left atrial appendage closure to patients with contraindication to oral anticoagulation. Circ Arrhythm Electrophysiol. 2019;12:e007257.
67. Calabrò P, Gragnano F, Niccoli G, Marcucci R, Zimarino M, Spaccarotella C, et al. Antithrombotic therapy in patients undergoing transcatheter interventions for structural heart disease. Circulation. 2021;144:1323–43.
68. Hindricks G, Potpara T, Dagres N, Arbelo E, Bax JJ, Blomström-Lundqvist C, et al. 2020 ESC Guidelines for the diagnosis and management of atrial fibrillation developed in collaboration with the European Association for Cardio-Thoracic Surgery (EACTS): the Task Force for the diagnosis and management of atrial fibrillation of the European Society of Cardiology (ESC) Developed with the special contribution of the European Heart Rhythm Association (EHRA) of the ESC. Eur Heart J. 2021;42:373–498.
69. Reddy VY, Sievert H, Halperin J, Doshi SK, Buchbinder M, Neuzil P, et al. Percutaneous left atrial appendage closure vs warfarin for atrial fibrillation: a randomized clinical trial. JAMA. 2014;312:1988–98.
70. Reddy VY, Doshi SK, Kar S, Gibson DN, Price MJ, Huber K, et al. 5-year outcomes after left atrial appendage closure: from the PREVAIL and PROTECT AF trials. J Am Coll Cardiol. 2017;70:2964–75.
71. Holmes DR Jr, Kar S, Price MJ, Whisenant B, Sievert H, Doshi SK, et al. Prospective randomized evaluation of the Watchman Left Atrial Appendage Closure device in patients with atrial fibrillation versus long-term warfarin therapy: the PREVAIL trial. J Am Coll Cardiol. 2014;64:1–12.
72. Mesnier J, Cepas-Guillén P, Freixa X, Flores-Umanzor E, Hoang Trinh K, O'Hara G, et al. Antithrombotic management after left atrial appendage closure: current evidence and future perspectives. Circ Cardiovasc Interv. 2023;16:e012812.
73. Nijenhuis VJ, Brouwer J, Delewi R, Hermanides RS, Holvoet W, Dubois CLF, et al. Anticoagulation with or without clopidogrel after transcatheter aortic-valve implantation. N Engl J Med. 2020;382:1696–707.

Correction to: Tips and Tricks for a Successful and Safe LAAO Procedure

Fabrizio Ugo, Ludovica Maltese,
and Francesco Rametta

Correction to:
Chapter 15 in: B. Cortese, S. Rigattieri (eds.), *High Bleeding Risk Patients in Interventional Cardiology*, https://doi.org/10.1007/978-3-031-87302-7_15

The original version of Chap. 15 was inadvertently published without the author name Dr. Francesco Rametta. The author name has now been included.

The updated version of this chapter can be found at
https://doi.org/10.1007/978-3-031-87302-7_15

B. Cortese, S. Rigattieri (eds.), *High Bleeding Risk Patients in Interventional Cardiology*,
https://doi.org/10.1007/978-3-031-87302-7_27

MIX
Papier aus verantwortungsvollen Quellen
Paper from responsible sources
FSC® C105338

If you have any concerns about our products,
you can contact us on
ProductSafety@springernature.com

In case Publisher is established outside the EU,
the EU authorized representative is:
Springer Nature Customer Service Center GmbH
Europaplatz 3, 69115 Heidelberg, Germany

Printed by Libri Plureos GmbH
in Hamburg, Germany